Myeloproliferative Neoplasms

CONTEMPORARY HEMATOLOGY

Judith E. Karp, MD, Series Editor

For other titles published in this series, go to
www.springer.com/series/7681

Myeloproliferative Neoplasms

Biology and Therapy

Edited by

Srdan Verstovsek

The University of Texas
M.D. Anderson Cancer Center
Houston, TX
USA

Ayalew Tefferi

Mayo Clinic
Rochester, MN
USA

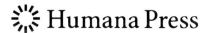 Humana Press

Editors
Srdan Verstovsek, MD, PhD
Department of Leukemia
The University of Texas
M.D. Anderson Cancer Center
Houston, TX
USA
sverstov@mdanderson.org

Ayalew Tefferi, MD
Division of Hematology
Mayo Clinic
Rochester, MN
USA
tefferi.ayalew@mayo.edu

Series Editor
Judith E. Karp, MD
The Sidney Kimmel Comprehensive Cancer
Center at Johns Hopkins
Division of Hematologic Malignancies
Baltimore, MD

ISBN 978-1-60761-265-0   e-ISBN 978-1-60761-266-7
DOI 10.1007/978-1-60761-266-7
Springer New York Dordrecht Heidelberg London

Library of Congress Control Number: 2010937641

Humana Press is part of Springer Science+Business Media (www.springer.com)

Preface

The year 2011 marks the golden anniversary of the first formal description of the classic myeloproliferative neoplasms (MPN) by William Dameshek (1900–1969) [1]. Dr. Dameshek underscored the histologic similarities between polycythemia vera (PV), essential thrombocythemia (ET), primary myelofibrosis (PMF), and chronic myelogenous leukemia (CML), and coined the term "myeloproliferative disorders (MPD)," in 1951 [2], to describe them. In 1960, Peter Nowell (1928) and David Hungerford (1927–1993) discovered the Philadelphia chromosome (Ph[1]) and its invariable association with CML [3]. In 1967, 1976, 1978, and 1981, Philip Fialkow (1934–1996) and colleagues used polymorphisms in the X-linked glucose-6-phosphate dehydrogenase (G-6-PD) locus to establish the stem cell-derived clonal nature of CML, PV, PMF, and ET, respectively [1]. The disease-causing mutation has since been determined for CML (*BCR-ABL1*) but not for PV, ET, or PMF [4].

Beginning in 2005, novel mutations involving *JAK2, MPL, TET2, ASXL1, IDH1, IDH2, CBL, IKZF1,* or *LNK* have been described in a subset of patients with *BCR-ABL1*-negative MPN [5]. With the exception of *JAK2*V617F, which occurs in approximately 95% of patients with PV and 60% of those with ET or PMF, these mutations are relatively infrequent and occur in a minority of patients with PV, ET, or PMF. Furthermore, none of these mutations, including *JAK2*V617F, has been shown to be a cardinal event in disease initiation or progression [5]. It is, therefore, not surprising that current efforts with anti-JAK2-targeted therapy have not produced the results that are usually seen with anti-*BCR-ABL1* (i.e., imatinib) therapy in CML. Nevertheless, JAK-STAT hyperactivation directly or indirectly contributes to the pathogenesis of certain MPN-associated disease aspects, and several anti-JAK ATP mimetics have accordingly been developed and currently undergoing clinical trials (*http://ClinicalTrials.gov*).

The above-mentioned development in the pathogenesis of PV, ET, and PMF has also played an essential part in the 2008 revision of the WHO classification system for MPN, which now includes eight separate entities: CML, PV, ET, PMF, systemic mastocytosis (SM), chronic eosinophilic leukemia-not otherwise specified (CEL-NOS), chronic neutrophilic leukemia (CNL), and "MPN unclassifiable (MPN-U)." The 2008 WHO revision also includes improved diagnostic criteria for PV, ET, and PMF, whereas *PDGFR*- or *FGFR1*-rearranged myeloid/lymphoid malignancies associated with eosinophilia were formally separated from CEL-NOS and excluded from the MPN category. As is the case with the classic *BCR-ABL1*-negative MPN, the genetic underpinnings of non-classic MPN remain unresolved, although certain mutations, such as *KIT*D816V in SM, are believed to contribute to disease pathogenesis and are reasonable targets to consider during new drug development.

The above-mentioned exciting developments in both classic (PV, ET, PMF) and non-classic (CEL-NOS, SM, CNL, MPN-U) *BCR-ABL1*-negative MPN are the focus of the current book, which provides a timely and comprehensive review of disease pathology, molecular pathogenesis, diagnosis, prognosis, and treatment. The experts in their respective fields have done an outstanding job in preparing a scientifically robust educational document that we regard as an essential reading for both practicing physicians and students of hematology.

Houston, TX   Srdan Verstovsek, MD, PhD
Rochester, MN   Ayalew Tefferi, MD

References

1. Tefferi A. The history of myeloproliferative disorders: before and after Dameshek. *Leukemia* 2008; 22: 3–13.
2. Dameshek W. Some speculations on the myeloproliferative syndromes. *Blood* 1951; 6: 372–375.
3. Nowell PC, Hungerford DA. Chromosome studies on normal and leukemic human leukocytes. *J Natl Cancer Inst* 1960; 25: 85–109.
4. Daley GQ, Van Etten RA, Baltimore D. Induction of chronic myelogenous leukemia in mice by the P210bcr/abl gene of the Philadelphia chromosome. *Science* 1990; 247: 824–830.
5. Tefferi A. Novel mutations and their functional and clinical relevance in myeloproliferative neoplasms: JAK2, MPL, TET2, ASXL1, CBL, IDH and IKZF1. *Leukemia* 2010; 24: 1128–1138.

Contents

Contributors

Omar Abdel-Wahab, MD
Human Oncology and Pathogenesis Program and Leukemia Service,
Memorial Sloan-Kettering Cancer Center, New York, NY, USA

Tiziano Barbui, MD
Research Foundation, Ospedali Riuniti di Bergamo, Bergamo, Italy

Giovanni Barosi, MD
Unit of Clinical Epidemiology and Centre for the Study
of Myelofibrosis, IRCCS Policlinico San Matteo Foundation, Pavia, Italy

Carlos E. Bueso-Ramos, MD, PhD
Department of Hematopathology, The University of Texas M.D. Anderson
Cancer Center, Houston, TX, USA

Francisco Cervantes, MD
Hematology Department, Hospital Clínic, IDIBAPS, University of Barcelona,
Barcelona, Spain

H. Joachim Deeg, MD
Clinical Research Division, Fred Hutchinson Cancer Research Center,
University of Washington, Seattle, WA, USA

Guido Finazzi, MD
Department of Hematology, Ospedali Riuniti di Bergamo, Bergamo, Italy

Jason Gotlib, MD, MS
Department of Medicine, Division of Hematology, Stanford University
School of Medicine and Stanford Cancer Center, Stanford, CA, USA

Juan-Carlos Hernández-Boluda, MD, PhD
Hematology Department, Hospital Clínico, Valencia, Spain

Daniella M.B. Kerbauy, MD, PhD
Hematology and Hemotherapy Service, Department of Clinical and
Experimental Oncology, UNIFESP/EPM, Sao Paulo, Brazil

Ross L. Levine, MD
Human Oncology and Pathogenesis Program and Leukemia Service,
Memorial Sloan-Kettering Cancer Center, New York, NY, USA

Ruben A. Mesa, MD
Professor of Medicine, Consultant of Hematology & Oncology, Mayo Clinic,
Scottsdale, AZ, USA

Animesh Pardanani, MBBS, PhD
Division of Hematology, Mayo Clinic, Rochester, MN, USA

John T Reilly, MD
Department of Haematology, Royal Hallamshire Hospital, Sheffield,
United Kingdom

Fabio P.S. Santos, MD
Department of Leukemia, The University of Texas M. D. Anderson Cancer
Center, Houston, TX, USA;
Department of Hematology, Hospital Israelita Albert Einstein, São Paulo, SP,
Brazil

Ayalew Tefferi, MD
Division of Hematology, Mayo Clinic, Rochester, MN, USA

James W. Vardiman, MD
Department of Pathology, The University of Chicago, Chicago, IL, USA

Srdan Verstovsek, MD, PhD
Department of Leukemia, The University of Texas M. D. Anderson Cancer
Center, Houston, TX, USA

Chapter 1

Diagnosis and Classification of the BCR-ABL1-Negative Myeloproliferative Neoplasms

Carlos E. Bueso-Ramos and James W. Vardiman

Keywords: Chronic neutrophilic leukemia • Polycythaemia vera • Primary myelofibrosis • Essential thrombocythaemia • Myeloproliferative neoplasm • Unclassifiable

Introduction

The myeloproliferative neoplasms (MPNs) are clonal hematopoietic stem cell disorders characterized by dysregulated proliferation and expansion of one or more of the myeloid lineages (erythroid, granulocytic, megakaryocytic, monocytic/macrophage, or mast cell). This dysregulation is thought to be a consequence of genetic abnormalities at the level of stem/progenitor cells. Most of the cases are initially diagnosed in a proliferative phase when maturation of the neoplastic cells in the bone marrow is effective and numbers of granulocytes, erythrocytes, and/or platelets in the peripheral blood are increased. Although their onset is often insidious, each MPN has the potential to progress to bone marrow failure due to myelofibrosis, ineffective hematopoiesis, and/or transformation to acute leukemia. Acute leukemia is defined as 20% or more blasts in the peripheral blood and/or bone marrow or by the appearance of a myeloid sarcoma in extramedullary tissue. In some patients, the initial proliferative stage is not apparent or is of very short duration, and the MPN is first recognized in a progressed stage. At diagnosis, splenomegaly and hepatomegaly are common and often become more prominent during the disease course. The organomegaly is caused by sequestration of excess blood cells in the spleen and liver, extramedullary hematopoiesis, or both.

In 2008, the World Health Organization (WHO) published a revised classification of the MPNs and altered the algorithms for their diagnosis [1]. In earlier diagnostic schemes, detection of the Philadelphia chromosome and/or *BCR-ABL1* fusion gene was used to confirm the diagnosis of chronic myelogenous leukemia (CML), whereas *BCR-ABL1*-negative MPNs were diagnosed mainly by their clinical and laboratory features, with little attention given to their histologic features. A number of nonspecific criteria such

S. Verstovsek and A. Tefferi (eds.), *Myeloproliferative Neoplasms: Biology and Therapy*, Contemporary Hematology, DOI 10.1007/ 978-1-60761-266-7_1, © Springer Science+Business Media, LLC 2011

as those suggested by the Polycythemia Vera Study Group for the diagnosis of polycythemia vera (PV) and essential thrombocythemia (ET) [2, 3] were necessary not only to distinguish the subtypes of MPN from each other but also to distinguish them from reactive granulocytic, erythroid, and/or megakaryocytic hyperplasia, which is often the major differential diagnosis for this group of neoplasms. The WHO revisions of the classification of MPNs were influenced by recently discovered genetic abnormalities that play a role in the pathogenesis of these neoplasms and can be used as diagnostic parameters, and by studies showing that the various subtypes of MPNs are characterized by histological features that contribute significantly to their diagnosis and classification [4, 5].

The genetic abnormalities that figure importantly in the WHO criteria include mutations or rearrangements of genes that encode protein tyrosine kinases involved in a number of cellular signal transduction pathways [6]. These genetic abnormalities result in constitutively activated protein tyrosine kinases that drive the myeloproliferative process and are described in detail in other chapters. In some MPNs, such as CML, in which the *BCR-ABL1* fusion gene results in constitutive activation of the *ABL*-derived tyrosine kinase, the genetic abnormality is associated with such consistent clinical, laboratory, and morphologic findings that it can be used as a major criterion for diagnosis. Other abnormalities, such as the Janus kinase 2 (*JAK2*) V617F mutation, are not specific for any single MPN, but their presence provides proof that the myeloid proliferation is neoplastic. The gene encoding JAK2, a cytoplasmic tyrosine kinase, is located on the short arm of chromosome 9 (9p24.1). It plays a critical role in intracellular signal transduction for surface receptors of erythropoietin, thrombopoietin, granulocyte colony-stimulating factor, granulocyte-macrophage colony-stimulating factor, and interleukins. These receptors are usually type 1 homodimeric receptors without endogenous tyrosine kinase activity. Binding of the cytokine to its membrane receptor induces conformational changes, leading to phosphorylation and activation of JAK2. The activated JAK2 phosphorylates the receptor's cytoplasmic domain, thus facilitating docking of downstream pathway proteins and initiation of signal transduction. Indeed, the discovery of *JAK2* V617F (exon 14) and similar activating mutations, such as those in *JAK2* exon 12 and myeloproliferative leukemia virus oncogene (*MPL*) W515L/K, has dramatically altered the diagnostic approach to the *BCR-ABL1*-negative MPNs, particularly PV, ET, and primary myelofibrosis (PMF). *JAK2* V617F is found in almost all patients with PV and in nearly half of those with ET or PMF, and thus it is not specific for any MPN [7–11]. In the few patients with PV that lack the mutation, most will demonstrate genetic abnormalities in the region of *JAK2* exon 12 [12], whereas 1–4% and 5–10% of patients with ET [13, 14] or PMF [15, 16] demonstrate activating mutations of the gene that encodes tyrosine kinase receptor MPL, respectively. Still, none of these mutations is specific for any MPN, nor does their absence exclude an MPN. The WHO diagnostic guidelines for PV, ET, and PMF combine genetic information with other key clinical and laboratory data and with histological features of the bone marrow biopsy (e.g. overall bone marrow cellularity, megakaryocyte morphology and topography, specific lineages involved in the proliferation, changes in the bone marrow stroma) to give criteria that are sufficiently robust to allow for the diagnosis and classification of these MPNs regardless of whether a mutation is present.

Appreciation of the role that constitutively activated protein tyrosine kinases play in the pathogenesis of CML, PV, ET, and PMF argued for inclusion of chronic myeloid proliferations with similar abnormalities in signal transduction proteins under the MPN umbrella. Thus systemic mastocytosis, which has many features in common with the MPNs and is almost always associated with the v-kit Hardy-Zukerman 4 feline sarcoma viral oncogene homolog *KIT* D816V gene mutation [17], is included in the MPN category in the revised WHO classification. On the contrary, although neoplasms with abnormal protein tyrosine kinase function due to translocations of platelet-derived growth factor receptor genes *PDGFRA* or *PDGFRB* or fibroblast growth factor receptor gene *FGFR1* are often associated with myeloproliferative features and marked eosinophilia resembling chronic eosinophilic leukemia (CEL), a substantial number exhibit a prominent lymphoblastic component as well and yet others have features of the myelodysplastic/myeloproliferative neoplasm (MDS/MPN) chronic myelomonocytic leukemia with eosinophilia [18–21]. To address this wide range of disease manifestations, cases with rearrangement of *PDGFRA*, *PDGFRB*, or *FGFR1* were assigned to a new subgroup of myeloid neoplasms distinct from the MPNs and are classified according to the genetic abnormality present. Cases of CEL that lack *PDGFRA*, *PDGFRB*, or *FGFR1* rearrangement remain within the MPN family, that is, CEL, not otherwise specified (CEL, NOS).

In summary, the WHO classification of MPNs, shown in Table 1.1, includes distinct entities that are defined by a combination of clinical, laboratory, genetic, and histologic features. Such a multidisciplinary and multiparameter approach is necessary for accurate diagnosis and classification, especially in the prodromal stages, because no single parameter, including any currently recognized genetic abnormality, is entirely specific. Although the majority of patients have genetic abnormalities that result in constitutive activation of protein tyrosine kinases involved in signal transduction pathways, for nearly half of them with ET and PMF, for most of them with CEL, NOS, and for the very rare chronic neutrophilic leukemia (CNL), the defining molecular and genetic defects remain unknown.

In this chapter, we concentrate mainly on the diagnostic criteria and morphologic features of the *BCR-ABL1*-negative disorders PV, ET, and PMF.

Table 1.1 WHO classification of myeloproliferative neoplasms (MPN) [1].

Chronic myelogenous leukemia (CML), *BCR-ABL1* positive
Chronic neutrophilic leukemia (CNL)
Polycythemia vera (PV)
Primary myelofibrosis (PMF)
Essential thrombocythemia (ET)
Chronic eosinophilic leukemia, not otherwise specified (CEL,NOS)[a]
Mast cell disease[b]
Myeloproliferative neoplasms, unclassifiable (MPN, U)

[a]Discussed in chapter 10
[b]Discussed in chapter 11

General Guidelines for Diagnosis and Classification of Myeloproliferative Neoplasms

The WHO diagnostic algorithms and classification for the MPNs are based on clinical, laboratory, morphologic, and genetic findings at the time of initial presentation, prior to any definitive therapy for the myeloid neoplasm (Fig. 1.1). When an MPN is suspected, the hemogram should be carefully correlated with a review of the peripheral blood film. Depending on the disease suspected, additional laboratory studies, such as serum erythropoietin, serum lactate dehydrogenase (LDH), and basic chemical profiles, including liver function studies, iron studies, and coagulation and platelet function studies, may be necessary for diagnosis and complete evaluation of the patient. Although some have argued that bone marrow specimens are not warranted for diagnosis of some MPNs [22], bone marrow histology is an important parameter in the WHO diagnostic guidelines. Furthermore, although molecular genetic studies for *JAK2* V617F, *BCR-ABL1*, and other genetic abnormalities may be performed successfully from peripheral blood, bone marrow specimens provide the best material for routine cytogenetic studies, which are strongly recommended for any patient suspected to have any myeloid neoplasm. The initial bone marrow biopsy specimen also provides a baseline against which future cytogenetic and histologic studies can be judged for evidence of disease progression.

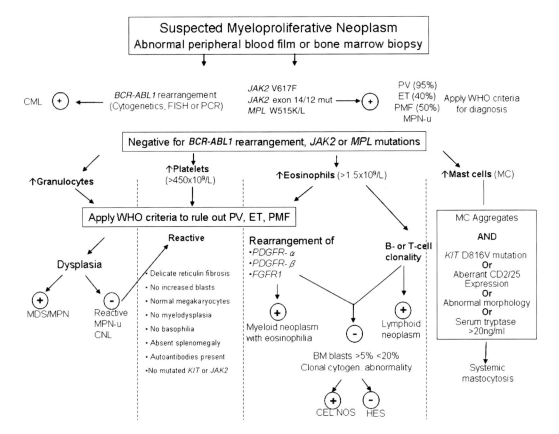

Fig. 1.1 Diagnostic work-up of myeloproliferative neoplasms. This diagram shows a simplified approach to the diagnosis of myeloproliferative neoplasms

The quality of the bone marrow specimen is key to an accurate interpretation, according to the WHO guidelines [23]. The biopsy gives the best information regarding marrow cellularity (Table 1.2), the proportion of hematopoietic cells, and their topography and maturation pattern, and allows for evaluation of the trabecular bone and marrow stroma, including vascularity and reticulin fiber content, all of which are important for diagnosis and classification. The biopsy also provides material for immunohistochemical studies, such as assessment

Table 1.2 Normal ranges of bone marrow cellularity for selected age groups, as adapted from the literature [24].

Age (years)	% Hematopoietic area
20–30	60–70
40–60	40–50
≥70	30–40

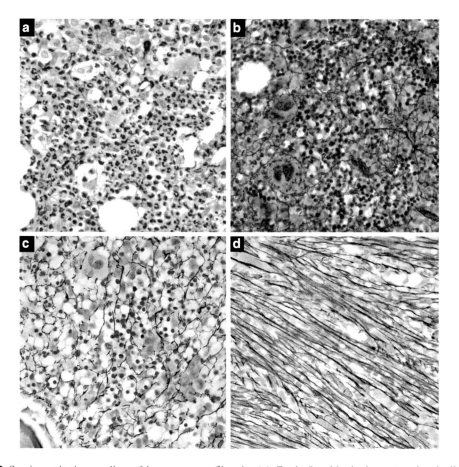

Fig. 1.2 Semiquantitative grading of bone marrow fibrosis. (**a**) Grade 0, with single scattered reticulin fibers consistent with the appearance of the normal bone marrow. (**b**) Grade 1, showing a loose meshwork of thin reticulin fibers with many intersections. (**c**) Grade 2, with a dense and diffuse increase in reticulin forming extensive intersections. (**d**) Grade 3, with dense reticulin fibers intermingled with bundles of collagen

Table 1.3 Consensus on the grading of myelofibrosis (MF) as adapted from the literature [24].

Grading[a]	Description
MF–0	Scattered linear reticulin with no intersections (cross-overs) corresponding to normal bone marrow
MF–1	Loose network of reticulin with many intersections, especially in perivascular areas
MF–2	Diffuse and dense increase in reticulin with extensive intersections, occasionally with only focal bundles of collagen and/or focal osteosclerosis
MF–3	Diffuse and dense increase in reticulin with extensive intersections with coarse bundles of collagen, often associated with significant osteosclerosis

[a]Fiber density should be assessed in hematopoietic (cellular) areas

of the number of CD34-positive cells, which may have additional diagnostic and prognostic value. To make an adequate assessment, the biopsy must be sizable and intact, without crush artifacts. It should be obtained at right angle to the cortical bone and be at least 1.5 cm in length (not including the cortical bone) with at least 10 totally or partially preserved intertrabecular areas. The marrow should be well fixed, thinly sectioned at 3–4 μm, and stained with hematoxylin and eosin and/or a similar stain that allows for detailed morphologic evaluation. A silver impregnation method for collagen type 3 in reticulin fibers is recommended, and marrow fibrosis should be graded according to a reproducible scoring system, such as the European consensus scoring system for marrow fibrosis (Table 1.3) [24]. A bone marrow aspirate should be obtained whenever possible, stained with Wright-Giemsa, and carefully evaluated and correlated with the biopsy. Often, particularly if there is any reticulin fibrosis, the aspirate is poorly cellular, and it can be misleading if not interpreted in context of the peripheral blood findings and the bone marrow biopsy. Touch preparations from the bone marrow biopsy are critical for assessment of cytology of the bone marrow cells if an aspirate cannot be obtained because of myelofibrosis. Finally, because these are serious diseases, the clinician, pathologist, cytogeneticist, and molecular diagnostician should confer jointly to discuss the findings in the case, to assure that all of the relevant information has been obtained and is correlated to reach a diagnostic conclusion, based on the WHO guidelines.

BCR-ABL1-Negative Myeloproliferative Neoplasms Polycythemia Vera, Primary Myelofibrosis, and Essential Thrombocythemia

Polycythemia Vera

Polycythemia is an increase in the number of red blood cells (RBCs) per unit volume of blood, usually defined as a greater-than-two-standard deviation increase from the age-, sex-, race-, and altitude of residence-adjusted normal value for hemoglobin (Hb), hematocrit, or red blood cell mass (RCM) [25, 26]. Polycythemia has multiple causes (Table 1.4). Usually polycythemia is a

Table 1.4 Causes of polycythemia.

"True" primary polycythemia
Congenital
Primary familial congenital erythrocytosis (*EPOR* mutation)
Acquired
Polycythemia vera
"True" secondary polycythemia
Congenital
VHL mutations, including Chuvash polycythemia
2,3-Bisphosphoglycerate mutase deficiency
High-oxygen-affinity hemoglobin
Congenital methemoglobinemia
HIF2alpha (*Hypoxia-inducible factor 2alpha*) mutation
PHD2 (*prolyl hydoxylase domain*) mutation
Acquired
Physiologically appropriate response to hypoxia
Cardiac, pulmonary, renal, and hepatic diseases, carbon monoxide poisoning, sleep apnea, renal artery stenosis, smoker's polycythemia, post-renal transplant[a]
Inappropriate production of EPO
Cerebellar hemangioblastoma, uterine leiomyoma, pheochromocytoma, renal cell carcinoma, hepatocellular carcinoma, meningioma, parathyroid adenoma
"Relative" or "Apparent" Polycythemia
Acute, transient hemoconcentration due to dehydration or other causes of contraction of plasma volume; red cell mass is not increased and is thus not a true polycythemia

[a] Cause for post-renal transplant is not entirely clear; in some cases it is likely due to chronically ischemic retained native kidney with endogenous EPO production plus increased sensitivity of the erythroid precursors to EPO

"true" increase in the RCM, but occasionally diminished plasma volume may lead to hemoconcentration and to "relative" or "apparent" polycythemia. True polycythemia may be "primary," in which an inherent abnormality of the erythroid progenitors renders them hypersensitive to factors that normally regulate their proliferation, or "secondary," in which the increase in RBCs is caused by an increase in serum erythropoietin related to tissue hypoxia or to its inappropriate secretion. Primary and secondary polycythemia may be either congenital or acquired.

The only acquired primary polycythemia is PV. It is a rare disorder with a reported annual incidence of 1–3 per 100,000 individuals in the western world, while the incidence is reportedly lower in Asia [26]. There is a familial predisposition. It is most frequent in patients who are in their sixties, and patients younger than 20 years are rarely encountered. Men are more likely to be affected than women. More than 90% of patients with PV demonstrate the acquired somatic mutation *JAK2* V617F, and most of the remainder has activating mutations of *JAK2* in the region of exon 12 – important findings that distinguish PV from other causes of polycythemia.

PV is a clonal proliferation not only of erythroid precursors but also of granulocytes and megakaryocytes and their precursors in the bone marrow (i.e. a panmyelosis), so that leukocytosis and thrombocytosis often accompany the increase in RBCs in the peripheral blood. Three phases of PV have been described: (1) a pre-polycythemic phase with borderline to mild erythrocytosis and often prominent thrombocytosis that is sometimes associated with thrombotic episodes, (2) an overt polycythemic phase, and (3) a post-polycythemic phase characterized by cytopenias, including anemia, and by bone marrow fibrosis and extramedullary hematopoiesis (post-polycythemia myelofibrosis) [26]. The natural history also includes a low incidence of evolution to acute leukemia, although some patients develop a myelodysplastic or blast phase related to prior cytotoxic therapy.

Diagnosis: Polycythemic Phase

The WHO criteria for the diagnosis of PV are listed in Table 1.5. The diagnosis is almost always made in the polycythemic phase. The most common initial symptoms (headache, dizziness, paresthesia, scotomata, erythromelalgia) are related to thrombotic events in the microvasculature, but thrombosis involving major arteries or veins occurs as well. Other symptoms include aquagenic pruritus, gout, and gastrointestinal hemorrhage. In 10–15% of patients, some of these manifestations occur up to 2 years prior to detection of an increase in the RCM [27]. Splanchnic vein thrombosis (Budd–Chiari syndrome) should always raise suspicion for an MPN, including PV, and may occur even when hematological findings are not characteristic of any MPN. In such "latent" or "pre-polycythemic" cases, the diagnosis can be substantiated if *JAK2* V617F is present, serum erythropoietin levels are decreased, and the bone marrow shows the typical morphologic features of PV (see later). The most prominent physical findings in PV include plethora in up to 80% of cases, splenomegaly in 70%, and hepatomegaly in 40–50%.

Blood and bone marrow findings: The major findings in the peripheral blood are the increased Hb, hematocrit, and erythrocyte count. The Hb level required for the diagnosis is >18.5 g/dL in men and 16.5 g/dL in women, or >17 g/dL in men or >15 g/dL in women if the Hb value is associated with an increase from baseline of at least a 2 g/dL that cannot be attributed to correction of iron deficiency (Table 1.5). More than 60% of patients have neutrophilia, and thrombocytosis is found in nearly 50%. The peripheral blood smear (Fig. 1.3a)

Table 1.5 WHO Diagnostic criteria for polycythemia vera (PV) [1].

Diagnosis requires the presence of both major criteria and one minor criterion or the presence of the first major criterion together with two minor criteria:

Major criteria

1. Hemoglobin >18.5 g/dL in men, 16.5 g/dL in women or other evidence of increased red cell volume[a]
2. Presence of *JAK2* V617F or other functionally similar mutation such as *JAK2* exon 12 mutation

Minor criteria

1. Bone marrow biopsy showing hypercellularity for age with trilineage growth (panmyelosis) with prominent erythroid, granulocytic, and megakaryocytic proliferation
2. Serum erythropoietin level below the reference range for normal
3. Endogenous erythroid colony formation *in vitro*

[a] Hemoglobin or hematocrit >99th percentile of method-specific reference range for age, sex, altitude of residence or Hemoglobin >17 g/dL in men, 15 g/dL in women if associated with a documented and sustained increase of at least 2 g/dL from an individual's baseline value that can not be attributed to correction of iron deficiency, or elevated red cell mass >25% above mean normal predicted value

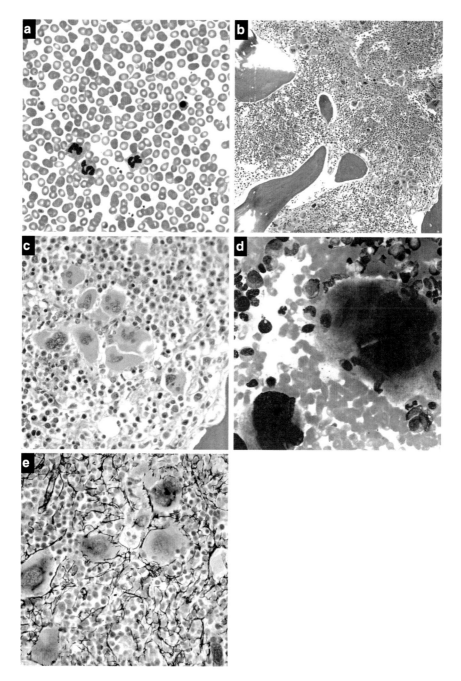

Fig. 1.3 Polycythemia vera and myelofibrosis. (**a**) Blood smear from a woman with polycythemia vera who presented with a Hb of 18 g/dL and splenomegaly. Laboratory studies showed a serum erythropoietin level below the reference range for normal. (**b**) The bone marrow is markedly hypercellular with trilineage hyperplasia and a marked increase in megakaryocytes. (**c**) High magnification of the biopsy specimen showing panmyelosis with a predominance of large hyperlobulated megakaryocytes. (**d**) Bone marrow aspirate smear showing large hyperlobulated megakaryocytes in a background of maturing normoblasts and left-shifted granulocytic elements. (**e**) Reticulin fibrosis in bone marrow trephine biopsy specimen

shows crowding of erythrocytes that are usually normochromic and normocytic, or microcytic and hypochromic if there is concomitant iron deficiency caused by gastrointestinal bleeding or phlebotomy. A mild "left shift" in neutrophils may be seen, with occasional immature granulocytes, but blasts are rarely encountered. Modest basophilia is common, and eosinophilia may be seen as well. Thrombocytosis is sometimes marked, and the diagnostic impression of ET is possible if the Hb value is only minimally elevated or if the disease is in the "latent" phase.

The characteristic bone marrow findings of PV are best observed in trephine biopsy specimens. The histopathological features of "pre-polycythemia" and of full-blown PV are similar and characterized by proliferation of the granulocytic, erythroid, and megakaryocytic lineages. The cellularity of the bone marrow ranges from 30 to 100% but is consistently hypercellular for the patient's age (Fig. 1.3b). The increase in cellularity may be particularly noticeable in the subcortical bone marrow, an area that is usually hypocellular, particularly in older patients. Although a modest "left shift" in granulopoiesis may be present, there is no increase in the percentage of myeloblasts. Erythropoiesis occurs in expanded erythroid islands throughout the marrow biopsy and is normoblastic except in cases in which iron deficiency leads to iron-deficient erythropoiesis, which can be best appreciated in bone marrow aspirate smears.

Megakaryocytes are increased in number (Fig. 1.3b–d). They vary from small to large in size, may be dispersed singly throughout the bone marrow or form loose clusters, and are often located abnormally next to the bony trabeculae (Fig. 1.3b). Although some megakaryocytes may be atypical, with abnormal nuclear cytoplasmic ratios and bizarre nuclei, the majority lacks significant atypia overall, in contrast to the megakaryocytes of PMF, nor are they as uniformly enlarged in size as those of ET (see comparison of PV, PMF, and ET megakaryocytes in Figs. 1.3–1.5). Reticulin fiber content is normal in most of the patients during diagnosis, but in as many as 20% of patients reticulin fibrosis is noted even in the polycythemic phase. Stainable iron is absent in the aspirated marrow of more than 90% of patients (the bone marrow biopsy is unreliable for assessment of iron if decalcified). Lymphoid nodules, sometimes sizable, are occasionally seen.

Patients who have PV with a *JAK2* exon 12 mutation have clinical features similar to those of patients with the *JAK2* V617F mutation, but in the bone marrow they have mainly erythroid proliferation, with less granulocytic and megakaryocytic expansion than observed in those patients with *JAK2* V617F [28].

Extramedullary tissues: The splenomegaly present in the polycythemic phase is due to the engorgement of the cords and sinuses with erythrocytes, with minimal evidence of extramedullary hematopoiesis. Similar changes are noted in the hepatic sinuses.

Additional laboratory studies: The WHO diagnostic criteria for PV (Table 1.5) require several laboratory studies. Major criteria for the diagnosis include documentation of increased Hb or RCM and the presence of *JAK2* V617F or a similar activating mutation, whereas the minor criteria include characteristic bone marrow histology, decreased serum erythropoietin, and endogenous erythroid colony (EEC) formation. Measurement of the erythropoietin level is an important initial test in the evaluation of polycythemia. Serum erythropoietin level is typically decreased in PV, in contrast to the elevated values often associated with secondary polycythemia. Although an elevated erythropoietin

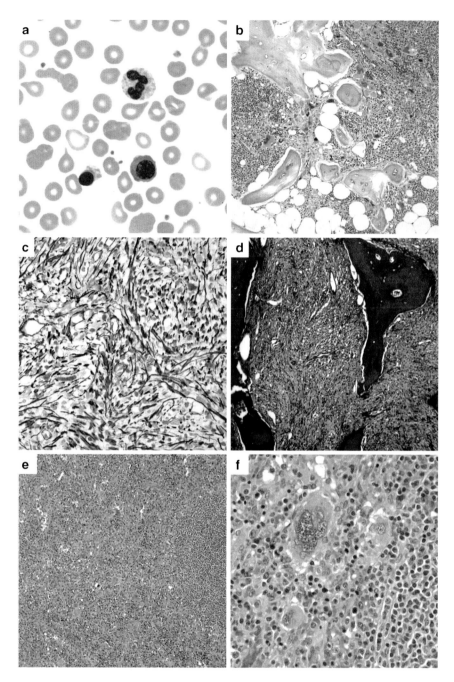

Fig. 1.4 Primary myelofibrosis, fibrotic stage. (**a**) Peripheral blood film from a man with primary myelofi-brosis who underwent splenectomy. Note the nucleated erythrocytes, hypochromasia, anisopoikilocytosis, and teardrop-shaped red blood cells (dacrocytes). Platelets range in size from tiny to large. (**b**) There is marked hypercellularity with a predominance of granulocytes precursors and atypical megakaryocytes. Note the dense small clusters of small and large megakaryocytes with maturation defects and abnormal translocation next to the trabecular bone. Osteosclerosis is present. (**c**) A reticulin stain shows a marked increase in reticulin fibers. (**d**) A trichrome stain shows an increase in collagen fibers. (**e**) The spleen shows expansion of the red pulp (*center*) and attenuated white pulp (*right*). Erythrocytes, granulocytes, and megakaryocytes are present in the sinusoids. (**f**) Megakaryocytes with abnormal nuclear: cytoplasmic ratios are conspicuous

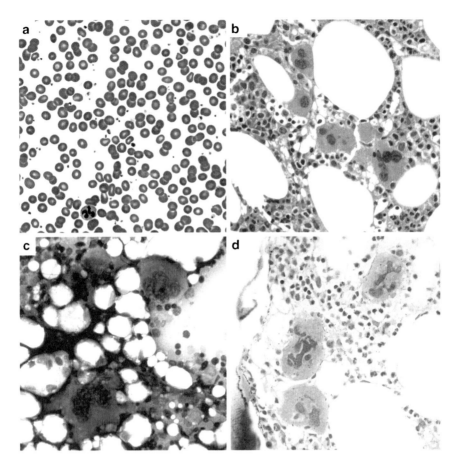

Fig. 1.5 Essential thrombocythemia in a 74-year-old woman. (**a**) Peripheral blood smear from a woman with a sustained platelet count >450 × 10⁹/L. Laboratory studies demonstrated the *JAK2* V617F clonal marker. (**b**) Bone marrow biopsy shows an increase in megakaryocytes, which occur in loose aggregates. Many megakaryocytes are unusually large with abundant mature cytoplasm and deeply lobulated staghorn nuclei. (**c**) Bone marrow aspirate smear with enlarged, mature megakaryocytes. (**d**) A reticulin stain shows the absence of relevant reticulin fibrosis

value speaks strongly against the diagnosis of PV, a normal erythropoietin value does not exclude PV or secondary erythrocytosis. When grown in vitro in semisolid medium, bone marrow cells isolated from patients with PV form EEC without the addition of exogenous erythropoietin. In contrast, precursors from healthy individuals and from patients with secondary polycythemia require erythropoietin for in vitro colony formation. But EEC formation is not specific for PV, and is seen in a number of cases of ET and PMF as well. Although testing for EECs provides information that can support the diagnosis of PV, the test is rarely available in clinical laboratories.

Although not included in the diagnostic criteria, routine cytogenetic studies at the time of diagnosis provide useful information and a baseline for future comparison. About 20% of patients with PV have abnormal karyotypes during diagnosis. The most common recurring abnormalities are +8, +9, del(20q), del(13q), and del(9p) [29]. Studies from *JAK2* V617F-positive patients with abnormal cytogenetics have revealed that the chromosomally abnormal cells are more likely to be homozygous for the *JAK2* mutation, but in some cases with mutated *JAK2*, individual cytogenetically abnormal cells in culture did not have the mutation, suggesting that in some instances the chromosome abnormality may precede acquisition of the mutation [30].

Abnormal findings on platelet function studies are common in PV, but they correlate poorly with bleeding or thromboses. However, patients with markedly elevated platelet counts ($1,000 \times 10^9$/L or more) may develop an acquired von Willebrand syndrome, which is associated with decreased functional activity of von Willebrand factor (vWF), and may predispose to bleeding. Most patients with PV have hyperuricemia, elevated histamine levels, and low serum ferritin, but none of these are specific for PV.

Disease Progression Including Post-Polycythemic Myelofibrosis and Acute Leukemia

Untreated patients with PV usually die within 1–2 years, because of thrombosis or hemorrhage. However, with proper management, survival times of 15 years or more are often reported, particularly in patients who are younger than 70 years at the time of diagnosis [27]. One of the most commonly recognized forms of disease progression is post-polycythemic myelofibrosis, which is a progressive and usually late complication that develops in approximately 15–20% of patients 10 years after the initial diagnosis of PV, and in 30–50% of those monitored for 15 years more [31, 32]. The criteria for diagnosis of post-polycythemic myelofibrosis are given in Table 1.6. It is characterized by myelofibrosis in the bone marrow (Fig. 1.3e) and extramedullary hematopoiesis in the spleen and liver, and sometimes in other sites. Usually there is anemia and a leukoerythroblastic blood smear with poikilocytosis, including teardrop-shaped forms (dacrocytes). The marrow cellularity decreases because of decreased erythropoiesis and granulopoiesis. Clusters of abnormal megakaryocytes often become the most prominent cellular component. Reticulin and overt collagen fibrosis of the marrow are frequent, and osteosclerosis may be prominent. Extramedullary hematopoiesis occurs in the sinuses of the spleen and liver, with particular prominence of the megakaryocytes [26].

Table 1.6 WHO Diagnostic criteria for post-polycythemic myelofibrosis (post-PVMF) [26].

Required criteria:

1. Documentation of a previous diagnosis of WHO-defined PV
2. Bone marrow fibrosis grade 2–3 (on 0–3 scale) or grade 3–4 (on 0–4 scale)

Plus two additional criteria required from the following list:

1. Anemia or sustained loss of either phlebotomy (in the absence of cytoreductive therapy) or cytoreductive treatment requirement for the erythrocytosis
2. Leukoerythroblastosis
3. Increasing splenomegaly defined as either an increase in palpable splenomegaly >5 cm from baseline (distance from the left costal margin) or the appearance of new splenomegaly
4. Development of at least two of the following constitutional symptoms: >10% weight loss in 6 months, night sweats, unexplained fever (>37.5°C)

There has been considerable controversy over factors that predispose to the development of post-polycythemic myelofibrosis, in particular whether cytoreductive therapy increases its incidence. However, recent data suggest that prior therapy is likely not the major risk factor. Rather, the allelic burden of the *JAK2* V617F mutation may be the most important predisposing factor, in that the incidence of post-polycythemic myelofibrosis is much higher in patients who are homozygous for the mutation at diagnosis than in those who are heterozygous [32, 33]. Additional factors reported to predict post-polycythemic myelofibrosis include an elevated serum LDH level and the presence of endogenous megakaryocytic colony formation at diagnosis [32].

Myelodysplastic syndromes and acute myeloid leukemia (AML) are infrequent and are usually late events in PV. The incidence of MDS/AML in patients with PV who have been treated only with phlebotomy is reportedly 1–2%, which is often assumed to be the incidence of MDS/AML in the "natural history" of the disease. However, the incidence of MDS/AML in some series reported in the literature ranges from 5 to 15% of patients monitored for 10 years or more [34, 35]. Greater patient age at diagnosis of PV and exposure to certain cytotoxic agents may increase the risk of MDS/AML. It is interesting that, in many cases, at the time of transformation to AML, the blasts do not carry the *JAK2* V617F mutation, suggesting that the blasts may originate from a pre-existent, *JAK2* non-mutated clone.

Differential Diagnosis Including Post-Polycy themic Myelofibrosis and Acute Leukemia

The causes of polycythemia are listed in Table 1.4. Most cases are acquired, either PV or secondary acquired polycythemia that is induced by hypoxia. Genetic testing for the *JAK2* V617F mutation and the study of serum erythropoietin levels should therefore be considered "up-front" tests for the diagnosis of PV and its differentiation from other causes of erythrocytosis. It should also be kept in mind that patients with an obvious cause of secondary polycythemia, such as chronic obstructive pulmonary disease, also may develop PV.

The only congenital primary polycythemia that has been well-characterized is primary familial and congenital polycythemia, which is caused by mutations in *EPOR*, the gene that encodes the erythropoietin receptor; this is a rare condition with an autosomal dominant inheritance pattern [36, 37]. Several mutations have been described that lead to truncation of the cytoplasmic portion of EPOR and a loss of the binding site for SHP1, a protein that normally downregulates erythropoietin-mediated activation of the signaling pathway. These mutations are hence activating mutations that lead to hypersensitivity of the erythroid precursors to erythropoietin, and serum erythropoietin levels are usually low or normal. There is erythroid proliferation with erythrocytosis, but no granulocytosis or thrombocytosis. However, *EPOR* mutations account for only a small number of the cases of primary familial and congenital polycythemia reported, and for the majority, the molecular defects are not known [36].

Most cases of secondary polycythemia are acquired and induced by hypoxia. Chronic obstructive lung disease, right-to-left cardiopulmonary shunt, sleep apnea, and renal disease that obstructs flow to the kidney are among the most frequent causes [37]. Chronic carbon monoxide poisoning causes tissue hypoxia and is responsible, in part, for "smoker's polycythemia," but nicotine further contributes by lowering plasma volume through its diuretic effect. However, inappropriate production of erythropoietin by a number of tumors, such as cerebellar hemangioblastoma, uterine leiomyoma, meningioma, and hepatocellular adenoma, among others, is a cause of secondary erythrocytosis that is sometimes overlooked.

Congenital secondary polycythemia should be considered in young patients or in patients with polycythemia of life-long duration. Two broad categories of defects are found in this category: those associated with increased Hb affinity for oxygen and those associated with mutations of genes that encode proteins in the oxygen-sensing/erythropoietin synthesis pathways. A number of Hb variants have increased affinity for oxygen and do not readily give up oxygen to the tissue, so that the oxygen dissociation curve is shifted "to the left." This is associated with tissue hypoxia, reduced P50, increased erythropoietin, and secondary erythrocytosis. Many of the abnormal Hbs with altered oxygen affinity are not detected by the usual electrophoretic screening tests, so that measurement of P50 is useful if these are suspected. A similar effect is observed in patients who have 2,3-bisphos-phoglycerate mutase deficiency, who are unable to release oxygen normally from their Hb, and who also have a shift to the left in the oxygen dissociation curve with reduced P50. The second category of congenital secondary poly-cythemias includes disorders in which mutations encoding proteins in the oxygen-sensing pathways result in increased synthesis of erythropoietin. The best known of these is Chuvash polycythemia, which affects individuals in the Chuvash region of Russia [36]. This inherited form of polycythemia results from a mutation in the von Hippel-Lindau (*VHL*) gene, which encodes the protein VHL. In contrast to normal VHL, the abnormal protein is unable to participate in the degradation of hypoxia-inducible factor-alpha, a transcription factor for erythropoietin synthesis, and thus erythropoietin production is not appropriately downregulated. A number of other mutations involving genes encoding proteins important in the regulation of erythropoietin synthesis have also been described [36].

Primary Myelofibrosis

Myelofibrosis is an increase in the amount and density of extracellular matrix proteins that provides the structural network upon which hematopoiesis occurs. This increase can vary from a focal, loose network of reticulin fibers to diffuse, dense, and markedly thickened fibers associated with collagen fibrosis and osteosclerosis [38].

Reactive myelofibrosis can occur in infections, inflammatory conditions, metabolic disorders, and neoplastic diseases, and secondary to exposure to various physical and chemical agents (Fig. 1.1). The underlying disease process is generally identified by the patient's medical history or by examining trephine biopsy sections. The fibrosis is confined to the areas involved by the primary disease. The trabecular bone may be normal or show increased osteoblastic and/or osteoclastic activity.

PMF is a clonal MPN characterized by proliferation of predominantly megakaryocytes and granulocytes and remodeling of bone marrow, including progressive myelofibrosis, exaggerated angiogenesis and, often, extramedullary hematopoiesis [1]. Two phases of the disease are recognized: (1) a pre-fibrotic or early stage, in which the marrow is hypercellular with absent or only slight reticulin fibrosis and minimal if any extramedullary hematopoiesis, often accompanied by peripheral blood thrombocytosis; and (2) the fibrotic stage, which is characterized by a usually hypocellular bone marrow with marked reticulin and/or collagen fibrosis and, often, osteosclerosis (Fig. 1.4). This latter stage often is associated with a leukoerythroblastic peripheral blood smear and with prominent hepatosplenomegaly due to extramedullary hematopoiesis. Progression from the pre-fibrotic to the fibrotic stage is stepwise [38].

In PMF, the megakaryocytic and granulocytic lineages have the most proliferative and/or survival advantage but, as in the other MPNs, all of the myeloid lineages and some B and T lymphocytes are derived from an abnormal bone marrow stem cell. In contrast, the fibroblasts are not derived from the neoplastic clone, but instead proliferate and deposit connective tissue in response to a number of cytokines that are abnormally produced and released [39, 40]. A large number of effectors, such as growth factors, their receptors, and subsequent downstream signaling factors, are involved in the changes of the histopathological phenotype [39, 40]. Fibrogenic factors include platelet-derived growth factor and transforming growth factor-beta, which are synthesized, packaged, and released by the neoplastic megakaryocytes and platelets. In addition to fibrosis, there is prominent neoangiogenesis (CD34+, CD105+) in the bone marrow and spleen. Serum levels of vascular endothelial growth factor are higher than normal in patients with PMF, and an increase in microvascular density (CD105+) in the bone marrow correlates with the degree of fibrosis and with *JAK2* V617F mutant allele burden [40]. Not only are cytokines that promote vascular proliferation and connective tissue deposition increased in PMF but so also are the plasma levels of macrophage inflammatory protein 1-beta, tissue inhibitor of metalloproteinase (TIMP-1), insulin-like growth binding factor-2, and tumor necrosis factor alpha-1 [41].

In an attempt to investigate the rule of abnormal megakaryopoiesis in the pathogenesis of PMF, several transgenic mouse models have been generated [42]. These models are based either on *JAK2* V617F or mutations that interfere with the extrinsic (thrombopoietin and its receptor *MPL*) and intrinsic (the GATA1 transcription factor) control of normal megakaryopoiesis. In animal models, mutated *MPL* bestows a more PMF-like phenotype than does *JAK2* V617F.

Diagnosis

The diagnostic criteria for PMF are shown in Table 1.7. PMF is a progressive disease, and the findings at diagnosis depend on the stage of disease in which the patient's symptoms are first recognized. Nearly 70% of patients are first encountered in the fibrotic stage, when the findings of leukoerythroblastosis, myelofibrosis, and splenomegaly are evident (Fig. 1.4). For the 20–25% of patients recognized in the early pre-fibrotic stage, the marked thrombocytosis often found at that time may lead to misclassification as ET. Thus, careful correlation of the clinical findings with laboratory data and careful examination of the peripheral blood and bone marrow biopsy are required to reach a correct diagnosis in the early stage.

Clinical Findings

The annual incidence of PMF reportedly ranges from 0.5 to 1.5 per 100,000 people. The median age at diagnosis is usually in the seventh decade, and less than 10% of patients are diagnosed before the age of 40 years [43].

The onset of PMF is usually insidious. Almost 25% of patients are asymptomatic when their illness is discovered by an abnormal routine blood count

Table 1.7 WHO diagnostic criteria for primary myelofibrosis [48].

Major criteria

1. Presence of megakaryocyte proliferation and atypia,[a] usually accompanied by either reticulin and/or collagen fibrosis or in the absence of significant reticulin fibrosis, the megakaryocyte changes must be accompanied by an increased bone marrow cellularity characterized by granulocytic proliferation and often decreased erythropoiesis (i.e. pre-fibrotic cellular-phase disease)

2. Not meeting WHO criteria for polycythemia vera,[b] *BCR-ABL1*+ chronic myelogenous leukemia,[c] myelodysplastic syndrome,[d] or other myeloid disorders

3. Demonstration of *JAK2* V617F or other clonal marker (e.g. *MPL*W515K/L) or in the absence of the above clonal markers, no evidence that bone marrow fibrosis is secondary to infection, autoimmune disorder or other chronic inflammatory condition, hairy cell leukemia or other lymphoid neoplasm, metastatic malignancy, or toxic (chronic) myelopathies[e]

Minor criteria

  1. Leukoerythroblastosis[f]

  2. Increase in serum lactate dehydrogenase level[f]

  3. Anemia[f]

  4. Palpable splenomegaly[f]

[a] Small to large megakaryocytes with an aberrant nuclear/cytoplasmic ratio and hyperchromatic, bulbous, or irregularly folded nuclei and dense clustering

[b] Requires the failure of iron replacement therapy to increase hemoglobin level to the polycythemia vera range in the presence of decreased serum ferritin. Exclusion of polycythemia vera is based on hemoglobin and hematocrit levels. Red cell mass measurement is not required

[c] Requires the absence of BCR-ABL1

[d] Requires absence of dyserythropoiesis and dysgranulopoiesis

[e] It should be noted that patients with conditions associated with reactive myelofibrosis are not immune to primary myelofibrosis and the diagnosis should be considered in such cases if other criteria are met

[f] Degree of abnormality could be borderline or marked

that shows anemia or marked thrombocytosis. Of symptomatic patients, more than half of them report only nonspecific symptoms such as fatigue. Hypercatabolic symptoms, including weight loss, night sweats, and low-grade fever, are common, as are symptoms related to hyperuricemia, such as gouty arthritis or renal stones. In the pre-fibrotic stage, symptoms such as fatigue, easy bruising, and weight loss are often reported, but palpable splenomegaly and hepatomegaly are usually absent or only minor to moderate in severity [44]. Patients whose disease is in this phase may present with bleeding and/or thrombosis, and because the platelet count is often markedly elevated, the clinical picture may overlap that of ET. Blood and bone marrow are always involved. In the advanced stages of the disease, extramedullary hematopoiesis involving spleen, liver, lymph nodes, kidney, adrenal gland (Fig. 1.4e, f), dura mater, gastrointestinal tract, lung, pleura, breast, and soft tissue becomes prominent. In the initial stages, randomly distributed CD34-positive progenitors are slightly increased in the bone marrow, but not in the peripheral blood. Only in the advanced stages do CD34-positive cells appear in the peripheral blood in large numbers.

During the fibrotic stage of PMF, symptoms related to anemia are common. Splenomegaly can be massive and may lead to early satiety, abdominal discomfort, or acute abdominal pain due to splenic infarct [45]. The splenomegaly is due to extramedullary hematopoiesis. Hepatomegaly is found in as many as 50% of patients whose disease is in the fibrotic stage, partly because of extramedullary hematopoiesis and partly because of portal vein hypertension. Ascites and variceal bleeding are common complications. The clinical findings in the fibrotic stage of PMF mimic those seen in post-polycythemic myelofibrosis and post-ET myelofibrosis; only through documentation of the initial disease can these entities be distinguished.

Laboratory Findings

Peripheral blood: The pre-fibrotic stage is characterized by modest anemia (mean Hb, 13 g/dL; range 7.0–15.5), mild leukocytosis (mean white blood cell [WBC] count, 14 × 10^9/L; range 5.6–32.7), and moderate to marked thrombocytosis (mean platelet count, 962 × 10^9/L; range 104–3,215). The most striking finding on the peripheral blood smear in this early stage is usually marked thrombocytosis. Mild neutrophilia and a "left shift" with occasional myelocytes may be present, but myeloblasts, nucleated RBCs, and dacrocytes are only rarely observed.

The hematological parameters worsen gradually as the disease progresses, and patients whose disease is in the fibrotic stage are more anemic (mean Hb, 11.5 g/dL; range 4.2–14.0) and have lower platelet counts (mean platelet count, 520 × 10^9/L; range 190–2,496) than those whose disease is in the pre-fibrotic stage. Although mild leukocytosis is common in the fibrotic period, severe leukopenia also may occur as bone marrow failure becomes more prominent owing to increasing myelofibrosis (mean WBC count ~14.0 × 10^9/L; range 1.0–62.2).

Leukoerythroblastosis, numerous dacrocytes, and large, abnormal platelets are evident in the fibrotic stage of the disease (Fig. 1.4a). Circulating megakaryocyte nuclei are frequently observed. Blasts can be seen on the peripheral blood smear during the fibrotic stage of disease, and can occasionally account for 5–9% of the WBCs. Blast percentages of 10–19% in the peripheral blood should arouse concern for an accelerated phase, and a bone marrow specimen is warranted for further evaluation [23].

Bone marrow: A bone marrow biopsy is essential for diagnosis of PMF (Fig. 1.4b). The biopsy should be processed to allow accurate assessment of cellularity, the relative numbers of cells in the various myeloid lineages and their degree of immaturity, and the amount/grade of fibrosis, as well as careful evaluation of megakaryocyte morphology. The bone marrow biopsy should always be stained for reticulin fibers, using a standard protocol to avoid technical variation. The reticulin fiber content should be evaluated by a semi quantitative grading system that is reproducible (See Table 1.3 and Fig. 1.2) [24]. An immunostain for CD34 or CD105 endothelial markers may provide additional information regarding neoangiogenesis, and the CD34 stain may highlight more blasts than suspected from routinely stained sections. A bone marrow aspirate and touch imprint will provide helpful information regarding blast percentages and maturation of the neoplastic populations.

In the pre-fibrotic stage, the bone marrow is hypercellular and shows an increase in the number of neutrophils, some hypersegmented, but often a decrease in erythropoiesis. The percentage of myeloblasts is not increased, which can be confirmed by immunohistochemical staining for CD34. The megakaryocytes are abnormal, forming dense clusters and translocation close to the trabecular bone. They vary from small to large forms, with an abnormal nuclear/cytoplasmic ratio and disorganized, plump, "cloud-like" or "balloon-like" nuclear lobulation (Fig. 1.4). Often the nuclei are hyperchromatic, and numerous bare megakaryocytic nuclei, which are immunoreactive with CD61 stain, are seen. Overall, the megakaryocytes of PMF, even in the early stages, have a pleomorphic and bizarre appearance that, when combined with the background of exuberant neutrophil proliferation, can distinguish pre-fibrotic stage PMF from ET, with which it is most frequently confused (Fig. 1.5). Reticulin fibers vary in quantity and thickness, but are often not increased except focally around the blood vessels. A stain for CD34 will demonstrate the increase in vascularity, but there are no clusters of blasts or significant increase in blasts. Lymphoid nodules are reportedly present in 24% of patients with PMF, most frequently in the pre-fibrotic stage [46]. In some of these cases, the B and T lymphocytes have been shown to be derived from the neoplastic clone [47].

As PMF progresses to the fibrotic stage, marrow cellularity gradually decreases, and reticulin or even collagen fibrosis of the marrow increases (Fig. 1.4). Islands of hematopoiesis are separated by loose connective tissue or fat and by dilatation of marrow sinuses. The sinuses, which are factor VIII positive and CD34 negative, are prominent and contain hematopoietic cells. Atypical megakaryocytes are often the predominant cells in the marrow in the fibrotic stage and occur in sizable clusters or sheets. New bone formation and osteosclerosis occur (Fig. 1.4).

The finding of 10–19% blasts in the bone marrow and/or blood support the diagnosis of "PMF in accelerated stage," and the finding of 20% or more is considered as evidence of transformation to AML. Patients may present for the first time with overt acute megakaryoblastic leukemia, their bone marrow or blood showing a background of fibrosis, osteosclerosis, and enlarged, atypical megakaryocytes that resemble those of PMF. In such cases, the best diagnosis is AML, with a comment suggesting molecular studies for *BCR-ABL1, JAK2* V617F mutation, and *MPL* W515L/K to confirm its possible origin from PMF or another MPN.

Extramedullary tissues: Many of the abnormalities observed in the peripheral blood, such as dacrocytes and leukoerythroblastosis, are due to abnormal release of cells from sites of extramedullary hematopoiesis. The most common sites of extramedullary hematopoiesis in PMF are the spleen and liver, but almost any organ can be affected. In the spleen, the red pulp is expanded by trilineage hematopoiesis in the sinuses (Fig. 1.4). Megakaryocytes are often the most prominent component and may show cytological atypia [48]. The red pulp cords may show fibrosis or contain megakaryocytes, normoblasts, and granulocytes. Hepatic sinuses also demonstrate extramedullary hematopoiesis. Fibrosis and cirrhosis of the liver are common, and they, along with the extramedullary hematopoiesis, play the major role in the pathogenesis of portal hypertension that can develop.

Extramedullary tissues also may be a site of transformation to a blast phase, and myeloid sarcoma should be considered in the differential diagnosis of any extramedullary lesion in a patient with PMF. Wright-Giemsa-stained smears and touch imprints from extramedullary tissue and immunohistochemical stains for CD34 are very helpful in excluding this possibility when examining extramedullary tissues from such cases.

The extramedullary hematopoiesis in PMF is composed of neoplastic cells, and is likely derived from hematopoietic stem cells and precursor cells that arise in the bone marrow. The structure of the marrow sinuses is distorted and compromised by the surrounding connective tissue increase, and immature bone marrow cells more readily gain access to the marrow sinuses and hence the circulation in patients with PMF [49]. CD34-positive cells are increased in the peripheral blood of patients with PMF, particularly in the fibrotic stage, when compared with other MPNs and with normal controls, and an increase in CD34-positive cells can also be demonstrated in the spleen.

Genetic Studies

Approximately, 50% of patients with PMF have the *JAK2* V617F mutation, whereas mutations of *MPL*, such as *MPL* W515L/K, are found in an additional 5%. These mutations are not specific for PMF. For MPNs for which pre-fibrotic PMF and ET represent the most probable diagnoses, a *JAK* 2V617F allele burden >50% favors a diagnosis of pre-fibrotic PMF [50].

The level and duration of *JAK2* V617F as well as additional molecular abnormalities (e.g. those in TET oncogene family member 2, *TET2*) may play a role in PMF. *TET2* is a homolog of the gene originally discovered at the chromosome Ten–Eleven Translocation site in a subset of patients with acute leukemia. Mutations and deletions of *TET2* located at chromosome 4q24 are found in bone marrow cells from 17% of patients with PMF (both *JAK2* V617F positive and negative). The frequency of mutations in MPNs increases with age but does not alter disease severity [51]. *JAK2* V617F may be dependent not only on the amount of heterozygous and homozygous mutant protein, but also on the various pathways regulating JAK2 activity, including MPL, JAK2, STAT, MAPK, and PI3K signaling pathways.

Clonal cytogenetic abnormalities are detected during diagnosis in about one third of patients with PMF, and the frequency increases over time [52–54]. These studies showed the favorable prognostic effect of isolated del(20q)/del(13q) in PMF. The prognostic value of other cytogenetic abnormalities is an area of active investigation. More than 90% of patients whose MPN transforms into MDS or AML have cytogenetic abnormalities that are often complex and include abnormalities of chromosome 5 and/or 7 [55]. Neither Philadelphia chromosome nor *BCR-ABL1* fusion gene is expressed in PMF.

Miscellaneous laboratory findings: Serum LDH level is increased in most patients with PMF, and the increase correlates with the degree of microvascular density in the bone marrow [56]. Nearly half of patients with PMF have some disturbance of the immune system.

Disease Progression/Prognosis

The natural evolution of PMF is progressive bone marrow fibrosis accompanied by bone marrow failure. An increase in spleen size can be very problematic, leading not only to pain and discomfort but also to worsening of cytopenias, portal hypertension, and hypercatabolic symptoms. Although splenectomy may benefit occasional patients, a significant number will develop more prominent hepatomegaly. Myeloid blast transformation occurs in ~5–20% of patients, at a median time of about 3 years after the initial recognition of PMF, and usually responds poorly to therapy. Transformation is almost always accompanied by karyotypic evolution [45].

The most important predictors of shortened survival at diagnosis include anemia (Hb <10 g/dL), advanced age (>65 years), circulating blasts (1% or greater), leukopenia (<4.0 × 10^9/L), leukocytosis (>25 × 10^9/L), presence of constitutional symptoms, and various cytogenetic abnormalities such as trisomy 8 [12, 57]. Survival time depends on the stage of the disease at diagnosis. Overall median survival of patients whose disease is diagnosed in the fibrotic stage is approximately 5 years, whereas 10-year and 15-year relative survival rates of 72% and 59% have been reported in patients whose disease was diagnosed in the pre-fibrotic stage, respectively[58]. The international prognostic scoring system for PMF is based on five independent predictors of inferior survival: age >65 years, Hb <10 g/dL, leukocyte count >25 × 10^9/L, circulating blasts ≥1%, and presence of constitutional symptoms [43]. The presence of 0, 1, 2, and ≥3 adverse prognostic factors defines low-, intermediate-1–, intermediate-2–, and high-risk disease.

Differential Diagnosis

The differential diagnosis of the fibrotic stage of PMF includes post-polycythemic myelofibrosis and post-ET myelofibrosis, but without a history of preceding PV or ET the distinction between these and the fibrotic stage of PMF is impossible. However, sometimes distinguishing other myeloid neoplasms, metastatic tumor, and even inflammatory diseases from PMF can be problematic (Fig. 1.6).

Pre-fibrotic PMF vs. ET: Distinguishing pre-fibrotic PMF from ET is a challenging diagnostic problem. Thrombocytosis, sometimes in excess of 1,000 × 10^9/L, is not uncommon in pre-fibrotic PMF. Because reported overall survival durations of ET and PMF differ, their distinction is important. The peripheral blood smear may support a diagnosis of pre-fibrotic PMF if neutrophilia, occasional immature granulocytes, basophilia, and rare dacrocytes are identified. In bone marrow biopsy specimens, however, in contrast to the clustered, highly atypical, and variably sized megakaryocytes of PMF, the megakaryocytes of ET are often more dispersed, uniformly large or giant, with abundant, mature cytoplasm and with deeply lobulated staghorn-like nuclei (Fig. 1.5). The neutrophilic proliferation that is often seen in the bone marrow specimens of pre-fibrotic PMF is absent in ET. Any appreciable reticulin fibrosis and increased vascularity is a strong argument in favor of PMF.

Acute panmyelosis with myelofibrosis: This subtype of AML is characterized in the peripheral blood by pancytopenia with minimal poikilocytosis and an absence of dacrocytes. The granulocytes are dysplastic and a few circulating blasts are common. There is minimal if any organomegaly (Fig. 1.1). The bone marrow is variably cellular with proliferation of erythroid, granulocytic, and megakaryocytic elements in variable proportions. Blasts constitute 20% or more of the marrow cells [59]. The megakaryocytes, of small and dysplastic morphology, are dispersed in the bone marrow. Immature megakaryocytes and megakaryoblasts may be present, and in most cases it is more difficult to distinguish acute panmyelosis with myelofibrosis from high-grade MDS or acute megakaryocytic leukemia than from PMF. However, differentiation from PMF in an accelerated or blast phase may be more problematic.

Myelodysplastic syndrome with myelofibrosis: Significant myelofibrosis may be found in 5–10% of cases of MDS, generally in those with excess blasts, and such cases have been collectively referred to as MDS with fibrosis (MDS-F) [60]. In contrast to patients with PMF, those with MDS-F lack significant organomegaly, and the blood and bone marrow demonstrate prominent

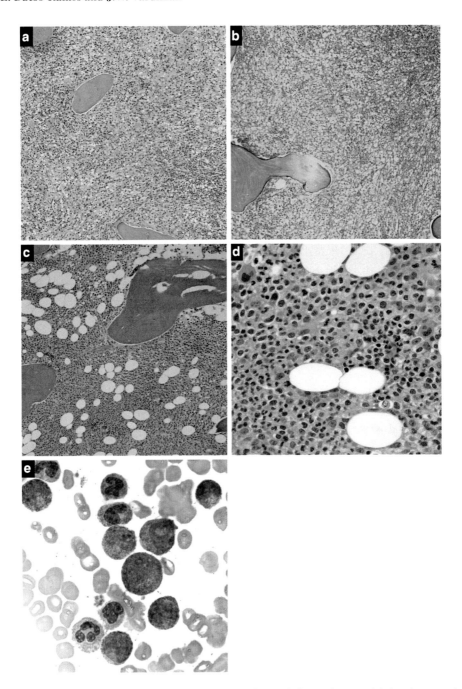

Fig. 1.6 Reactive myelofibrosis and hematopoietic effects of growth factor therapy. (**a**) Autoimmune (reactive) myelofibrosis with a hypercellular bone marrow biopsy specimen and increased numbers of megakaryocytes of normal morphology dispersed in the marrow. (**b**) Marked reticulin fibrosis in trephine biopsy specimen (reticulin stain). (**c**) The bone marrow biopsy of a man who had undergone hematopoietic growth factor therapy. Note the hypercellular bone marrow trilineage hyperplasia. (**d**) High magnification of the biopsy specimen showing granulocytic predominance and mature megakaryocytes of normal morphology. (**e**) Bone marrow aspirate smear showing left-shifted granulopoiesis with increased cytoplasmic granulation and Dohle bodies

multilineage dysplasia (Fig. 1.1). In the bone marrow, the megakaryocytes are small, dysplastic forms, in contrast to the pleomorphic, bizarre, and often enlarged forms of PMF. Cellular bone marrow aspirates are not obtainable, but the blasts can be identified on biopsy touch imprints and by immunostaining of the bone marrow biopsy for CD34.

Autoimmune myelofibrosis: Patients with autoimmune disorders such as systemic lupus erythematosus may develop myelofibrosis (Fig. 1.6). These patients often present with peripheral blood cytopenias, particularly anemia, and may have mild poikilocytosis with rare dacrocytes. The bone marrow varies from hypocellular to nearly 100% cellular, with marked reticulin fibrosis and increased numbers of dispersed megakaryocytes of normal morphology (Fig. 1.6). There is usually erythroid hyperplasia and interstitial aggregates of T and B lymphocytes. A slight increase in polytypic plasma cells is often seen in a perivascular distribution. Splenomegaly is absent [61].

Essential Thrombocythemia

Essential thrombocythemia is an MPN that involves primarily the megakaryocytic lineage [4]. It is characterized by sustained thrombocytosis ($\geq$450 $\times$ 10^9/L) in the peripheral blood and increased numbers of large, mature megakaryocytes with staghorn-like nuclei in a normocellular bone marrow (Fig. 1.5). The marked thrombocytosis is associated with abnormal platelet function and increased risk of thrombosis and hemorrhage. The WHO published a revised set of diagnostic criteria for ET in 2008 [62] (Table 1.8). The clonal nature of ET was elucidated from sex-linked G6PD studies, identifying ET as a clonal stem cell disorder.

Subsequent investigations utilizing polymerase chain reaction and DNA methylation of X-linked genes have shown that the majority of patients with ET have monoclonal hematopoiesis. The *JAK2* V617F mutation is present in approximately 50% of cases, and the *MPL* W515K/L in 1–2%. These mutations lead to constitutive activation of pathways that stimulate megakaryocyte proliferation and platelet production. The cause of the proliferation in the remaining cases is currently unknown. The finding of a *BCR-ABL1* fusion gene excludes the diagnosis.

Serum level of thrombopoietin, the major megakaryocytic growth and differentiation factor, has been reported to be inappropriately normal or elevated. Circulating levels of thrombopoietin are regulated by the extent of its binding to MPL. As megakaryocyte and platelet mass increase, levels of thrombopoietin fall as a result of this binding. Normally as the MPL–thrombopoietin complex is destroyed as platelets are removed from the circulation, thrombopoietin levels increase to stimulate more platelet production [63]. The binding of thrombopoietin with MPL on the megakaryocyte normally initiates conformational changes of MPL and activation of the JAK kinase constitutively bound to the cytoplasmic domain of MPL. This initiates signaling through the STAT, PI3K, and MAPK pathways to stimulate proliferation, endoreduplication, and expansion of the megakaryocytic mass.

In patients with ET and mutated *JAK2* V617F or *MPL* W515K/L, the normal pathway of stimulation by thrombopoietin is constitutively activated because of the mutation, and megakaryocyte proliferation and platelet production are either independent of, or hypersensitive to, thrombopoietin. A similar, albeit unknown, defect is presumably present in the remaining cases of ET. The reason that the *JAK2* V617F mutation leads to ET in some patients and in others to PV or PMF is not clear, although it has been noted that patients with ET tend to have lower allele burden of the mutated *JAK2* than patients with PV or PMF [64, 65].

Diagnosis

There is no unique test that specifically identifies ET, so all other causes for thrombocytosis must be excluded before diagnosis. Although the *JAK2* V617F mutation is found in about half of the patients with ET and the *MPL* W515K/L mutation in another 1–2%, these mutations are not specific [11]. Still, when one of these mutations is present it confirms the clonal nature of the thrombocytosis. Patients with reactive thrombocytosis infrequently experience bleeding or thromboses, but patients with clonal megakaryocytic proliferations associated with thrombocytosis are at increased risk for these events. In cases of ET that do not demonstrate a mutation or a clonal chromosomal marker, additional studies are necessary to exclude not only reactive causes of the thrombocytosis but also other neoplastic causes. The diagnostic criteria for ET are given in Table 1.8.

Clinical findings: Essential thrombocythemia is a rare disorder, with an estimated incidence of about 0.6–2.5 per 100,000 persons per year [66]. The disease can occur at any age, including in children; most cases occur in the sixth decade of life, although a second peak, particularly in women, occurs at approximately 30 years of age [67].

Approximately 30–50% of patients with ET are asymptomatic at diagnosis, and the disease is discovered when a blood count is obtained for routine screening or for evaluation of another illness. The remaining patients have symptoms that are related to microvascular occlusive events (headache, transient ischemic attacks, dizziness, visual disturbances, erythromelalgia, or seizure), major vascular occlusive events (stroke, myocardial infarct, deep venous thrombosis, Budd–Chiari syndrome), or, less commonly, hemorrhage from mucosal surfaces

Table 1.8 WHO Diagnostic Criteria for Essential Thrombocythemia (ET).

Diagnosis requires meeting all four criteria

1. Sustained platelet count $\geq 450 \times 10^9/L$[a]
2. Bone marrow biopsy specimen showing proliferation mainly of the megakaryo-cytic lineage with increased numbers of enlarged, mature megakaryocytes. No significant increase or left-shift of neutrophil granulopoiesis or erythropoiesis
3. Not meeting WHO criteria for polycythemia vera[b], primary myelofibrosis[c], *BCR-ABL1* positive CML[d] or myelodysplastic syndrome[e] or other myeloid neoplasm
4. Demonstration of *JAK2* V617F or other clonal marker, or in the absence of *JAK2* V617F, no evidence of reactive thrombocytosis[f]

[a] Sustained during the work-up process
[b] Requires the failure of iron replacement therapy to increase hemoglobin level to the poly-cythemia vera range in the presence of decreased serum ferritin. Exclusion of polycythemia vera is based on hemoglobin and hematocrit levels and red cell mass measurement is not required
[c] Requires the absence of relevant reticulin fibrosis, collagen fibrosis, peripheral blood leukoerythrob-lastosis, or markedly hypercellular marrow accompanied by megakaryocyte morphology that is typical for primary myelofibrosis – small to large megakaryocytes with an aberrant nuclear/cytoplasmic ratio and hyperchromatic, bulbous or irregularly folded nuclei and dense clustering
[d] Requires the absence of BCR-ABL1
[e] Requires absence of dyserythropoiesis and dysgranulopoiesis
[f] Causes of reactive thrombocytosis include iron deficiency, splenectomy, surgery, infection, inflammation, connective tissue disease, metastatic cancer, and lymphoproliferative disorders. However, the presence of a condition associated with reactive thrombocytosis does not exclude the possibility of ET if other criteria are met

(epistaxis, gastrointestinal bleeding) [68]. Splenomegaly and/or hepatomegaly are present in only a minority of patients and are usually not marked.

Peripheral blood: Thrombocytosis is the most striking abnormality found on the hemogram, and counts may range from 450×10^9/L to more than $2,000 \times 10^9$/L [1]. The peripheral blood smear in ET will characteristically show platelet anisocytosis, ranging from small to giant platelets. Hypogranular platelets are not common (Fig. 1.5a). Platelet anisocytosis correlates with an elevation in platelet distribution width. Enumeration of platelets in whole blood counters can be problematic because of variations in platelet size and spontaneous platelet aggregation. Large platelets and platelet aggregates may not be counted as platelets, resulting in significant underestimation of platelet counts. Review of a peripheral blood film is mandatory to avoid errors in platelet counting. Other abnormal morphological findings may include minimal leukocytosis with WBC counts usually in the range of $8–15 \times 10^9$/L [4], although the WBC count may be elevated in patients who have experienced hemorrhage. Generally, the leukocyte differential is unremarkable; basophilia and immature granulocytes are infrequent, and leukoerythroblastosis is not observed at the time of diagnosis. Mild anemia may be present, but anisocytosis is absent, and dacrocytes are not observed. Hypochromia and microcytosis may be present in patients with a history of bleeding. Morphologic findings reflective of hyposplenism include the presence of Howell–Jolly bodies, Pappenheimer bodies (siderotic granules), target cells, and acanthocytes.

Bone marrow: A bone marrow biopsy is essential in distinguishing ET from the other MPNs, including the pre-fibrotic stage of PMF, and from reactive causes of thrombocytosis. In patients with ET, bone marrow is typically normocellular or slightly hypercellular (Fig. 1.5b). The most striking abnormality is the increase in the number and size of the megakaryocytes. They may occur in loose clusters and/or be singly dispersed in the marrow. There are large to giant megakaryocytes with abundant, mature cytoplasm and deeply lobulated and hyperlobulated staghorn nuclei (Fig. 1.5b, c) [62]. No significant population of bizarre megakaryocytes with increased nucleus/cytoplasm ratio or marked pleomorphism is observed in ET. If such forms are encountered frequently, a diagnosis of PMF should be considered rather than ET. In most cases, the myeloid/erythroid precursor ratio is normal, but if there has been hemorrhage, there may be some erythroid proliferation. Granulocytic proliferation is uncommon, and if present should raise doubts about the diagnosis of ET. Blasts are not increased in number and there is no evidence of myelodysplasia. The network of reticulin fibers is normal to only mildly increased [62], and the trabecular bone is normal (Fig. 1.5d). On the aspirate smears, there are huge multilobulated megakaryocytes with abundant cytoplasm, often associated with large aggregates of platelets. Stainable iron is normal. The presence of increased angiogenesis, marked decrease of c-MPL expression in megakaryocytes (less than 50% positive by immunohistochemical stain), and proliferation of large to giant megakaryocytes in normocellular bone marrow is highly sensitive and specific for distinguishing ET from reactive thrombocytosis [69].

Extramedullary tissues: Splenic enlargement is uncommon at the time of diagnosis and, if present, may be largely due to pooling and sequestration of platelets; extramedullary hematopoiesis is not present or minimal.

Genetic studies: Nearly 50% of patients with ET have *JAK2* V617F mutation and 1–2% have mutated *MPL*. Bone marrow karyotype is frequently normal; cytogenetic abnormalities are detected in less than 10% of cases at the time of diagnosis [70]. The most frequent abnormalities, such as del(20q) and trisomy 8, are not specific and can be found in any myeloid neoplasm. Cytogenetic abnormalities are more common when ET evolves to acute leukemia, perhaps as a result of cytotoxic therapy. Cytogenetic studies may be helpful in excluding ET as the reason for thrombocytosis in some cases. The discovery of del(5q) as a sole abnormality would suggest the diagnosis of MDS associated with thrombocytosis rather than ET, whereas t(3;3)(q21;q26.2) or inv(3)(q21q26.2) would indicate MDS or AML rather than ET. Detection of Philadelphia chromosome or *BCR-ABL1* fusion gene indicates that the diagnosis is CML, not ET. Moreover, each of these disorders is associated with characteristic megakaryocyte morphology that differs from the large, hyperlobulated megakaryocytes seen in ET.

Miscellaneous laboratory studies: Patients with ET usually have abnormal findings on platelet function studies, but correlation between an abnormal result and ability to predict hemorrhagic or thrombotic episodes is poor. There is evidence of abnormal platelet activation by unknown mechanisms [71]. Higher platelet counts tend to be associated with a greater probability of hemorrhage, however, most likely because of an acquired von Willebrand syndrome. This is associated with loss of large vWF multimers and vWF function. Serum uric acid levels may be elevated in 25–30% of patients with ET, and serum potassium and phosphorus levels are sometimes falsely elevated because of platelet lysis in uncentrifuged serum specimens. Serum ferritin level is almost always normal [62].

Disease Progression/Prognosis

The natural history of ET is that of an indolent disorder with long symptom-free intervals punctuated by episodes of thrombosis or hemorrhage. Progression to post-ET myelofibrosis occurs in a minority of patients after years of follow-up [72]. Similarly, a small number of patients, less than 5%, show transformation to acute leukemia, and the majority of those reported have been treated previously with cytotoxic agents. Overall, median survival times of 10–15 years have been reported, and in the large majority of patients, life expectancy is near normal [58].

Differential Diagnosis

The clinical history, physical findings, and a few ancillary laboratory studies are often sufficient to distinguish between reactive and neoplastic causes of thrombocytosis. A history of chronic thrombocytosis and hemorrhagic or thrombotic episodes, and the findings of splenomegaly and clustering of large hyperlobated megakaryocytes in bone marrow, would favor ET, whereas the lack of these findings plus evidence of an underlying inflammatory disease, such as an elevated C-reactive protein, would favor reactive thrombocytosis. Nevertheless, if an underlying cause to explain the thrombocytosis is not readily identified, studies for the *JAK2* V617F mutation should be performed, and a bone marrow specimen obtained and examined for the characteristic features of ET or another myeloid neoplasm, as well as for marrow involvement by a disorder that might lead to reactive thrombocytosis.

The most frequently encountered myeloid neoplasms that are typically associated with thrombocytosis and could be confused with ET include the polycythemic stage of PV, the pre-fibrotic stage of PMF, and CML. Each of these diseases has been characterized in the preceding sections and tables in this chapter. It should be remembered that some cases of CML, particularly those with the p230 oncoprotein, may initially display marked thrombocytosis and minimal leukocytosis.

The provisional MDS/MPN entity refractory anemia with ring sideroblasts and thrombocytosis (RARS-T) is another diagnostic consideration. It resembles ET in that it is characterized by a platelet count $\geq 450 \times 10^9/L$ and proliferation of megakaryocytes in the bone marrow that morphologically resembles those of ET or PMF [73]. However, RARS-T demonstrates ineffective erythroid proliferation with dyserythropoiesis and ring sideroblasts that account for 15% or more of the erythroid precursors. There is marked anemia. Nearly half of cases of RARS-T have the *JAK2* V617F mutation. It is a myeloid neoplasm with both myelodysplastic and myeloproliferative features at the molecular and clinical levels, and it may develop from RARS through the acquisition of somatic mutations of *JAK2*, *MPL*, or other as-yet-unknown genes [74].

Other myeloid neoplasms associated with thrombocytosis: Elevated platelet counts are uncommon in MDS or AML, but in some specific instances, the platelet count may be markedly elevated. Myelodysplastic syndromes associated with del(5q) as the sole abnormality, and MDS and AML with t(3;3)(q21;q26.2) or inv(3)(q21q26.2), are frequently associated with thrombocytosis. In the case of MDS with del(5q), in contrast to the normocellular bone marrow with hyperlobulated megakaryocyte nuclei of ET, there is hypercellular bone marrow with small hypolobulated megakaryocytes. The MDS and AML cases associated with t(3;3) or inv(3) are characterized by numerous CD61-positive, factor VIII-positive dysplastic micromegakaryocytes.

Other *BCR-ABL1*-Negative Myeloproliferative Neoplasms

The *BCR-ABL1*-negative MPNs include not only PV, ET, and PMF, but also CNL; CEL, NOS (i.e. eosinophilic leukemia lacking *PDGFRA*, *PDGFRB*, or *FGFR1* abnormalities); mastocytosis; and MPNs that lack the criteria for any of the other recognized MPNs and are therefore considered as MPN, unclassifiable. The diagnosis and management of all cases of eosinophilic leukemia and mastocytosis are described in later chapters. CNL and MPN, unclassifiable, are discussed in this section.

Chronic Neutrophilic Leukemia

CNL is a rare MPN characterized by a sustained proliferation of mature neutrophilic granulocytes in the bone marrow with leukemic involvement of the peripheral blood and infiltration of the spleen and liver [75]. Although some data suggest that CNL arises in a pluripotent stem cell with involvement of lymphoid as well as myeloid lineages, other data indicate that the lineage involvement in CNL may be limited to the granulocytes [76, 77]. Mononuclear cells isolated from the blood and bone marrow of patients with CNL reportedly give rise to colonies of mature granulocytes without added growth factors. The abnormalities in signal transduction that account for the endogenous colony formation are not known, but *JAK2* V617F mutations have been reported in a few cases [78, 79]. However, CNL is so rare that not enough cases have been studied to reliably assess its cell of origin, underlying biology, or even incidence. Fewer than 150 cases are reported in the literature, and likely less than 50% of those meet the WHO criteria for its diagnosis [80].

Diagnosis

The WHO criteria for CNL are found in Table 1.9. Although CNL usually affects older adults, it has been reported in adolescents as well. The sexes are nearly equally affected [75]. Many patients are asymptomatic when a routine blood count reveals neutrophilia, whereas others complain of fatigue, gout, or pruritus. The most consistent physical finding is splenomegaly and/or hepatomegaly. A bleeding tendency of uncertain origin has been reported in 25–30% of cases [81].

Blood and bone marrow: The WBC count is 25×10^9/L or greater (median, 50×10^9/L). Segmented neutrophils and bands account for 80% or more of the WBCs, whereas the sum of immature granulocytes (promyelocytes, myelocytes, and metamyelocytes) is usually less than 5% and always less than 10% of the WBCs [75]. Myeloblasts are almost never seen in the blood during diagnosis. Toxic granulation in the neutrophils is common but not invariable, and there is no significant dysplasia (Fig. 1.7a). Monocytes constitute $<1 \times 10^9$/L, and significant basophilia and eosinophilia are not observed. The platelet count is usually normal or slightly reduced, and marked thrombocytopenia

Table 1.9 WHO Diagnostic criteria for chronic neutrophilic leukemia [75].

1. Peripheral blood leukocytosis, WBC $\geq 25 \times 10^9$/L
Segmented neutrophils and bands are >80% of white blood cells
Immature granulocytes (promyelocytes, myelocytes, metamyelocytes) are <10% of white blood cells
Myeloblasts are <1% of white blood cells
2. Hypercellular bone marrow biopsy
Neutrophilic granulocytes increased in percentage and number
Myeloblasts are <5% of nucleated bone marrow cells
Neutrophilic maturation pattern normal or shifted to segmented forms
Megakaryocytes normal
3. Hepatosplenomegaly
4. No identifiable cause for physiologic neutrophilia, or if present, proof of clonality of myeloid cells
No infectious or inflammatory process
No underlying tumor
5. No Philadelphia chromosome or *BCR-ABL1* fusion gene
6. No rearrangement of *PDGFRA*, *PDGFRB* or *FGFR1*
7. No evidence of PV, ET, or PMF
8. No evidence of MDS or of MDS/MPN
No granulocytic dysplasia
No myelodysplastic changes in other myeloid lineages
Monocytes $<1 \times 10^9$/L

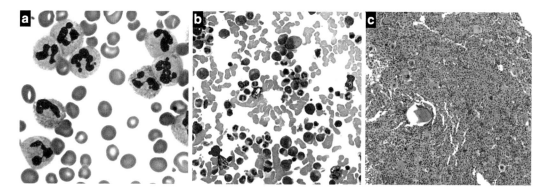

Fig. 1.7 Chronic neutrophilic leukemia. (**a**) Peripheral blood smear showing marked mature neutrophilia. (**b**) Increased granulocytic precursors in the bone marrow aspirate smear. (**c**) Prominent neutrophilia in the bone marrow biopsy specimen with left-shift and increased medium-sized megakaryocytes

or thrombocytosis is uncommon. Platelet function study results have been reported to be abnormal, although only a fraction of patients described in the literature have been tested.

The bone marrow in CNL is hypercellular because of neutrophil proliferation, with a myeloid/erythroid precursor ratio often 20:1 or more (Fig. 1.7b, c). Percentages of blasts and promyelocytes are not increased at diagnosis, but the percentages of myelocytes, metamyelocytes, bands, and segmented neutrophils are increased [75]. The neutrophils may show reactive changes with toxic granules, but there is no significant dysplasia. The percentage of erythroid precursors is decreased, but those present are usually normoblastic. Megakaryocytes are morphologically normal, but mild megakaryocytic proliferation may be observed. Reticulin fibrosis is uncommon.

Extramedullary tissues: Splenomegaly and hepatomegaly are due to tissue infiltration by neutrophils. In the spleen, the infiltration assumes the usual leukemic pattern with infiltration in the red pulp cords and sinuses, whereas in the liver, the sinuses, portal areas, or both may be infiltrated [75].

Genetic studies: Cytogenetic abnormalities, including trisomy 8, trisomy 9, trisomy 21, del(20)q, and del(11q), have been reported in 20–25% of patients. Although a cytogenetic abnormality is helpful in proving the clonality of the proliferation, none have been recognized to be specific for CNL. By definition, there is no *BCR-ABL1* fusion gene and no rearrangement of *PDGFRA*, *PDGFRB*, or *FGFR1*. As previously noted, the *JAK2* V617F mutation has been reported in CNL [78, 79], but its incidence is unknown owing to the limited number of cases studied.

Disease Progression

Published reports indicate that CNL follows a progressive disease course. Often acceleration of the disease is associated with increasing neutrophilia and worsening anemia and thrombocytopenia. Transformation to a blast phase reportedly occurs in 10–15% of patients. By report, intracranial hemorrhage as a cause of death occurs in a disproportionate number of patients. Whether this reflects an underlying coagulation or platelet defect or is instead simply associated with progressive disease or with the therapy for the disease is not clear [80].

Differential Diagnosis

When considering the diagnosis of CNL, the major diagnostic challenge is to exclude reactive neutrophilia due to an underlying infection, inflammatory disorder, and/or nonhematopoietic or hematopoietic neoplasm, including other myeloid neoplasms. The clinical history and physical findings are critical. If no underlying disorder is apparent to explain the neutrophilia and there is no genetic evidence supporting the neoplastic origin of the neutrophils, observation of the patient for an appropriate period is recommended prior to rendering a diagnosis of CNL.

In the older literature, nearly 30% of reported cases of CNL were associated with plasma cell neoplasms, and in virtually none of the reported cases was there documented evidence of neutrophil clonality. Neutrophilia associated with plasma cell tumors is likely reactive and driven by cytokines released from the neoplastic plasma cells or accessory bone marrow cells. The WHO specifically recommends that a diagnosis of CNL should not be made when another neoplastic process, such as myeloma, is present, unless the neutrophils are documented to be clonal. Some epithelial tumors and sarcomas excrete cytokines that stimulate neutrophil production, so nonhematopoietic tumors should be excluded as well (Fig. 1.6c–e). The other disorders to be considered in the differential diagnosis of CNL are CML, *BCR-ABL1* positive (particularly when associated with the variant p230 BCR-ABL1 fusion protein); chronic myelomonocytic leukemia; and atypical CML, *BCR-ABL1* negative. The features distinguishing these entities and CNL are shown in Table 1.10.

Myeloproliferative Neoplasm, Unclassifiable

The designation myeloproliferative neoplasm, unclassifiable (MPN, U) should be applied only to patients who have definite clinical, laboratory, and morphologic features of an MPN, but fail to meet the criteria for any of the specific MPN entities (Fig. 1.8). Most of the cases fall into one of the three categories: (1) early stages of PV, PMF, or ET in which the clinical, laboratory, and morphologic manifestations are not yet fully developed, (2) myelofibrotic, accelerated, or blast phase of any MPN in which the underlying disease is not clear or was never previously recognized, and (3) patients with convincing evidence of an MPN in whom a coexisting inflammatory, metabolic, or neoplastic process obscures the diagnosis [73]. The designation should *NOT* be used if (1) the laboratory data necessary for classification are incomplete or were never obtained, (2) the size or quality of the bone marrow specimens is inadequate for complete evaluation, or (3) the patient has received prior growth factor therapy or cytotoxic therapy. The finding of a *BCR-ABL1* fusion gene or rearrangement of *PDGFRA*, *PDGFRB*, or *FGFR1* precludes the diagnosis of MPN, U. Although *JAK2* V617F is most often observed in MPNs, it has been described in AML, MDS, and MDS/MPN as well [11] and cannot be used as the sole evidence to designate a case as MPN, U if other data are not supportive.

If a case does not have features of one of the well-defined MPN entities, the possibility (or probability) that it is not an MPN at all must be seriously considered. Reactive bone marrow responses to a number of inflammatory and infectious agents must be kept in mind, particularly when considering CNL and CEL, NOS. Marrow fibrosis with osteosclerosis may

Table 1.10 Comparison of major features of the myeloid neoplasms, including CNL.

	CML, CP, BCR-ABL1+	CNL	CMML-1, 2	aCML, BCR-ABL1-
Ph chromosome	~95%	0	0	0
BCR-ABL1 fusion gene	100	0	0	0
Principle proliferating cells	Granulocytes, megakaryocytes	Granulocytes	Monocytes, +/-granulocytes	Granulocytes
Monocytes (peripheral blood)	Usually <3%	<1 × 10^9/L	>1 × 10^9/L; >10%	<1 × 10^9/L; <10%
Basophils (peripheral blood)	>2%	<2%	<2%	<2%
Dysplasia	Absent/minimal	Absent, "toxic" changes frequent	Often	Always dysgranulopoiesis, often trilineage dysplasia
Blasts (peripheral blood)	<10%	<1%	<20%	<20%
Immature granulocytes (peripheral blood)	Often >20%	<10%	Usually <20%	10–20%
Megakaryocytes	Usually normal or increased numbers with "dwarf" morphology	Normal or increased numbers with normal morphology	Decreased, normal or occasionally increased numbers with variable but often dysplastic morphology	Normal, decreased or rarely increased numbers, often with dysplastic morphology

CML, CP, *BCR/ABL1*+ = CML, chronic phase; *CNL*, chronic neutrophilic leukemia; *CMML-1, 2* chronic myelomonocytic leukemia 1 and 2; aCML, *BCR-ABL1* = atypical chronic myeloid leukemia

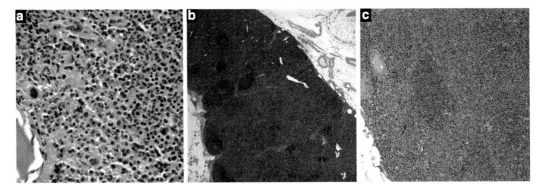

Fig. 1.8 Myeloproliferative neoplasm, unclassifiable. 59-year-old man who presented with splenomegaly, lymphadenopathy and a white blood cell count of 80 × 10⁹/L, increased granulocytic precursors, Hb of 12.6 g/dL and a platelet count of 98 × 10⁹/L. Laboratory studies showed diploid male karyotype. Molecular studies were negative for *BCR-ABL1*, *JAK2* mutation, *MPL* mutation, and *KIT* mutation. (**a**) Bone marrow biopsy demonstrates hypercellular bone marrow with granulocytes proliferation and atypical megakaryocytes. No significant dysplasia, fibrosis, basophilia, or monocytosis was identified. (**b**) Lymph node biopsy that is diffusely infiltrated by myeloid cells, leaving only a few remnants of normal follicles. (**c**) The infiltrate is parafollicular in distribution. Numerous granulocytes and megakaryocytes are present

be found in a number of inflammatory and neoplastic conditions as well, including chronic osteomyelitis, Paget's disease, metabolic bone diseases, osteosclerotic myeloma, hairy cell leukemia, metastatic carcinoma, and lymphoma.

When a diagnosis of MPN, U is made, the report should indicate why a more definitive diagnosis cannot be made. If one or more specific MPNs can be excluded on the basis of the laboratory, clinical, and/or morphologic data, then that should be stated as well, and additional studies or recommendations to classify the case should be recommended, even if it is only a suggestion to repeat the studies after an appropriate interval of time. Sharing the case with colleagues, particularly with the clinical staff responsible for the care of the patient, is important, and sending the case for an expert opinion should be considered as well.

Conclusion

In summary, the fourth edition of the WHO classification of myeloid neoplasms manifests the advances in biomarker development that are revolutionizing the way we study, diagnose, and treat myeloid neoplasms since the third edition was published in 2001. It is expected that additional updates and revisions to this classification will be needed as progress on the etiology, pathophysiology, disease progression, and therapeutic development continues to occur rapidly [82].

Acknowledgment We thank Kathryn Hale from Scientific Publications at the University of Texas M.D. Anderson Cancer Center for her editorial review of the manuscript and La Kisha Rodgers for her secretarial support.

References

1. Vardiman JW, Thiele J, Arber DA, et al. The 2008 revision of the World Health Organization (WHO) classification of myeloid neoplasms and acute leukemia: rationale and important changes. *Blood* 2009; 114: 937–51.
2. Berlin NI. Diagnosis and classification of the polycythemias. *Semin Hematol* 1975; 12: 339–51.
3. Murphy S. Therapeutic dilemmas: balancing the risks of bleeding, thrombosis, and leukemic transformation in myeloproliferative disorders (MPD). *Thromb Haemost* 1997; 78: 622–6.
4. Thiele J, Kvasnicka HM. Chronic myeloproliferative disorders with thrombocythemia: a comparative study of two classification systems (PVSG, WHO) on 839 patients. *Ann Hematol* 2003; 82: 148–52.
5. Thiele J, Kvasnicka HM, Vardiman J. Bone marrow histopathology in the diagnosis of chronic myeloproliferative disorders: a forgotten pearl. *Best Pract Res Clin Haematol* 2006; 19: 413–37.
6. De Keersmaecker K, Cools J. Chronic myeloproliferative disorders: a tyrosine kinase tale. *Leukemia* 2006; 20: 200–5.
7. James C, Ugo V, Le Couedic JP, et al. A unique clonal JAK2 mutation leading to constitutive signalling causes polycythaemia vera. *Nature* 2005; 434: 1144–8.
8. Baxter EJ, Scott LM, Campbell PJ, et al. Acquired mutation of the tyrosine kinase JAK2 in human myeloproliferative disorders. *Lancet* 2005; 365: 1054–61.
9. Kralovics R, Stockton DW, Prchal JT. Clonal hematopoiesis in familial polycythemia vera suggests the involvement of multiple mutational events in the early pathogenesis of the disease. *Blood* 2003; 102: 3793–6.
10. Levine RL, Wadleigh M, Cools J, et al. Activating mutation in the tyrosine kinase JAK2 in polycythemia vera, essential thrombocythemia, and myeloid metaplasia with myelofibrosis. *Cancer Cell* 2005; 7: 387–97.
11. Jones AV, Kreil S, Zoi K, et al. Widespread occurrence of the JAK2 V617F mutation in chronic myeloproliferative disorders. *Blood* 2005; 106: 2162–8.
12. Scott LM, Tong W, Levine RL, et al. JAK2 exon 12 mutations in polycythemia vera and idiopathic erythrocytosis. *N Engl J Med* 2007; 356: 459–68.
13. Beer PA, Campbell PJ, Scott LM, et al. MPL mutations in myeloproliferative disorders: analysis of the PT-1 cohort. *Blood* 2008; 112: 141–9.
14. Vannucchi AM, Antonioli E, Guglielmelli P, et al. Characteristics and clinical correlates of MPL 515W>L/K mutation in essential thrombocythemia. *Blood* 2008; 112: 844–7.
15. Pardanani AD, Levine RL, Lasho T, et al. MPL515 mutations in myeloproliferative and other myeloid disorders: a study of 1182 patients. *Blood* 2006; 108: 3472–6.
16. Guglielmelli P, Pancrazzi A, Bergamaschi G, et al. Anaemia characterises patients with myelofibrosis harbouring Mpl mutation. *Br J Haematol* 2007; 137: 244–7.
17. Longley BJ, Tyrrell L, Lu SZ, et al. Somatic c-KIT activating mutation in urticaria pigmentosa and aggressive mastocytosis: establishment of clonality in a human mast cell neoplasm. *Nat Genet* 1996; 12: 312–4.
18. Golub TR, Barker GF, Lovett M, Gilliland DG. Fusion of PDGF receptor beta to a novel ets-like gene, tel, in chronic myelomonocytic leukemia with t(5;12) chromosomal translocation. *Cell* 1994; 77: 307–16.
19. Cools J, DeAngelo DJ, Gotlib J, et al. A tyrosine kinase created by fusion of the PDGFRA and FIP1L1 genes as a therapeutic target of imatinib in idiopathic hypereosinophilic syndrome. *N Engl J Med* 2003; 348: 1201–14.
20. Abruzzo LV, Jaffe ES, Cotelingam JD, et al. T-cell lymphoblastic lymphoma with eosinophilia associated with subsequent myeloid malignancy. *Am J Surg Pathol* 1992; 16: 236–45.

21. Macdonald D, Reiter A, Cross NC. The 8p11 myeloproliferative syndrome: a distinct clinical entity caused by constitutive activation of FGFR1. *Acta Haematol* 2002; 107: 101–7.

22. Spivak JL. Polycythemia vera: myths, mechanisms, and management. *Blood* 2002; 100: 4272–90.

23. Vardiman J, Brunning RD, Arber DA. Introduction and overview of the classification of the myeloid neoplasms. In: Swerdlow SH, Campo E, Harris NL, et al. *WHO Classification of Tumours of Hematopoietic and Lymphoid Tissues. 4th ed.* IARC: Lyon, France, 2008: pp 18–30.

24. Thiele J, Kvasnicka HM, Facchetti F, et al. European consensus on grading bone marrow fibrosis and assessment of cellularity. *Haematologica* 2005; 90: 1128–32.

25. Hollowell JG, van Assendelft OW, Gunter EW, et al. Hematological and iron-related analytes–reference data for persons aged 1 year and over: United States, 1988–94. *Vital Health Stat 11* 2005: 1–156.

26. Thiele J, Kvasnicka HM, Orazi A, Tefferi A, Birgegard G. Polycythemia vera In: Swerdlow SH, Campo E, Harris NL, et al. (eds). *WHO Classification of Tumours of Haematopoietic and Lymphoid Tissues. 4th ed.* IARC: Lyon, France, 2008: pp 40–43.

27. Polycythemia vera: the natural history of 1213 patients followed for 20 years. Gruppo Italiano Studio Policitemia. *Ann Intern Med* 1995; 123: 656–64.

28. Percy MJ, Scott LM, Erber WN, et al. The frequency of JAK2 exon 12 mutations in idiopathic erythrocytosis patients with low serum erythropoietin levels. *Haematologica* 2007; 92: 1607–14.

29. Reilly JT. Pathogenetic insight and prognostic information from standard and molecular cytogenetic studies in the BCR-ABL-negative myeloproliferative neoplasms (MPNs). *Leukemia* 2008; 22: 1818–27.

30. Wang X, LeBlanc A, Gruenstein S, et al. Clonal analyses define the relationships between chromosomal abnormalities and JAK2V617F in patients with Ph-negative myeloproliferative neoplasms. *Exp Hematol* 2009; 37: 1194–200.

31. Najean Y, Dresch C, Rain JD. The very-long-term course of polycythaemia: a complement to the previously published data of the Polycythaemia Vera Study Group. *Br J Haematol* 1994; 86: 233–5.

32. Alvarez-Larran A, Bellosillo B, Martinez-Aviles L, et al. Postpolycythaemic myelofibrosis: frequency and risk factors for this complication in 116 patients. *Br J Haematol* 2009; 146: 504–9.

33. Vannucchi AM, Antonioli E, Guglielmelli P, et al. Clinical profile of homozygous JAK2 617V>F mutation in patients with polycythemia vera or essential thrombocythemia. *Blood* 2007; 110: 840–6.

34. Finazzi G, Caruso V, Marchioli R, et al. Acute leukemia in polycythemia vera: an analysis of 1638 patients enrolled in a prospective observational study. *Blood* 2005; 105: 2664–70.

35. Passamonti F, Rumi E, Arcaini L, et al. Leukemic transformation of polycythemia vera: a single center study of 23 patients. *Cancer* 2005; 104: 1032–6.

36. Gordeuk VR, Stockton DW, Prchal JT. Congenital polycythemias/erythrocytoses. *Haematologica* 2005; 90: 109–16.

37. Patnaik MM, Tefferi A. The complete evaluation of erythrocytosis: congenital and acquired. *Leukemia* 2009; 23: 834–44.

38. Klco JM, Vij R, Kreisel FH, Hassan A, Frater JL. Molecular pathology of myeloproliferative neoplasms. *Am J Clin Pathol* 2010;133: 602–15.

39. Lataillade JJ, Pierre-Louis O, Hasselbalch HC, et al. Does primary myelofibrosis involve a defective stem cell niche? From concept to evidence. *Blood* 2008; 112: 3026–35.

40. Bock O, Muth M, Theophile K, et al. Identification of new target molecules PTK2, TGFBR2 and CD9 overexpressed during advanced bone marrow remodelling in primary myelofibrosis. *Br J Haematol* 2009; 146: 510–20.

41. Ho CL, Lasho TL, Butterfield JH, Tefferi A. Global cytokine analysis in myelo-proliferative disorders. *Leuk Res* 2007; 31: 1389–92.

42. Varricchio L, Mancini A, Migliaccio AR. Pathological interactions between hematopoietic stem cells and their niche revealed by mouse models of primary myelofibrosis. *Expert Rev Hematol* 2009; 2: 315–34.

43. Passamonti F, Cervantes F, Vannucchi AM, et al. A dynamic prognostic model to predict survival in primary myelofibrosis: a study by the IWG-MRT (International Working Group for Myeloproliferative Neoplasms Research and Treatment). *Blood* 2010;115: 1703–8.

44. Thiele J, Kvasnicka HM, Boeltken B, et al. Initial (prefibrotic) stages of idiopathic (primary) myelofibrosis (IMF) - a clinicopathological study. *Leukemia* 1999; 13: 1741–8.

45. Tefferi A. Myelofibrosis with myeloid metaplasia. *N Engl J Med* 2000; 342: 1255–65.

46. Cervantes F, Pereira A, Marti JM, Feliu E, Rozman C. Bone marrow lymphoid nodules in myeloproliferative disorders: association with the nonmyelosclerotic phases of idiopathic myelofibrosis and immunological significance. *Br J Haematol* 1988; 70: 279–82.

47. Reeder TL, Bailey RJ, Dewald GW, Tefferi A. Both B and T lymphocytes may be clon-ally involved in myelofibrosis with myeloid metaplasia. *Blood* 2003; 101: 1981–3.

48. Thiele J, Kvasnicka HM, Tefferi A, et al. Primary myelofibrosis. In: Swerdlow SH, Campo E, Harris NL, et al. (eds). *WHO Classification of Tumours of Hematopoietic and Lymphoid Tissues. 4th ed.* IARC: Lyon, France, 2008: pp 44–47.

49. Wolf BC, Banks PM, Mann RB, Neiman RS. Splenic hematopoiesis in poly-cythemia vera. A morphologic and immunohistologic study. *Am J Clin Pathol* 1988; 89: 69–75.

50. Hussein K, Bock O, Theophile K, et al. JAK2(V617F) allele burden discriminates essential thrombocythemia from a subset of prefibrotic-stage primary myelofibro-sis. *Exp Hematol* 2009; 37: 1186–93 e7.

51. Tefferi A, Pardanani A, Lim KH, et al. TET2 mutations and their clinical correlates in polycythemia vera, essential thrombocythemia and myelofibrosis. *Leukemia* 2009; 23: 905–11.

52. Tam CS, Abruzzo LV, Lin KI, et al. The role of cytogenetic abnormalities as a prognostic marker in primary myelofibrosis: applicability at the time of diagnosis and later during disease course. *Blood* 2009; 113: 4171–8.

53. Hussein K, Pardanani AD, Van Dyke DL, Hanson CA, Tefferi A. International Prognostic Scoring System-independent cytogenetic risk categorization in primary myelofibrosis. *Blood* 115: 496–9.

54. Hidaka T, Shide K, Shimoda H, et al. The impact of cytogenetic abnormalities on the prognosis of primary myelofibrosis: a prospective survey of 202 cases in Japan. *Eur J Haematol* 2009; 83: 328–33.

55. Mesa RA, Li CY, Ketterling RP, et al. Leukemic transformation in myelofibrosis with myeloid metaplasia: a single-institution experience with 91 cases. *Blood* 2005; 105: 973–7.

56. Boveri E, Passamonti F, Rumi E, et al. Bone marrow microvessel density in chronic myeloproliferative disorders: a study of 115 patients with clinicopathological and molecular correlations. *Br J Haematol* 2008; 140: 162–8.

57. Hussein K, Van Dyke DL, Tefferi A. Conventional cytogenetics in myelofibrosis: literature review and discussion. *Eur J Haematol* 2009; 82: 329–38.

58. Kvasnicka HM, Thiele J. The impact of clinicopathological studies on staging and survival in essential thrombocythemia, chronic idiopathic myelofibrosis, and polycythemia rubra vera. *Semin Thromb Hemost* 2006; 32: 362–71.

59. Orazi A, O'Malley DP, Jiang J, et al. Acute panmyelosis with myelofibrosis: an entity distinct from acute megakaryoblastic leukemia. *Mod Pathol* 2005; 18: 603–14.

60. Steensma DP, Hanson CA, Letendre L, Tefferi A. Myelodysplasia with fibrosis: a distinct entity? *Leuk Res* 2001; 25: 829–38.

61. Pullarkat V, Bass RD, Gong JZ, Feinstein DI, Brynes RK. Primary autoimmune myelofibrosis: definition of a distinct clinicopathologic syndrome. *Am J Hematol* 2003; 72: 8–12.

62. Thiele J, Kvasnicka HM, Orazi A, Tefferi A, Gisslinger H. Essential thrombocythaemia. In: Swerdlow SH, Campo E, Harris NL, et al. (eds). *WHO Classification of Tumours of Hematopoietic and Lymphoid Tissues. 4th ed.* IARC: Lyon, France, 2008: pp 48–50.

63. Kaushansky K. Historical review: megakaryopoiesis and thrombopoiesis. *Blood* 2008; 111: 981–6.

64. Hussein K, Bock O, Theophile K, et al. JAK2 (V617F) allele burden discriminates essential thrombocythemia from a subset of prefibrotic-stage primary myelofibrosis. *Exp Hematol.* 2009; 37: 1186–93.

65. Scott LM, Scott MA, Campbell PJ, Green AR. Progenitors homozygous for the V617F mutation occur in most patients with polycythemia vera, but not essential thrombocythemia. *Blood* 2006; 108: 2435–7.

66. Jensen MK, de Nully Brown P, Nielsen OJ, Hasselbalch HC. Incidence, clinical features and outcome of essential thrombocythaemia in a well defined geographical area. *Eur J Haematol* 2000; 65: 132–9.

67. Finazzi G, Harrison C. Essential thrombocythemia. *Semin Hematol* 2005; 42: 230–8.

68. Gisslinger H. Update on diagnosis and management of essential thrombocythemia. *Semin Thromb Hemost* 2006; 32: 430–6.

69. Mesa RA, Hanson CA, Li CY, et al. Diagnostic and prognostic value of bone marrow angiogenesis and megakaryocyte c-Mpl expression in essential thrombocythemia. *Blood* 2002; 99: 4131–7.

70. Steensma DP, Tefferi A. Cytogenetic and molecular genetic aspects of essential thrombocythemia. *Acta Haematol* 2002; 108: 55–65.

71. Elliott MA, Tefferi A. Thrombosis and haemorrhage in polycythemia vera and essential thrombocythemia. *Br J Haematol.* 2005; 128: 275–290.

72. Cervantes F, Alvarez-Larran A, Talarn C, Gomez M, Montserrat E. Myelofibrosis with myeloid metaplasia following essential thrombocythaemia: actuarial probability, presenting characteristics and evolution in a series of 195 patients. *Br J Haematol* 2002; 118: 786–90.

73. Kvasnicka HM, Bain BJ, Thiele J, et al. Myeloproliferative neoplasm, unclassifiable. In: Swerdlow SH, Campo E, Harris NL, et al. (eds). *WHO Classification of Tumours of Haematopoietic and Lymphoid Tissues. 4th ed.* IARC: Lyon, France, 2008: pp 64–65.

74. Malcovati L, Della Porta MG, Pietra D, et al. Molecular and clinical features of refractory anemia with ringed sideroblasts associated with marked thrombocytosis. *Blood* 2009; 114: 3538–45.

75. Bain BJ, Brunning RD, Vardiman J, Thiele J. Chronic neutrophilic leukaemia. In: Swerdlow SH, Campo E, Harris NL, et al. (eds). *WHO Classification of Tumours of Haematopoietic and Lymphoid Tissues. 4th ed.* IARC: Lyon, France, 2008: pp 38–39.

76. Bohm J, Kock S, Schaefer HE, Fisch P. Evidence of clonality in chronic neutrophilic leukaemia. *J Clin Pathol* 2003; 56: 292–5.

77. Yanagisawa K, Ohminami H, Sato M, et al. Neoplastic involvement of granulocytic lineage, not granulocytic-monocytic, monocytic, or erythrocytic lineage, in a patient with chronic neutrophilic leukemia. *Am J Hematol* 1998; 57: 221–4.

78. Mc Lornan DP, Percy MJ, Jones AV, Cross NC, Mc Mullin MF. Chronic neutrophilic leukemia with an associated V617F JAK2 tyrosine kinase mutation. *Haematologica* 2005; 90: 1696–7.

79. Kako S, Kanda Y, Sato T, et al. Early relapse of JAK2 V617F-positive chronic neutrophilic leukemia with central nervous system infiltration after unrelated bone marrow transplantation. *Am J Hematol* 2007; 82: 386–90.

80. Elliott MA, Hanson CA, Dewald GW, et al. WHO-defined chronic neutrophilic leukemia: a long-term analysis of 12 cases and a critical review of the literature. *Leukemia* 2005; 19: 313–7.
81. Shigekiyo T, Miyagi J, Chohraku M, et al. Bleeding tendency in chronic neutrophilic leukemia. *Int J Hematol* 2008; 88: 240–2.
82. Abdel-Wahab O, Manshouri T, Patel J, et al. Genetic analysis of transforming events that convert chronic myeloproliferative neoplasms to leukemias. *Cancer Res.* 2010; 70: 447–52.

Chapter 2

Genetics of the Myeloproliferative Neoplasms

Omar Abdel-Wahab and Ross L. Levine

Keywords: JAK2V617F • JAK2 exon 12 • JAK2 • MPL • TET1 • TET2 • ASXL1 • ASXL2 • 46/1 Haplotype • SNP • microRNA • Epigenetics • Genetics • Genomics • Familial MPN • 20q- • Hopscotch

Introduction

The myeloproliferative neoplasms (MPNs) are clonal disorders of hematopoiesis characterized by the production of mature appearing cells within the blood stream. The MPNs were initially grouped together by William Dameshek in 1951, who noted the pathogenetic and clinical similarity of the different MPN [1]. However, it was not until the last 5 years that researchers have begun to elucidate the genetic basis for this group of diseases. Beginning with the 2005 discovery of the *JAK2*-V617F mutation, different MPNs have been the source of multiple gene discovery efforts [2–5]. This has led to the exciting discovery of a series of mutations in patients with MPN in known genes as well as in novel genes not previously known to be involved in pathogenesis of human disease.

In many ways, the history of genetic discoveries in the MPNs has mirrored the history of genomic technology development [6]. Early studies of the genetic underpinnings of MPNs relied on seminal X-inactivation studies, which demonstrated the clonal, stem cell origin of the different MPNs. Later, completion of the Human Genome Project as well as greater access to Sanger sequencing promoted candidate-based sequencing approaches, which were partially responsible for the discovery of activating mutations in *JAK2* and *MPL* [2, 3, 7–10]. Sequencing of the human genome provided a high-resolution genome-wide map of common SNPs, which, in turn, promoted greater analysis of single nucleotide polymorphisms (SNPs) in the international HapMap project and the SNP database (dbSNP). These efforts allowed the identification of a germline SNP, which confers heritable risk of MPN development and the first specific genetic evidence of a germline cause for MPNs [11–13]. More recently, the use of array-based technologies, including SNP arrays and comparative genomic hybridization arrays (aCGH), has led to the identification of somatic mutations in *TET2* and *ASXL1* in MPNs [14–18].

S. Verstovsek and A. Tefferi (eds.), *Myeloproliferative Neoplasms: Biology and Therapy*,
Contemporary Hematology, DOI 10.1007/ 978-1-60761-266-7_2,
© Springer Science+Business Media, LLC 2011

In this review, we discuss the somatic as well as germline genetic aberrations that contribute to the pathogenesis of the different MPNs. Despite the insights into the genetic basis of these diseases that has emerged in recent years, it has become increasingly clear that there are yet additional unidentified genetic events, which contribute to MPN development. To this end, we also review recent data on the role of additional genetic and epigenetic abnormalities in MPN pathogenesis, including the role of micro-RNAs, epigenetic regulation, and post-translational modifications that may promote or influence the MPN phenotype.

Somatic Mutations in MPN Pathogenesis

Early Evidence for Clonal Disorder

The classic MPNs include the disorders such as polycythemia vera (PV), essential thrombocytosis (ET), and primary myelofibrosis (MF). The earliest insights into the genetic causes for the MPNs were made in 1976–1981, when a series of studies demonstrated that all three classic MPNs represented clonal disorders derived from a genetically aberrant hematopoeitic progenitor cell [19–21]. Each of these studies took advantage of the ability to identify polymorphisms in the X chromosome gene glucose-6-phosphate dehydrogenase (*G-6-PD*) within female patients heterozygous for the gene. By demonstrating that the granulocytes, platelets, and red blood cells from patients with PV, MF, and then ET contained only one of the two possible G-6-PD alleles, while all other tissues of the body contained both G-6-PD alleles, the clonal nature of these disorders was proven. Moreover, several patients in these initial studies harbored additional karyotypic abnormalities, which were present only in the myeloid compartment and not in other tissues of the body as further evidence for the existence of clonal somatic abnormalities present in MPNs [19–21]. Despite further extensive X-chromosome inactivation studies as well as efforts to identify somatic genetic abnormalities in MPNs based on gross cytogenetic abnormalities, no specific gene involved in MPN pathogenesis was identified until over 20 years later.

JAK2 and MPL Mutations: Constitutive Tyrosine Kinase Activation in MPN Pathogenesis

JAK2 Mutations in MPNs
The initial specific mutation identified in MPN pathogenesis was the *JAK2V617F* mutation. The *JAK2V617F* mutation is a somatic guanine to thymidine substitution, which results in a substitution of valine for phenylalanine at codon 617 of *JAK2*. *JAK2* encodes a cytoplasmic nonreceptor tyrosine kinase, which is downstream of both type I and type II cytokine receptors [2–5]. The *JAK2V617F* mutation is present in the vast majority of patients with PV, most patients with ET and MF and a minority of patients with other myeloid disorders (Table 2.1).

The *JAK2V617F* mutation was discovered independently by four different groups in 2005 and their findings were all published in April to March of 2005 [2–5]. James et al. identified the *JAK2V617F* mutation based on the elegant demonstration that chemical or short interfering RNA (siRNA)

Table 2.1 Frequency of the *JAK2V617F* allele in myeloid disorders.

Disease	Frequency
Polycythemia vera	81–99%
Essential thrombocytosis	41–72%
Primary myelofibrosis	39–57%
Chronic myelomonocytic leukemia	3–9%
Myelodysplasia[a]	3–5%
Acute myeloid leukemia[b]	<5%

[a]*JAK2V617F* mutations are enriched in the MDS subtype, RARS-T (refractory anemia with ringed sideroblasts and thrombocytosis) and occur in 40–50% of RARS-T patients
[b]*JAK2V617F* mutations are most common in AML evolved from a preceding MPN and account for 30–50% of such secondary AML patients

mediated inhibition of JAK2 in primary patient samples led to abolishment of endogenous erythroid colony (EEC) formation in PV samples [3]. Given this finding, they hypothesized that mutations resulting in aberrant *JAK2* activity may be present in MPNs and sequenced *JAK2* leading to the discovery of the frequent somatic mutation of *JAK2* in patients with MPN. Baxter and colleagues utilized a candidate gene sequencing approach to identify the *JAK2V761F* mutation [2]. On the basis of the hypothesis that the classic MPN might bear a mutation in a tyrosine kinase such as that found in the related disorder chronic myelogenous leukemia (CML), Levine et al. utilized high-throughput DNA sequencing of tyrosine kinases in MPNs to identify the *JAK2V617F* mutation [5]. In contrast, Kralovics et al. utilized prior knowledge that ~30% of patients with MPN harbored a region of loss of heterozygosity (LOH) on chromosome 9p [4]. They then hypothesized that *JAK2* may be implicated in MPN patients, based on its location in the minimally duplicated region at 9p. This led to sequencing of *JAK2* in patients with MPN and the discovery of the *JAK2V617F* mutation.

All of these four initial publications reported that the *JAK2V617F* mutation was most commonly found in PV (81–99% of cases) followed by ET (41–72%) and MF (39–57%) and could be present as a heterozygous or homozygous mutation. Moreover, they each demonstrated that homozygous *JAK2V617F* mutation rise as a result of duplication of the mutant allele by mitotic recombination [also referred to as uniparental disomy (UPD)]. For reasons that are still unclear, the frequency of *JAK2V617F* homozygosity differs amongst the MPN with homozygosity for *JAK2V617F* occurring in ~30% of MPN patients compared with only ~2–4% of patients with ET [2–5].

A subset of the initial four publications documenting the *JAK2V617F* mutation also provided some functional insight into the *JAK2V617F* mutation. Levine et al. and James et al. both demonstrated that the *JAK2V617F* mutation results in constitutive tyrosine kinase phosphorylation and showed that expression of JAK2V617F, but not wild-type JAK2, in Ba/F3 cells coexpressing the erythropoietin receptor resulted in transformation to factor-independent growth of Ba/F3 cells [3, 5]. Importantly, James et al. also reported that expression of the *JAK2V617F* allele in vivo via retroviral murine retroviral bone marrow transplantation (BMT) into C57 Bl/6 mice resulted in significant erythrocytosis.

Although the initial discovery of an activating mutation in a kinase downstream of myeloid cytokine receptors in PV, ET, and MF was a major insight into MPN pathogenesis, and a number of questions immediately arose with the discovery of *JAK2V617F*. First question was how a single recurrent mutation could be responsible for the development of three phenotypically disparate disorders. At least three publications of the phenotype of mice undergoing retroviral bone BMT with the *JAK2V617F* allele demonstrated that the genetic background of recipient mice clearly affected the hematopoietic phenotype (Table 2.2) [22–25]. For instance, transplantation of the *JAK2V617F* allele into Balb/C mice resulted in polycythemia and leukocytosis, while transplantation into C57 Bl/6 mice most commonly results in isolated polycythemia with modest changes in the white blood cell count. This provided the earliest genetic evidence that the genetic background upon which the *JAK2V617F* mutation is introduced may influence the disease phenotype. Moreover, transplantation of *JAK2V617F* into either background did not result in thrombocytosis in mice suggesting that additional inherited or acquired genetic events might be necessary for development of ET and/or MF.

An additional question that arose immediately after the initial discovery of *JAK2V617F* relates to the pathogenetic relevance of gene dosage. Specifically, given that some patients who are heterozygous vs. others who are homozygous for the *JAK2V617F* allele, it is important to ascertain whether there are functional differences based on mutational gene dosage. As stated earlier, the initial genetic studies identified homozygous *JAK2V617F* mutations more often in PV than in ET, suggesting homozygous *JAK2V617F*-mutant progenitors might be biased toward the erythroid lineage. Given this finding, Tiedt et al. generated conditional *JAK2V617F* transgenic mouse models to investigate the effects of varying wild-type *JAK2* to *JAK2V617F* ratios in MPN phenotype (Table 2.2) [26]. The resultant cross of their *JAK2V617F* transgenic mice with mice expressing Cre-recombinase under the control of the hematopoiesis specific *Vav* promoter (VavCre;FF1) led to the expression of *JAK2*-V617F, which was lower than the endogenous wild-type *JAK2*. These VavCre;FF1 mice developed thrombocytosis and neutrophilia most closely resembling human ET. In contrast, conditional expression of the *JAK2V617F* transgene using the interferon-inducible MxCre resulted in the expression of *JAK2V617F* approximately equal to wild-type *JAK2*, which resulted in polcythemia, leukocytosis, and variable thrombocytosis most reminiscent of human PV. As discussed earlier, retroviral BMT assays result in much higher levels of *JAK2V617F* and a PV-like phenotype without thrombocytosis. In total, the results of these genetic experiments suggest that the phenotype of MPN progenitor cells are affected by the level of *JAK2V617F* expression such that lower *JAK2V617F*:wild-type *JAK2* levels result in megakaryocytic expansion and thrombocytosis, while higher *JAK2V617F*:wild-type *JAK2* levels result in a more marked erythrocytosis over thrombocytosis. A second study reporting creation of *JAK2V617F* transgenic mice under the Vav promoter confirmed that low-level *JAK2V617F* expression results in thrombocytosis (Table 2.2) [27]. Despite the utility of the current retroviral transplant and transgenic models, more accurate genetic "knock-in" models in which *JAK2V617F* is expressed from the endogenous promoter will further elucidate differences in heterozygous vs. homozygous states of the *JAK2V617F* mutation on hematopoiesis. Moreover, it remains unclear whether the differences between cells homozygous and heterozygous for *JAK2V617F* result from increased expression of the mutant JAK2 kinase, from the absence

Table 2.2 Murine models of *JAK2V617F*-positive MPN.

Disease model	Strain	Expression of *JAK2V617F*:*JAK2* wildtype	Polycythemia	Leukocytosis	Megakaryocytic hyperplasia	Thrombocytosis	Myelofibrosis
Retroviral BMT[a]	Balb/C	>>	+	+	+	-	+
Retroviral BMT	C57/Bl6	>>	+	-	+	-[b]	+/-
Transgenic							
VavCre;FF1	C57/Bl6	<	-	+	+	+	+
MxCre;FF1	C57/Bl6	=	+	+	+	+	+
Transgenic							
VavCre Line B	C57/Bl6	<	+	-	+	+	+
VavCre Line A	C57/Bl6	>	+	+	+	+	+

Evidence that host genetic variation and *JAK2V617F* gene dosage influence MPN phenotype

[a]Bone marrow transplantation (BMT)

[b]In one study, a subset of mice with reduced *JAK2V617F* expression in a murine BMT developed transient thrombocytosis

of expression of wild-type JAK2, or a combination of both factors and whether the differences in signaling between cells homozygous and heterozygous for *JAK2V617F* are quantitative and/or qualitative in nature.

The genetic studies of the effect of *JAK2V617F* gene dosage on hematopoeisis raised the question of what stage in the hematopoeitic hierarchy does the *JAK2* mutation arises. Although the clonal nature of MPNs had been known for more than 20 years, it had not been previously known whether the *JAK2V617F* mutation arises at the level of a self-renewing hematopoietic stem cell (HSC), in nonself renewing multipotent progenitors, or even in myeloid-erythroid progenitors (MEP). This question was addressed by Jamieson et al., who utilized progenitor FACS analysis and methylcellulose cultures to identify that the *JAK2V617F* mutation occurred in cells with an HSC surface immunophenotype (cells that are CD34+ CD38– CD90+ Lin–) [28]. Moreover, it was noted that HSCs from patients with PV had increased numbers of common myeloid progenitors as well as a skewed differentiation potential toward an erythroid fate. Later work from the same group elucidated that enforced expression of *JAK2V617F* specifically led to upregulation of the erythroid transcription factor GATA-1 and decreased expression of the myeloid transcription factor PU.1 [29]. Interestingly, this was shown in both primary patient samples as well as by transduction of *JAK2V617F* into umbilical cord blood stem/progenitor cells. Use of these transduced cells further demonstrated that expression of *JAK2V617F* at the stem/progenitor cell level led to skewed differentiation toward an erythroid lineage.

Despite these insights into the effects of *JAK2V617F* on signaling, hematopoesis, and gene dosage effects of the mutation, the exact mechanism by which the valine to phenylalanine substitution at residue 617 leads to aberrant signaling of *JAK2* has yet to be fully elucidated. The Jak kinases have seven homologous domains (JH1–7), which includes the catalytic kinase domain (JH1) and a catalytically inactive pseudokinase domain (JH2). It is hypothesized that the JH2 domain serves autoinhibitory function and that the valine-to-phenylalanine substitution at codon 617 might abrogate autoinhibition and result in constitutive tyrosine kinase activity. Although this hypothesis seems logical, yet it has to be proven functionally [30]. Moreover, it has been shown that substitution of other residues (tryptophan, methionine, isoleucine, and leucine) instead of phenylalanine at position 617 leads to the same constitutive activation of *JAK2*. Despite this the valine-to-phenylalanine substitution is the exclusive mutation identified at codon 617 in humans with MPNs implying that this particular amino acid substitution may be critical to myeloid transformation [31]. Moreover, it has recently been shown that the *JAK2V617F* mutation can be acquired multiple times in multiple different clones on different strands of DNA in patients with polyclonal ET.

ET, unlike PV and MF, is frequently found as an oligoclonal or polyclonal disease based on X-chromosome inactivation patterns [8]. Using a technique of allele-specific restriction enzyme digestion to determine whether the heterozygous JAK2 mutation could be detected as occurring on different strands of DNA in cells from the same individual, Lambert et al. demonstrated that several ET patients had clones with the *JAK2V617F* mutation occurring on different strands of DNA [32]. This again raises the question of why the particular 617F residue is so critical, so much such that it has been acquired several times independently in different hematopoeitic stem/progenitor cells within the same individual. Lastly, a recurring mutation in the pseudokinase domains of *JAK2* has also recently been discovered in patients with Down Syndrome acute lymphoblastic leukemia (ALL) with a recurring mutation at codon R683 in 18–25% of cases (Fig. 2.1) [33]. Why mutations at R683 result in lymphoid transformation and V617F mutations result in MPNs is not understood.

Given that a small number of PV patients and a significant proportion of ET and MF patients do not have evidence of the *JAK2617F* mutation, a number of candidate gene resequencing efforts in MPNs were performed following the discovery of the *JAK2V617F* mutation. This led to the discovery of a series of mutations in the thrombopoietin receptor gene *MPL* in 2006 as well as a series of mutations in exon 12 of *JAK2* in 2007 [9, 10].

JAK2 exon 12 mutations were discovered by Scott et al. through systematic resquencing of all coding exons of *JAK1, JAK2, JAK3, TYK2, STAT5A*, and *STAT5B* in *JAK2V617F*-negative PV patients [10]. Four novel somatic mutations in exon 12 of *JAK2* were identified including the K539L allele as well as three additional alleles that were small deletions or insertions at codons 538–543 (Fig. 2.1). These four mutations were functionally validated to lead

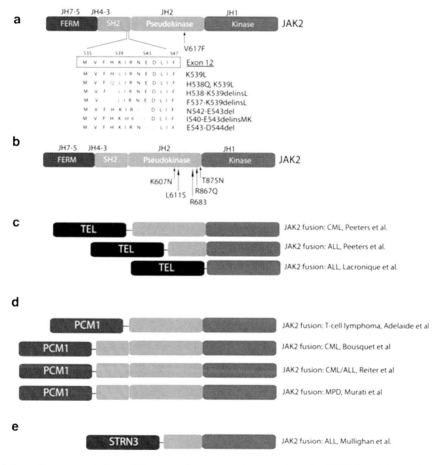

Fig. 2.1 Schematic representation of the most frequent point mutations in *JAK2* found in myeloproliferative neoplasms (**a**) and the acute leukemias (**b**). In addition the TEL-, PCM1-, and STRN3-JAK2 fusions involved in various blood cancers are shown in (**c**), (**d**), and (**e**), respectively. The TEL-JAK2 fusions involve the entire JH1 kinase domain with various lengths of the JH2 pseudokinase domain. The PCM1-JAK2 fusions all involve the JH1 and JH2 domains and variable amounts of the SH2 domain. A recent translocation between exon 9 of the striatin gene *STRN3* to exon 18 of *JAK2* (**e**) was recently discovered by transcriptome sequencing in ALL

to constitutive activation of *JAK2* through transformation of Ba/F3 cells to factor independent growth. The *JAK2K539L* allele was also shown to result in erythrocytosis and a PV phenotype in a murine BMT assay.

Since the original description of *JAK2* exon 12 mutations, several additional mutations in exon 12 of *JAK2* have also been described including the H538Q allele [34]. Interestingly, clinical analysis of patients bearing the *JAK2* exon 12 mutations suggested that exon 12 mutations are most commonly associated with a phenotype of isolated erythrocytosis without associated leukocytosis or thrombocytosis [10]. This provides further evidence that different mutations in *JAK2* may result in varying clinical phenotypes via mechanisms that are not currently identified.

In addition to the activating point mutations in *JAK2* in MPNs, a number of chromosomal translocations involving *JAK2* have been found in leukemias and rarely in classic MPNs. A fusion of *JAK2* to *TEL* (translocation ETS leukemia or *ETV6*) was the first described *JAK2* somatic alteration identified in human malignancy [35]. All described *TEL-JAK2* fusion proteins include the JH1 kinase domain of *JAK2*, and occasional translocations have also been found to include the JH2 pseudokinase domain [35, 36] (Fig. 2.1). The *TEL-JAK2* fusion results in constitutive kinase activity of *JAK2*, which is transforming in Ba/F3 assay and in in vivo models. The second most frequently reported *JAK2* translocation fuses *JAK2* to *PCM1* [37–40]. The *PCM1* gene encodes a centrosomal protein, pericentriolar material 1. Unlike the *TEL-JAK2* fusion, all *PCM1-JAK2* fusions identified to date contain both the kinase and pseudokinase domains of *JAK2*. Lastly, a recent translocation between *JAK2* and the striatin gene was recently discovered in a patient with ALL, using next generation transcriptome sequencing [41].

In the original description of *JAK2* exon 12 mutations, it was thought that exon 12 mutations occur exclusively in patients who do not bear the *JAK2V617F* mutation. However, it has been more recently shown that rare PV patients may actually bear both *JAK2V617F* as well as exon 12 mutations. In a report by Li et al., it was identified that a single patient had both the *JAK2V617F* mutation and an exon 12 mutation [34]. Clonal analysis demonstrated that the *JAK2V617F* and *JAK2* exon 12 mutations had occurred in independent clones suggesting that the two mutations possibly have overlapping effects on cell behavior and/or indicate the presence of a MPN predisposition allele. Moreover, in the same report, clonal analysis of several patients with the *JAK2V617F* mutation revealed the presence of endogenous erythroid colonies, which were negative for any mutation of *JAK2*. Several other authors have corroborated this last finding, strongly suggesting the possibility of transforming mutations in MPN patients, which precede acquisition of mutations in *JAK2* and *MPL* and illustrate the clonal heterogeneity present within MPN patients.

Somatic mutations in *MPL* were originally discovered by Pikman et al. during candidate gene resequencing of *EPO-R, MPL*, and *GCSF-R* [9]. A series of somatic mutations in *MPL* have now been identified including *MPLW515L, MPLW515K, MPLS505N, MPLA506T, MPLA519T* (Fig. 2.2). *MPL* mutations may occur in as many as 8% of ET and MF patients, although the actual frequency of *MPL* mutations in MPN patients has not been as extensively studied as the prevalence of *JAK2V617F* [42]. As with *JAK2* exon 12 mutations, mutations in *MPL* were originally thought to occur only in patients without the *JAK2V617F*

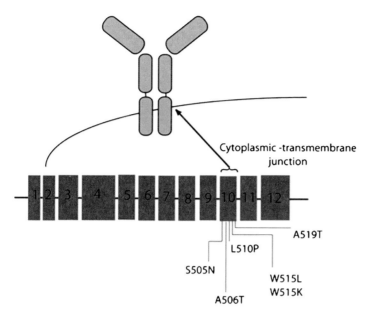

Fig. 2.2 Schematic representation of the thrombopoietin receptor Mpl and the exons of *Mpl*. The most common recurring mutations of *Mpl* occur in exon 10, which encodes the cytoplasmic–transmembrane junction

mutation; however, several reports have identified MPN patients with concurrent *JAK2* mutations as well as *MPL* mutations [43]. Interestingly, whenever clonality studies have been performed on such patients, it is clear that when *MPL* mutations occur concurrently with *JAK2V617F* mutations, the *MPL* and *JAK2* mutations occur exclusively in independent clones, suggesting overlapping effects of these mutations on cell growth/phenotype [43]. This is in contrast with cytogenetic alterations, including deletion of 20q and gains of portions of chromosome 8 and 9, which have been documented to occur concurrently with *MPL/JAK2* mutations in MPN clones [43].

As with the *JAK2* mutations described earlier, *MPL* mutations have been clearly shown to be transforming in Ba/F3 assays [9]. In addition, murine BMT assays with *MPLW515K/L* result in a completely penetrant MPN with marked thrombocytosis, splenomegaly, and fibrosis of the bone marrow recapitulating human ET and MF.

TET2 and ASXL1 Mutations in MPNs: Epigenetic Events in MPN Pathogenesis?

Evidence for Additional Mutations Beyond JAK2 and MPL

Although the discovery of mutations in *JAK2* and *MPL* were extremely enlightening, several lines of evidence made it clear that mutations in genes other than *JAK2* and *MPL* must be present in the MPNs. First was the aforementioned question of how a single mutation in *JAK2*, which appeared to be sufficient for MPN pathogenesis, could result in the development of three phenotypically variable diseases. One attractive hypothesis to this question was that additionally acquired or inherited genetic modifiers outside of *JAK2* or *MPL* could be present and modify the MPN phenotype resulting in the *JAK2V617F* mutation.

EST marker	PAC Clone (Accession #)	Associated gene	Accession #	Expression BM	Expression CD34+	Function
AA568401	dJ661I20 (AL031669)			+		
stSG3021	dJ1121H13 (AL049812)	RPTPrho	AF043644	+	+	Receptor protein tyrosine phosphatase
SGC32867	dJ862K6 (AL031681)	SFRS6	U30828	-	-	Pre-mRNA splicing factor
WI-6622	dJ138B7 (Z98752)	h-l(3)mbt	U89358	+	+	Chromosome condensation during mitosis
AA053121	dJ138B7 (Z98752)	SGK2	AF169034	+	+	Serum- and glucocorticoid-induced protein kinase
SHGC-36858	dJ399F1	CGI-53	AF151811	+	-	Gene of unknown function downregulated by delta-opioid agonist
WI-7535	dJ399F1	M.m NGD5	L38481	+	+	
stSG53114	dJ399F1	MYBL2	X13293	+		Transcription factor involved in cell cycle
AA910031	dJ1030M6 (AL035089)	X.1 D7	X13856	-	-	Oocyte maturation in Xenopus
stSG8966	dJ49SO3 (AL121587)			-	-	
sts-T63166	dJ49SO3 (AL121587)			+	-	
stSG20384	dJ1108D11 (AL034419)			-	-	
stSG40369	dJ1108D11 (AL034419)	CAGF9	U80736	+	-	Glutamine rich protein
AA716165	dJ1108D11 (AL034419)			-	-	
AA993161	dJ1108D11 (AL034419)			-	-	
AI081352	dJ1183I21 (AL035447)			-	-	

Fig. 2.3 Schematic representation of the long arm of chromosome 20 and the commonly deleted regions (CDR) found in MDS, MPN, and the 1.7 Mb overlapping deleted regions of overlap (termed the Myeloid CDR). The 16 transcribed genes within the myeloid CDR are shown in the accompanying table along with the expressed sequence tag (EST) marker and one PAC containing each EST marker. Of the 16 transcribed genes, 8 are expressed in bone marrow cells, of which 5 are also expressed in CD34+ cells. Adapted from Bench et al. [68]

Evidence for the presence of additional genetic events in MPNs came from the fact that despite the discovery of *JAK2* and *MPL* mutations, a significant proportion of ET and MF patients still had no identifiable known mutations. Moreover, clonal analysis of patients with *JAK2/MPL* mutations consistently demonstrated the presence of occasional patients with *JAK2* wildtype EEC – clear evidence that an additional aberration responsible for erythropoietin-independent growth may be present in some MPN patients [44]. Clonality analysis of patients with both a cytogenetic abnormality in conjunction with the *JAK2V617F* mutation also revealed that occasional patients could be identified, where cytogenetically abnormal clones with and without the *JAK2V617F* mutation could be identified [43]. This was first described in a patient with loss of the long arm of chromosome 20 (20q-) in addition to the *JAK2V617F* mutation and suggested that loss of a gene on 20q might be responsible for the cytokine-independent growth of *JAK2* wild-type clones (Fig. 2.3).

Since the discovery of the *JAK2V617F* mutation in 2005, a number of reports have consistently reported that leukemic blasts of acute myeloid leukemia (AML) derived from a *JAK2V617F* MPN are frequently *JAK2* wild-type [45, 46]. This suggests that the MPN and AML clones could arise from two different progenitor cells or that an ancestral clone bearing an abnormality preceding the *JAK2V617F* mutation could be present giving rise to both the MPN and the AML.

Lastly, the discovery of *JAK2* and *MPL* mutations led to intense scrutiny of possible genetic causes for familial cases of MPNs. Although the germline *MPLS505N* mutation was identified in familial ET kindred in Japan [47], thus far no heritable mutations in *JAK2* have been described. Given that some heritable genetic abnormality must be present to account for *JAK2/MPL* wild-type familial MPN cases, additional novel mutations in MPN pathogenesis have been speculated to exist for some time.

Somatic Mutations in TET2

Mutations in the gene *TET2* (ten-eleven translocation two) were originally published in papers by Delhommeua et al. and Langemeijer et al. in 2009 and identified mutations in *TET2* in MPNs, myelodysplastic syndromes (MDS), and AML (Table 2.3 and Fig. 2.4) [16, 18]. However, the earliest description

Table 2.3 Frequency of *TET2* mutations in myeloid disorders.

Disease[a]	Frequency
Polycythemia vera	9.8–16%
Essential thrombocytosis	4.4–5%
Primary myelofibrosis	7.7–17%
Systemic mastocytosis	20–30%
Chronic myelomonocytic leukemia	20–58%
Myelodysplasia	10–26%
De novo acute myeloid leukemia	12–24%
Secondary acute myeloid leukemia	15–25%

[a]No formal study of *TET2* mutations in CML has been published but evaluation of a small number of BCR-ABL positive accelerated and blast-crisis phase CML and ALL has documented existence of *TET2* mutations in DNA from patients with BCR-ABL positive disease

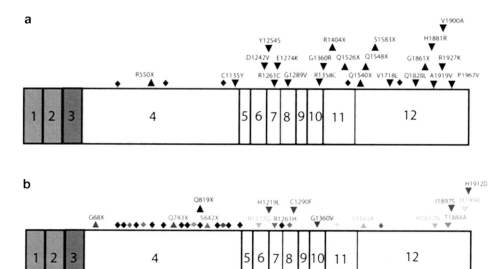

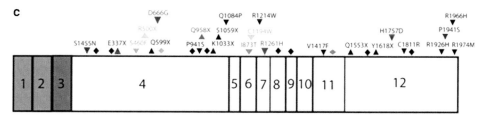

Fig. 2.4 Schematic representation of *TET2* and mutations found in 354 MPN (**a**), 144 MDS (**b**), and 46 CMML (**c**), samples. Mutations in *TET2* have been found in every exon and occur as missense (*down arrowheads*), nonsense (*up arrowheads*), and frameshift mutations (*diamonds*). This diagram also illustrates that the frequency of TET2 mutations as well as the frequency of bi- and tri-allelic *TET2* mutations (which are color-coded) are more common in MDS and CMML than in classic MPNs. Adapted from Abdel-Wahab et al. [14]

of the *TET2* mutation was made public, based on the observations in MPN patients in a late-breaking abstract by Delhommeau et al., at the December 2008 meeting of the American Society of Hematology. It was noted in this abstract that the majority of *JAK2V617F* mutant PV patients (~85%) reveal expansion of CD34+CD38+ committed progenitor cells over CD34+CD38-mutlipotent progenitors in ex vivo liquid cultures. In contrast, a minority (~15%) of *JAK2V617F* mutant PV patients reveal expansion of the more immature multipotent progenitor cells (CD34+ CD38-) over CD34+CD38+ cells. Hypothesizing that a novel genetic abnormality might be responsible for this immunophenotypic difference in the 2 patient subsets, the authors performed SNP arrays (Affymetrix 500K) and array CGH (Agilent 244K) on a small number of these patient samples. They remarkably found that 3 of 5 *JAK2V617F* mutant PV patients with expansion of CD34+CD38- cells had evidence of LOH at the genomic locus 4q24. One of these 5 patients had a deletion of a 325 kB region of DNA at 4q24- with the only gene present in this region being *TET2*. This then led to sequencing of *TET2* in these patient samples and identification of *TET2* mutations in MPNs.

Prior to the discovery of *TET2* mutations, karyotypic abnormalities at 4q24 had been described in patients with MDS and AML by Viguie et al. [48] In this report, four patients with 4q24 rearrangements (t(3;4)(q26;q24), t(4;5)(q24;p16), t(4;7)(q24;q21), del(4)(q23;24)) were described, and the karyotypic abnormality was present in both myeloid and lymphoid lineages. Moreover, one patient who developed concomitant lymphoma also had the 4q24 rearrangement in the malignant lymphoid cells. Consistent with this observation, both Delhommeau and Langemeijer found evidence of 4q24 LOH in MDS and AML [16, 18].

Sequencing of *TET2* has led to the identification *TET2* mutations in every myeloid disorder investigated to date (Table 2.3) [14, 16, 18, 49–53]. Mutations in *TET2* have been found in all coding regions and can appear as missense, nonsense, or frameshift mutations (Fig. 2.3). In addition, mutations in *TET2* are not uncommonly biallelic (i.e., involving both copies of *TET2*). Taken together, these data suggest that mutations in *TET2* represent loss-of-function mutations.

TET2 is a member of the *TET* family of genes, the first member of which to be described was *TET1*. *TET1* (ten-eleven translocation 1), located on chromosome 10, was originally identified in cases of adult and pediatric AML as a translocation with the gene *MLL* (located on chromosome 11) [54]. Although *TET1* was the original gene member identified in hematologic malignancies, no sequence alterations in *TET1* or *TET3* have been identified to date [14]. In a landmark publication in 2009, the function of *TET1* was first described (Fig. 2.5) [55]. Tahiliani et al. were interested in the identification of human enzymes, which modify bases of nucleic acids as a means to understand how catalytic modifications of DNA bases affect the genetic code. As such, they undertook a bioinformatics approach to identify human homologs of the trypanosome proteins JBP1 and JBP2, which are known to oxidize the 5-methyl group of thymine [56]. Such enzymes were not previously known to exist in higher organisms. Surprisingly, they found that the *TET* family of genes was human homologues of these trypanosome enzymes. Further characterization of *TET1* revealed that it is an 2-oxoglutarate- and iron(II)-dependent dioxygenase, which serves to oxidize the 5-methyl group of cytosine leading to the formation of 5-hydroxymethylcytosine. The exact function of this modification is not yet known but it is hypothesized to affect gene expression

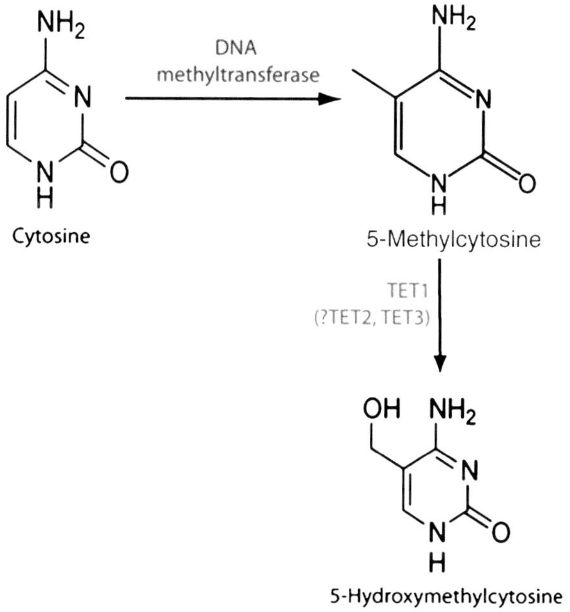

Fig. 2.5 Recently discovered enzymatic function of TET1 to mediate hydroxymethylation of 5-methylcytosine. TET2 and TET3 are also predicted to contain the 2-oxoglutarate and Fe(II)-dependent enzymatic domain seen in TET1 but their enzymatic function has not been formally demonstrated

by (1) serving as an intermediate step to promote demethylation of DNA, (2) affecting recruitment of methyl-binding proteins to DNA, (3) recruiting proteins to DNA, which specifically recognize the hydroxy-methylcytosine mark.

It has been shown that mutations in *TET2* lead to decreased *TET2* gene expression in granulocytes of diseased patients [18]. Although it is predicted that *TET2* and *TET3* share the catalytic domain of *TET1*, *TET2* and *TET3* have not been formally shown to share the catalytic activity of *TET1* to oxidize 5-methyl group of cytosines. This question is critical as both *TET1* and *TET2* appear to be expressed in myeloid cells and it is known whether decreased *TET2* expression and/or function by mutation can be compensated by expression of *TET1*.

The fact that *TET2* is expressed at the level of the CD34+ stem/progenitor cell and that *TET2* mutations are found in all myeloid disorders to date suggests that *TET2* mutations might be an early event in MPN pathogenesis [16, 18, 50]. Initial clonality studies of a small cohort of *JAK2V617F* mutant MPN patients with a *TET2* mutation revealed that *TET2*-mutant/*JAK2*-mutant and *TET2*-mutant/*JAK2*-wildtype clones could be identified but not *TET2*-wildtype/*JAK2*-mutant clones – clear support of the hypothesis that *TET2* mutations occur as a "pre-JAK2" event [16]. Subsequent studies, however, have no repeated cases where *TET2* mutations are clearly acquired after *JAK2* mutations, suggesting that mutations in *TET2* may not represent the earliest genetic aberration in all patients with *TET2*-mutant MPNs.

Although it is clear that *TET2* mutations can arise at the level of the stem/progenitor cell, the effect of *TET2* mutations on hematopoeitic function and transformation is not yet known. The accumulating genomic data have proven that *TET2* alterations do not seem to associate with any particular phenotype of myeloid disease [14, 51–53]. Moreover, *TET2* mutations can occur in concert with *JAK2, KIT, MLL, Flt3*, and *CEBPa* mutations but are not enriched in patients with these recurrent somatic alterations. One single report describes a possibly significant association of *TET2* mutation with *NPM1* alterations in AML but this finding has not been reproduced [57].

Preliminary evidence of the functional importance of *TET2* myelopoiesis comes from xenograft studies in the initial reports of *TET2* mutations by Delhommeau and colleagues [16]. They noted that injection of *JAK2V617F*-positive CD34 cells from MPN subjects with (*n* = 2) versus without *TET2* mutations (*n* = 3) into NOD-SCID mice revealed a more efficient engraftment of *TET2* mutant cells over *TET2* wildtype CD34+ cells. Moreover, the resulting hematopoiesis was skewed toward increased frequency of myeloid progenitors over lymphoid progenitors. Further experiments in more genetically uniform human and murine HSPCs are needed to confirm and expand this data given that unknown additional genetic factors beyond *TET2* and *JAK2* alleles in these 5 samples may have influenced the results.

The effect of *TET2* alterations on clinical outcome in myeloid malignancies has been the subject of much debate. Thus far *TET2* mutations have not been shown to influence survival or prognosis in any MPN (including PV, ET, and systemic mastocytosis) [51–53]. Moreover, *TET2* mutations do not appear to influence the number or type of karyotypic abnormalities found in MPN patients [58]. At the same time, *TET2* mutations have been shown to cause a negative effect on overall survival in AML [14, 18]. In two separate reports, *TET2* mutations were found to lead to significantly decreased overall survival in AML, which was independent of other prognostic factors including age, cytogenetic status, and other genetic alterations (*Flt3, NPM1, MLL, CEBPa*). This is in striking contrast with a report of a similar number of patients with MDS from the Francophone Study Group, which reported an overall survival of 76.9% in *TET2* mutant MDS patients (95% CI, 49.2–91.3%) vs. 18.3% (95% CI, 4.2–41.1%) in *TET2* wild-type MDS patients (*p*=0–005) [59]. In a multivariate analysis including age, IPSS, *TET2* mutational status, and transfusions, the absence of a *TET2* mutation was associated with a 4.1-fold increased risk of death (95% CI, 1.4–12-fold, *p*=0.009) suggesting that *TET2* mutations were an independent favorable prognostic factor. Clinical analysis of larger numbers of patients with MDS and larger number of more genetically uniform and uniformly treated AML patients will be needed to clarify these findings.

It has been hypothesized for some time from empirical clinical observations that alteration of DNA methylation must be important in the pathogenesis of myeloid malignancy as the use of DNA methyltransferase inhibitors, particularly in MDS, has been an important therapeutic development. The possibility exists that *TET2* mutations at the level of the stem/progenitor cell might result in increased likelihood of hematopoeitic transformation and aberrant myelopoiesis due to alterations in DNA methylation. How mutations in *TET2* might influence response to DNA methyltransferase inhibitors such as decitabine or 5-azacitidine is currently unknown. Moreover, if alterations in *TET2* precede *JAK2* mutations and promote neoplasia at the level of the stem/progenitor cell, it is not clear how *TET2* mutations might affect response to treatment of MPN patients with *JAK2* inhibitors.

Somatic Mutations in ASXL1

Shortly after the discovery of *TET2* mutations in myeloid cancers, somatic mutations were identified in another putative epigenetic modifier in myeloid malignancies, Additional Sex Combs Like 1 (*ASXL1*). Mutations in *ASXL1* were originally identified in aCGH studies of MDS samples [17]. Gelsi-Boyer et al. performed Agilent 244K CGH arrays on several patients with MDS and noted deletions in one patient at 20q11. In this particular patient, the 20q deletions involved only two possible genes – *ASXL1* and *DNMT3B*. Sequencing efforts of both genes followed and mutations in *ASXL1* were found in 4/35 patients with MDS (11%). Further sequencing of *ASXL1* by this group and others led to reports of *ASXL1* mutations at a similar frequency and spectrum of myeloid malignancies as *TET2* mutations (Table 2.4) [15, 17, 60].

ASXL1 is one of the three mammalian homologs of the *Additional sex combs* gene in *Drosophilia*. The genes are named for the fact that deletion of the *Additional sex combs* gene in *Drosophilia* leads to homeotic transformations. This occurs because *ASXL1* members appear to regulate the expression of both Polycomb group (PcG) and Trithorax group (TxG) proteins in *Drosophilia* and mammals [61, 62]. The *ASXL* family members can simultaneously promote and/or repress PcG and TxG members, and the exact mechanism of *ASX/PcG/ TxG* interactions is not well-understood. *ASXL1* was more recently found to be a coactivator of retinoic acid-mediated transcriptional activity in a yeast-two hybrid screen [61]. All three *ASXL* family members are characterized by an amino-terminal homology domain, two proximal interaction domains for nuclear receptors, and a C-terminal plant homeodomain (PHD) (Fig. 2.6) [61–63]. The PHD domain has been recognized in more than 100 human proteins (including MLL, JARID1, and TIF1) and appears to be a motif necessary for binding to modified histones. The exact motif at which the PHD domain of *ASXL1* binds is not known but two commonly recognized motifs, which PHD domains have been shown to recognize, include histone H3 tri-methylated on lysine 4 (H3K4me3) and histone H3 tri-methylated lysine 9 (H3K9me3).

The accumulating genetic data on *ASXL1* has suggested that *ASXL1* mutations are predominantly found as nonsense and frameshift alterations in exon 12 (Fig. 2.5) [15, 17, 60]. The mutations found have all been heterozygous, can be found at the level of CD34+ cells, and may overlap with *TET2* and *JAK2* mutations in MPNs (Table 2.4). Of note, none of the published genetic reports have included paired normal tissue and as a result many potential missense mutations

Table 2.4 Frequency of the *ASXL1* mutations in myeloid disorders[a].

Disease	Frequency
Classic MPN[b]	-7.8%[a]
Chronic myelomonocytic leukemia	11–36.4%
Myelodysplasia	17–43%
Acute myeloid leukemia	-17.8%[a]

[a]None of the published studies of *ASXL1* mutations in patient samples have included paired normal tissue. As such, possible missense mutations have been censored from analysis

[b]Classic MPN includes the disease PV, ET, and MF. No large genetic studies of *ASXL1* mutations in MPN patients have been performed to elucidate the percentage of *ASXL1* mutations separately in each of the three classic MPNs

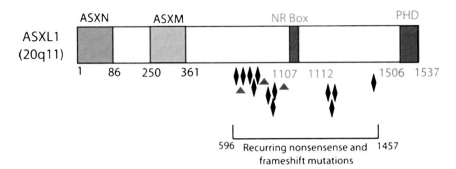

Fig. 2.6 Schematic representation of the domains of ASXL1 and recurring mutations. The conserved domains of ASXL1 include the amino terminal domains ASX Homology N (ASXN) and M (ASXM), which contain nuclear receptor co-regulator binding (NR) motifs; an additional NR motif is located toward the C-terminal region (NR box). A PHD (plant homeodomain) finger is located at the C-terminus. All identified mutations in ASXL1 are nonsense (*red triangles*) or frameshift (*diamonds*) recurring mutations occurring between amino acids 596 and 1,457. It is hypothesized that mutations in ASXL1 serve to truncate the protein before the PHD domain while leaving the ASXN and ASXM domains in place

in *ASXL1* have been censored from the literature. Nonetheless, the finding of recurrent nonsense and frameshift mutations at this particular location of *ASXL1* is striking and suggests that the mutations in *ASXL1* may serve to truncate the PHD domain of *ASXL1* while leaving the nuclear interacting domains intact (Fig. 2.5).

The initial excitement over the finding of widespread and recurrent *ASXL1* mutations in myeloid malignancies may have been quelled by the recent reports of a somatic *ASXL1* knockout mouse, which had minimal hematopoietic defects [62, 63]. This model, created by Fisher et al. placed a PGK promoter-drive neomycin expression cassette into exon 5 of *ASXL1* interrupting the reading frame of *ASXL1* (this allele is referred to as *Asxl1*^*tm1BC*) and leading to truncation of nuclear interacting domains as well as the PHD domain. Mice homozygous for this allele (*Asxl1*^*tm1BC /tm1BC*) had incompletely penetrant perinatal lethality; however, neither did they develop any overt hematologic malignancy nor did they observe defects in number or function of multipotent progenitors. Potential reasons for the fact that no clear hematopoietic phenotype was seen in the *Asxl1*^*tm1BC /tm1BC* mice include the possibility that (1) other *ASXL* genes exist, which have overlapping expression and redundant function, and (2) the *ASXL1* mutations found in humans are actually gain-of-function mutations poorly modeled by a mice lacking *ASXL1* expression altogether. Of note, *ASXL2* is expressed in hematopoieitic tissue and no mutations have been found in *ASXL2* in myeloid malignancies to date, leading credence to the possibility of *ASXL2* compensation in a state of total *ASXL1* loss.

Thus far no studies have examined whether mutations in *ASXL1* are associated with any particular outcome. Moreover, it is not known whether mutations in *ASXL1* affect response to chromatin-modifying therapies such as histone deactetylase inhibitors.

Genetics of Leukemic Transformation of MPNs

As stated earlier, it has been known since the discovery of the *JAK2V617F* mutation that *JAK2*-wildtype AML may arise from a preceding *JAK2V617F* MPN [45, 46]. The largest series to date reported by Theocharides et al. identified

JAK2V617F mutations in 17/27 samples at MPN diagnosis, yet 9 of these 17 *JAK2*-mutant patients presented with *JAK2V617F*-negative blasts during transformation to sAML. Since then, a number of studies have investigated potential genes, which might be altered at leukemic transformation of MPNs [45, 46, 49, 64]. The majority of these studies have been hampered by the relatively low number of samples and the lack of paired material from the MPN and leukemic state. Nonetheless, aggregate data from these studies have implicated mutations in *p53, TET2, NRAS, RUNX1,* and *CBL* at leukemic transformation. Reports from four groups have identified that a sizeable percentage of patients acquire *TET2* mutations in the leukemic state when not originally present in the MPN state [45, 46, 49, 64]. In contrast, analysis of paired samples revealed that *ASXL1* mutations seem to be present in both members of the pair and are not enriched in the leukemic state compared with the MPN phase of disease [65]. The functional relevance of this finding is not yet clear given that the molecular function of *TET2* and *ASXL1* mutations in hematopoiesis is not yet understood. Lastly, one recent report identified deletions in *Ikaros* in a small number of patients at the time of leukemic transformation of MPNs [66]. This is a particularly intriguing finding as deletions of *Ikaros* appear to be a near-obligate requirement in lymphoid leukemia transformation of CML (but not myeloid leukemic transformation of CML) [67].

The Possibility of Additional Mutated Genes in MPNs

Despite the discovery of mutations in four genes (*JAK2, MPL, TET2,* and *ASXL1*) in patients with MPN over the last 5 years, there is a significant proportion of patients with ET and PV without evidence of mutations in any of the aforementioned genes. This has motivated continued interest in gene discovery efforts in MPNs, and there are several intriguing possible genetic alterations being actively investigated. Longest suspected are the genes located in regions that are occasionally involved in gross cytogenetic alterations in MPN patients. The most common cytogenetic alteration in MPN is the deletion of the long arm of chromosome 20 (20q-). 20q- is found in 10% of PV patients, 4% of MDS patients, and 1–2% of AML patients [68]. It has been previously demonstrated that 20q-/*JAK2* wildtype EEC clones may be grown from 20q-/JAK2V617F mutant MPN patients bolstering the hypothesis that a novel tumor suppressor sufficient for EPO-independent growth may exist on 20q in MPNs.

Careful mapping of the commonly deleted region (CDR) in all three diseases has led to identification of a deleted region, which overlaps in all three conditions (termed as the "Myeloid CDR") [68]. The "myeloid CDR" spans 2 Mb and contains 16 known genes. Out of these 16 genes, 6 are expressed within normal CD34+ cells and as such these 6 genes have been the subject of intense investigation (Fig. 2.3). So far, mutations have not been reported in any of these 6 genes, and thus it is assumed that the gene involved in 20q-myeloid malignancies is a tumor suppressor gene affected by haploinsufficiency. A systematic RNA-interference strategy to identify the gene target in the 20q-CDR, as was done in 5q-MDS [69], has not been performed to date. Moreover, potentially important micro-RNAs within the noncoding region of 20q-, as with miR-145 in 5q-MDS [70], have not been identified.

In addition to the possibility of novel tumor suppressor gene on 20q, at least 4 new genes have been recently identified in myeloid malignancies related to

MPNs. This includes the genes *UTX* and *CBL* in MDS and CMML as well as *IDH1* and *IDH2* in AML [65, 71–76]. Thus far, no large-scale sequencing efforts of any of these genes have been published in the classic MPNs and the possibility that one or more of these genes may be mutated in some proportion of MPNs exists.

Inherited Genetic Events in MPN Pathogenesis

Evidence for Germline Mutations in MPN

The existence of families with MPNs has long suggested the presence of germline susceptibility genes, which predispose to MPN development. As mentioned earlier, mutations in *JAK2* were quickly evaluated and discarded as a potential cause for familial MPN as (1) no germline mutations in *JAK2* have been identified, and (2) there is repeated evidence of *JAK2* wild-type clones in members of familial MPN kindreds. There have been several studies of kindreds with familial MPNs (Table 2.5) [44, 77–80]. Familial MPNs are loosely defined as families where at least two relatives within the pedigree have an MPN. This must be distinguished from inherited disorders with Mendelian transmission and single hematopoietic lineage transmission (this includes the conditions known as "Hereditary Erythrocytosis" and "Hereditary Thrombocytosis.").

The single largest report of the familial aggregation of MPNs comes from a population-based study in Sweden, which examined the risk of MPN development in relative of citizens diagnosed with an MPN, was reported [81]. This study found that first-degree relatives of MPN patients have a three-to-sevenfold increased risk of developing an MPN compared with members of the population without a family history of MPN. This risk was specific to PV [RR = 5.7; 95% confidence interval (CI) 3.5–9.1], ET (RR = 7.4; CI 3.7–14.8), and MPN NOS (RR = 7.5; CI 2.7–20.8) but not CML where the relative risk was 1.9 with a p-value of 0.09. From the accumulated studies of families with MPNs, it seems that in most kindreds the inheritance pattern appears to be consistent with an autosomal dominant trait with decreased penetrance (Table 2.5). However, no clear cytogenetic or genetic locus was associated with germline predisposition toward MPN until the discovery of a risk SNP within *JAK2* itself in 2009.

The Germline JAK2 Haplotype

In 2009, three independent reports were published simultaneously of a germline haplotype block (commonly referred to as "46/1") that includes *JAK2* itself and is associated with development of both the *JAK2V617F* mutation and MPN. This haplotype block is markedly enriched in MPN patients and tagged by a SNP (rs10974944) located within an intron between exons 12 and 13 of *JAK2* [11–13]. All these three studies demonstrated that heterozygotes for this haplotype were significantly more likely to acquire the *JAK2V617F* mutation in *cis* with the predisposition SNP allele than on the other chromosome. Genotypes at rs10974944 exist as homozygous for the major allele (CC), heterozygous (GC), or homozygous for the minor allele (GG). The frequency of the GG/GC genotypes is much higher in MPN compared with matched controls (OR = 3.1, $P = 4.1 \times 10{-}20$) consistent with the G allele functioning as a dominant MPN predisposition allele and increasing the likelihood of developing an MPN to three-to-fourfold [11–13].

Table 2.5 Studies on Familial Myeloproliferative Neoplasms[a].

Reference	# Families	# Patients	Inheritance pattern	Findings
Rumi et al. [80]	20	43	AD, decreased penetrance	Identified evidence of clonal hematopoiesis without JAK2 mutations in some familial MPN kindred members suggesting JAK2V617F as a secondary event in familial MPN
Kralovics et al. [44]	6	13	AD, decreased penetrance	Excluded linkage between familial PV and candidate loci including c-mpl, EPO-R, 20q, 13q, 5q, and 9p
Rumi et al. [79]	35	75	AD, decreased penetrance	Found evidence of anticipation of disease-onset with successive generations in familial MPN
Bellanne-Chantelot et al. [99]	72	174	AD, decreased penetrance	Found evidence of MPN kindreds with and without JAK2V617F mutation
Hussein et al. [58]	1	2	NE	Suggested JAK2V617F as a secondary event in familial MPN
Pardanani et al. [77]	2	6	NE	Noted 2 siblings with MPN: 1 with JAK2V617F mutant PV and the other with JAK2 wild-type ET
Pietra et al. [78]	2	4	NE	Identified somatic JAK2 exon 12 mutations in familial MPN cases suggesting possible genetic predisposition for both JAK2V617F and exon 12 mutants in familia MPN
Abdel-Wahab et al. [14]	48	28	NE	Examined TET2 mutations MPN kindreds and identified only somatic TET2 mutations
Saint-Martin et al. [100]	42	61	NE	As above. Also noted that TET2 mutations were associated with leukemic transformation in this small cohort

[a]Adapted from Rumi et al. [101]

The *JAK2V617F* mutation and rs10974944 are contained in the same haplotype block, which is distinct from the promoter and 5' exons of *JAK2*. The mechanism by which a germline genetic variant in the 46/1 haplotype block could result in increased risk of developing the *JAK2V617F* mutation and MPN development is not known. Potential mechanisms were investigated in the three aforementioned studies, in which negative results included genotype-specific differences in (1) *JAK2* expression, (2) nonsynonymous alterations within the haplotype block, (3) alterations in the 3' UTR, and (4) differential splicing of *JAK2* [11–13].

The current proposed hypotheses as to how the 46/1 haplotype confers risk of *JAK2V617F* and MPN development includes two commonly cited hypotheses. First is the hypothesis that the haplotype confers an increased frequency of mutations at the *JAK2* locus, and those mutations that result in a selective growth advantage manifest as a clonal disorder. This hypothesis is strongly supported by the examples described earlier of MPN patients that have acquired the *JAK2* mutation multiple times in independent clones. However, this so-called "hyper-mutability" hypothesis is hindered by the fact that no mechanism has been proposed to explain the mechanism by which the haplotype would increase the frequency of mutations at a distant nucleotide. Moreover, the haplotype is also enriched in *JAK2V617F*-negative MPN [82, 83].

The second hypothesis is the idea that the *JAK2V617F* mutation is equally likely to occur in different haplotypes but cells in which the mutation occurs on the risk haplotype gain a stronger growth advantage. This so-called "fertile ground" hypothesis is hindered only by the fact that the mechanism by which the haplotype might confer a growth advantage has not been proposed or identified. The recent discovery of the haplotype also increasing the risk of *JAK2* exon 12 and *MPL* mutations has been cited to favor the fertile ground hypothesis over the hypermutability hypothesis [84, 85]. Nevertheless, the possibility still exists that the haplotype is in linkage with a yet unidentified functional variant, which influences disease pathogenesis.

In addition to the above evidence for a germline genetic cause for MPN pathogenesis, there also exists the possibility that clustering of MPNs may also occur because of yet unidentified environmental exposures, which may increase the risk of developing *JAK2V617F*. The most intriguing suggestion of a possible environmental link and MPNs comes from recent epidemiologic data from three counties in eastern Pennsylvania where the incidence of PV is almost triple that of other areas in the United States [86]. Most of these cases have clustered in specific regions of these counties with clear evidence of *JAK2V617F*-positivity of many of the cases and no evidence for consanguity in the region. So far, no clear etiologic environmental exposure has been identified, and the area is under investigation by several federal agencies.

Novel Genetic Alterations in MPN: The Possibility of Epigenetic Alterations, Regulatory RNAs, and Post-translational Modifications

Although the study of the genetic causes of MPNs has been extremely insightful and resulted in the identification of multiple novel alleles, less explored thus far has been the possibility of disease-modifying alterations outside of coding nucleotides. This includes the possibility of epigenetic modifications, differential expression of microRNAs (miRNAs), and post-translational modifications, which might modify the phenotype of disease produced in patients with *JAK2* mutations. Such "post-genetic" alterations could also possibly be responsible for establishing clonal hematopoeisis prior to acquisition of mutations in *JAK2.*

There has been increasing interest in the study of epigenetic regulation of the JAK-STAT pathway in MPNs, partly based on several important observations of the JAK-STAT pathway in *Drosophilia.* In *Drosophilia*, the JAK-STAT pathway is simpler than in mammals with only a single JAK member (termed Hopscotch*)* with a single downstream STAT (STAT92E). Studies of the JAK-STAT pathway in *Drosophilia* have proven that the Hopscotch ligand, *Unpaired*, is under direct epigenetic transcriptional regulation by PcG proteins. Thus, inactivation of PcG allows excessive expression of *Unpaired* with inappropriate activation of Hopscotch and resultant tumors in eye and wing imaginal discs of *Drosophilia* [87]. Similar epigenetic control of JAK-STAT pathway members in mammals has not been demonstrated so clearly. However, there are at least two reports, which suggest that *SOCS3*, a negative regulator of JAK2 signaling, is hypermethylated in MPNs [88, 89]. In one study, however, *SOCS3* promoter hypermethylation was restricted to patients with MF and not to those with PV or ET, and it was not clear whether *SOCS3* promoter hypermethylated cases had decreased *SOCS3* expression by qRT-PCR. Although there is increasing evidence that epigenetic alterations exist in patients with MPN, specific gene targets of epigenetic alteration that might explain MPN pathogenesis have not been elucidated.

In addition to the search for epigenetic regulation of JAK-STAT pathway members in MPN, it has recently been discovered that JAK2 itself may potentially affect chromatin state. Here again, studies of JAK-STAT pathway in *Drosophilia* have been prescient as it has been known since 2006 that Hopscotch overactivation globally disrupts heterochromatic gene silencing and destabilizes heterochromatin in *Drosophilia* [90]. However, the exact mechanism by which Hopscotch affects chromatin structure in *Drosophilia* is still not clear. Equally exciting and unresolved is the recent discovery by Dawson et al. that JAK2 can be found in the nucleus and appears to phosphorylate histone H3 among all core histones [91]. This was confirmed through evidence of (a) decreased H3 phosphorylation in the presence of at least two different JAK2 inhibitors and (b) phosphorylation of H3Y41 only after JAK2 transfection in JAK2-null gamma-2A cells. The authors then demonstrate that phosphorylation of H3Y41 results in displacement of HP1-alpha. They then posit that HP1-alpha displacement results in overexpression of *lmo2*, an oncogene with a known role in leukemogenesis. There are many questions yet to be answered regarding the possible role of intranuclear JAK2, such as: (1) how is JAK2 entering the nucleus given that it has no classic nuclear localization sequence? (2) how is the kinase activity of JAK2 relevant to its nuclear function given that this activity has always been known to require expression of a cytoplasmic cytokine receptor? and (3) are there are any nuclear targets of JAK2 kinase activity besides histones?

miRNAs are short (~22 nucleotides), phylogenetically-conserved, nonprotein coding RNAs, which regulate gene expression through sequence-specific base pairing with target mRNA. An increasing body of work has demonstrated that miRNAs have an important role in both normal and malignant hematopoiesis. As such, a number of groups have hypothesized that differential expression of a single miRNA or a cluster of miRNAs could result in abnormal clonal hematopoesis preceding acquisition of the *JAK2V617F* mutation in MPNs. To date, the study of miRNAs in MPNs has been nascent and has largely relied on the use of comparison of miRNA gene expression profiling of MPN hematopoietic subsets compared with that of normal subjects. Although this has resulted in a list of miRNAs, which are potentially differentially expressed in MPN relative to normal individuals, functional validation of any of these candidate miRNAs has not been performed. This is critical as the target genes of miRNAs range from 1 to >100 with many of miRNA target genes being only predicted putative targets.

One of the best examples of the possible involvement of a miRNA in the pathogenesis comes from O'Connell et al. who noted that lipopolysaccharide injection of mice resulted in transient induction of miR-155 followed by granulocyte/monocyte expansion [92]. They then validated this finding by overexpressing miR-155 in a murine BMT assay, which resulted in a clear MPN phenotype with neutrophilia, splenomegaly, and extramedullary hematopoiesis. To ascertain whether miR-155 had a role in human myeloid disease, the authors compared miR-155 expression by qRT-PCR in bone marrow cells of AML patients with that of controls. Although they noted increased miR-155 expression in AML, the expression if miR-155 in other myeloid malignancies, including MPNs, was not assessed.

There have been at least four studies of miRNAs expression profiling in MPN patients relative to controls published thus far with the goal of identifying miRNAs differentially regulated in the patients with MPN relative to normal individuals (Table 2.6) [93–96]. The list of miRNAs found to be differentially expressed in patient with MPN relative to control in these different studies to date only share one miRNA, namely *miR-150*. This is a potentially important finding as miR-150 has been recently recognized to regulate

Table 2.6 Results of micro-RNA gene expression profiling (GEP) experiments in MPN subjects relative to normal controls.

Reference	Study design	GEP platform	Findings
Bruchova et al. [94]	Liquid culture of mononuclear cells from PV and normal patients. GEP at days 1, 14, and 21	CombiMatrix MicroRNA Custom Array	PV-specific difference in miR-*150* expression (decreased in PV)
Guglielmelli et al. [95]	miRNA gene expression in MF granulocytes compared with PV/ET and normal subjects	Quantification of 156 mature miRNAs by qRT-PCR	miR-*31*, *-150*, *-95* decreased in MF relative to PV/ET/controls; miR-*34a*, *-342*, *-326*, *-105*, *-149*, and *-147* in all MPN compared with controls
Bruchova et al. [93]	Comparison of GEP from hematopoietic subsets from 5 PV and 5 controls	CombiMatrix MicroRNA Custom Array	The following miRNAs were decreased in PV subsets relative to controls: reticulocytes- miR-*150*, *-30b*, *-30c*; granulocytes: *let7a*. Multiple miRNAs found to be upregulated in PV relative to controls as well.
Slezak et al. [96]	Comparison of GEP from granulocytes from 6 MPN and 5 controls	827 custom microRNA array	miR-*133a* and *-1* most significantly downregulated in MPN subjects relative to controls

lineage fate in MEPs [97]. In a series of in vitro and in vivo experiments by Lu et al. it was shown that overexpression of *miR-150* in MEP cells promotes development of megakaryocytic cells over erythroid cells. Thus, it is possible that downregulation of miR-150 in MEPs of MPN patients with predominant erythrocytosis over thrombocytosis could be a result of differential expression of *miR-150*. Additional functional work to validate findings miRNA gene-expression studies along with improved understanding of miRNA network in normal hematopoiesis will hopefully improve our understanding of the possible role of miRNAs in MPNs.

In addition to regulation at the genetic, epigenetic, and post-transcriptional levels, there exists the possibility that post-translational modifications may be important in creating the MPN phenotype. Some precedent for this already exists with the discovery by Zhao et al. that the presence of JAK2V617F influences the deamidation state of the proapoptotic protein Bcl-XL [98]. It is currently thought that when a cell encounters DNA damage, the activity of the amiloride-sensitive sodium-hydrogen exchanger isoform 1 (NHE1) increases. This increases the intracellular pH, which leads to nonenzymatic deamidation of Bcl-XL. This post-translational modification results in a conversion of an asparagine residue into isoaspartic acid, which, in turn, reduces the ability of Bcl-XL to inhibit the Bcl-2 homology 3 (BH3)-only family of proapoptotic proteins, thereby promoting apoptosis. Evaluation of this pathway in primary MPN samples revealed that DNA damage-induced Bcl-XL deamidation was inhibited in *JAK2V617F* bearing granulocytes but not in granulocytes from normal individuals or in lymphoid cells from diseased individuals with lower levels of *JAK2V617F* allele burden. Further cell line experiments suggest that the V617F mutation in *JAK2* somehow affects the DNA damage response and ultimately affects deamidation of Bcl-XL. Thus far no further clear examples of post-translational regulation of the MPNs have been suggested.

Conclusion: A Multi-Step Model of MPN Pathogenesis

The discovery of gain-of-function mutations in *JAK2* and *MPL* in MPNs led to initial enthusiasm that *JAK2/MPL* mutations were the disease-initiating events in MPN, and were responsible for the onset of disease as well as clonal hematopoiesis. The fact that *JAK2/MPL* mutations were transforming in in vitro as well as in vivo assays supported this "single-hit" model of MPN pathogenesis. However, careful genetic analysis of isolated clones from *JAK2/MPL* mutant MPN patients as well as familial MPN kindreds provided clear evidence that alterations other than *JAK2* mutation must be present.

The fact that clonal hematopoiesis can exist in members of MPN kindreds before *JAK2* development as well as the fact that *JAK2* wild-type leukemic blasts were found derived from *JAK2V617F* mutant MPN samples suggest that genetic alteration(s) can precede acquisition of *JAK2/MPL* mutations. The discovery of mutations in *TET2*, *ASXL1*, and the strong, yet unidentified germline genetic risk haplotype for MPNs, has led to the hypothesis that these genetic alterations can in fact establish clonal hematopoiesis without causing overt disease (Fig. 2.7). In this multi-step model of MPN pathogenesis, it is proposed that a genetic alteration, somatic or inherited, occurs in a hematopoietic stem/progenitor cell. This state of clonal hematopoiesis may

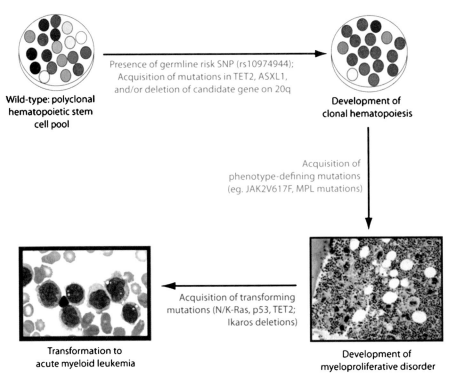

Fig. 2.7 Hypothesized multi-step model of MPN pathogenesis. Prior to the acquisition of mutations that activate the JAK-STAT pathway, it is proposed that genetic abnormalities may occur, which establishes a state of clonal hematopoiesis. The events that establish clonal hematopoiesis could occur as a poorly understood effect from the presence of the MPN risk haplotype, acquisition of mutations in *TET2* or *ASXL1*, and/or loss of an unidentified gene located on 20q. Establishment of clonal hematopoiesis is thought to increase the likelihood of acquisition of phenotype-defining mutations (such as mutations in *JAK2* and *MPL*). Later, stepwise acquisition of disease-transforming genetic events promotes transformation from a chronic MPN state to a state of acute myeloid leukemia. No canonical genetic events have been identified at leukemic transformation of MPNs, but genes that are enriched in MPN state compared with leukemic state in paired samples include mutations in p53, TET2, and N/K-Ras. It has also recently been observed that Ikaros deletions may occur at leukemic transformation

not yield an overt clinical phenotype but likely increases the likelihood of *JAK2/MPL* mutation acquisition; clones that acquire activating mutations in the JAK-STAT mitogenic pathway gain further clonal advantage. The finding that mutations in *TET2* and *ASXL1* can occur years before the clinical onset of MPN phenotype has led to strong interest that mutations in either of these genes could establish clonal hematopoiesis. However, definitive evidence that alterations in *TET2* and *ASXL1* lead to clonal hematopoiesis has not been shown, and mutations in *TET2* have now been found to occur at all stages in MPN pathogenesis (before or after *JAK2V617F* acquisition) making it clear that *TET2* mutations are not a canonical "pre-JAK2" event [64, 65]. This has led some authors to speculate that disease pathogenesis in MPNs is heterogenous with some patients acquiring *JAK2/MPL* mutations as the initiating and sole event whereas others develop nonphenotype defining "pre-JAK2" mutations first [7]. The realization that the JAK2 haplotype leads to increased acquisition of both *JAK2* and *MPL* mutations suggests germline genetic variation is relevant to MPN pathogenesis. At the same time, functional data to support the role of the JAK2 haplotype and other germline MPN alleles in MPN pathogenesis does not yet exist.

Despite knowledge of specific genetic alterations in MPNs over the last 5 years, it is clear that yet more unidentified genetic and "post-genetic" events must occur in MPN patients. A significant proportion of ET and MF patients present without any known MPN disease alleles. Moreover, a full explanation for the intriguing MPN risk haplotype has not been identified, and the identity of which genes within recurrent cytogenetic alterations identified in MPN patients contribute to transformation is not known. Moreover, systematic evaluation of the epigenome, regulatory non-coding RNAs, and post-translational regulatory events in MPNs are just now being performed.

Improvements in next-generation sequencing technologies as well as increased access to these technologies will allow groups to better characterize the MPN genome. This will, in turn, hopefully provide a full catalogue of the somatic mutations, chromosomal rearrangements, and copy-number alterations, which exist in MPNs. In parallel, increasing use of transcriptome sequencing will likely promote efforts to identify alterations present at the transcriptional level, which may or may not be identified at the level of DNA. At the same time, improvements in the understanding and throughput of technologies to catalogue epigenetic alterations will hopefully allow for a better understanding of the methylation and chromatin states of MPN genomes. Although much progress has been made in improving our understanding of the pathogenesis of the different MPNs, there is much more work to be done!

References

1. Dameshek W. Some speculations on the myeloproliferative syndromes. Blood. 1951;6:372–375.
2. Baxter EJ, Scott LM, Campbell PJ, et al. Acquired mutation of the tyrosine kinase JAK2 in human myeloproliferative disorders. Lancet. 2005;365:1054–1061.
3. James C, Ugo V, Le Couedic JP, et al. A unique clonal JAK2 mutation leading to constitutive signalling causes polycythaemia vera. Nature. 2005;434:1144–1148.
4. Kralovics R, Passamonti F, Buser AS, et al. A gain-of-function mutation of JAK2 in myeloproliferative disorders. N Engl J Med. 2005;352:1779–1790.
5. Levine RL, Wadleigh M, Cools J, et al. Activating mutation in the tyrosine kinase JAK2 in polycythemia vera, essential thrombocythemia, and myeloid metaplasia with myelofibrosis. Cancer Cell. 2005;7:387–397.
6. Kahvejian A, Quackenbush J, Thompson JF. What would you do if you could sequence everything? Nat Biotechnol. 2008;26:1125–1133.
7. Kralovics R. Genetic complexity of myeloproliferative neoplasms. Leukemia. 2008;22:1841–1848.
8. Levine RL, Belisle C, Wadleigh M, et al. X-inactivation-based clonality analysis and quantitative JAK2V617F assessment reveal a strong association between clonality and JAK2V617F in PV but not ET/MMM, and identifies a subset of JAK2V617F-negative ET and MMM patients with clonal hematopoiesis. Blood. 2006;107:4139–4141.
9. Pikman Y, Lee BH, Mercher T, et al. MPLW515L is a novel somatic activating mutation in myelofibrosis with myeloid metaplasia. PLoS Med. 2006;3:e270.
10. Scott LM, Tong W, Levine RL, et al. JAK2 exon 12 mutations in polycythemia vera and idiopathic erythrocytosis. N Engl J Med. 2007;356:459–468.
11. Jones AV, Chase A, Silver RT, et al. JAK2 haplotype is a major risk factor for the development of myeloproliferative neoplasms. Nat Genet. 2009;41:446–449.

12. Kilpivaara O, Mukherjee S, Schram AM, et al. A germline JAK2 SNP is associated with predisposition to the development of JAK2(V617F)-positive myeloproliferative neoplasms. Nat Genet. 2009;41:455–459.

13. Olcaydu D, Harutyunyan A, Jager R, et al. A common JAK2 haplotype confers susceptibility to myeloproliferative neoplasms. Nat Genet. 2009;41:450–454.

14. Abdel-Wahab O, Mullally A, Hedvat C, et al. Genetic characterization of TET1, TET2, and TET3 alterations in myeloid malignancies. Blood. 2009;114:144–147.

15. Carbuccia N, Murati A, Trouplin V, et al. Mutations of ASXL1 gene in myeloproliferative neoplasms. Leukemia. 2009;23:2183–2186.

16. Delhommeau F, Dupont S, Della Valle V, et al. Mutation in TET2 in myeloid cancers. N Engl J Med. 2009;360:2289–2301.

17. Gelsi-Boyer V, Trouplin V, Adelaide J, et al. Mutations of polycomb-associated gene ASXL1 in myelodysplastic syndromes and chronic myelomonocytic leukaemia. Br J Haematol. 2009;145:788–800.

18. Langemeijer SM, Kuiper RP, Berends M, et al. Acquired mutations in TET2 are common in myelodysplastic syndromes. Nat Genet. 2009;41:838–842.

19. Adamson JW, Fialkow PJ, Murphy S, Prchal JF, Steinmann L. Polycythemia vera: stem-cell and probable clonal origin of the disease. N Engl J Med. 1976;295:913–916.

20. Fialkow PJ, Faguet GB, Jacobson RJ, Vaidya K, Murphy S. Evidence that essential thrombocythemia is a clonal disorder with origin in a multipotent stem cell. Blood. 1981;58:916–919.

21. Jacobson RJ, Salo A, Fialkow PJ. Agnogenic myeloid metaplasia: a clonal proliferation of hematopoietic stem cells with secondary myelofibrosis. Blood. 1978;51:189–194.

22. Bumm TG, Elsea C, Corbin AS, et al. Characterization of murine JAK2V617F-positive myeloproliferative disease. Cancer Res. 2006;66:11156–11165.

23. Lacout C, Pisani DF, Tulliez M, Gachelin FM, Vainchenker W, Villeval JL. JAK2V617F expression in murine hematopoietic cells leads to MPD mimicking human PV with secondary myelofibrosis. Blood. 2006;108:1652–1660.

24. Wernig G, Mercher T, Okabe R, Levine RL, Lee BH, Gilliland DG. Expression of Jak2V617F causes a polycythemia vera-like disease with associated myelofibrosis in a murine bone marrow transplant model. Blood. 2006;107:4274–4281.

25. Zaleskas VM, Krause DS, Lazarides K, et al. Molecular pathogenesis and therapy of polycythemia induced in mice by JAK2 V617F. PLoS One. 2006;1:e18.

26. Tiedt R, Hao-Shen H, Sobas MA, et al. Ratio of mutant JAK2-V617F to wild-type Jak2 determines the MPD phenotypes in transgenic mice. Blood. 2008;111:3931–3940.

27. Xing S, Wanting TH, Zhao W, et al. Transgenic expression of JAK2V617F causes myeloproliferative disorders in mice. Blood. 2008;111:5109–5117.

28. Jamieson CH, Gotlib J, Durocher JA, et al. The JAK2 V617F mutation occurs in hematopoietic stem cells in polycythemia vera and predisposes toward erythroid differentiation. Proc Natl Acad Sci U S A. 2006;103:6224–6229.

29. Geron I, Abrahamsson AE, Barroga CF, et al. Selective inhibition of JAK2-driven erythroid differentiation of polycythemia vera progenitors. Cancer Cell. 2008;13:321–330.

30. Saharinen P, Takaluoma K, Silvennoinen O. Regulation of the Jak2 tyrosine kinase by its pseudokinase domain. Mol Cell Biol. 2000;20:3387–3395.

31. Dusa A, Staerk J, Elliott J, et al. Substitution of pseudokinase domain residue Val-617 by large non-polar amino acids causes activation of JAK2. J Biol Chem. 2008;283:12941–12948.

32. Lambert JR, Everington T, Linch DC, Gale RE. In essential thrombocythemia, multiple JAK2-V617F clones are present in most mutant-positive patients: a new disease paradigm. Blood. 2009;114:3018–3023.

33. Bercovich D, Ganmore I, Scott LM, et al. Mutations of JAK2 in acute lymphoblastic leukaemias associated with Down's syndrome. Lancet. 2008;372:1484–1492.

34. Li S, Kralovics R, De Libero G, Theocharides A, Gisslinger H, Skoda RC. Clonal heterogeneity in polycythemia vera patients with JAK2 exon12 and JAK2-V617F mutations. Blood. 2008;111:3863–3866.

35. Lacronique V, Boureux A, Valle VD, et al. A TEL-JAK2 fusion protein with constitutive kinase activity in human leukemia. Science. 1997;278:1309–1312.

36. Peeters P, Raynaud SD, Cools J, et al. Fusion of TEL, the ETS-variant gene 6 (ETV6), to the receptor-associated kinase JAK2 as a result of t(9;12) in a lymphoid and t(9;15;12) in a myeloid leukemia. Blood. 1997;90:2535–2540.

37. Adelaide J, Perot C, Gelsi-Boyer V, et al. A t(8;9) translocation with PCM1-JAK2 fusion in a patient with T-cell lymphoma. Leukemia. 2006;20:536–537.

38. Bousquet M, Quelen C, De Mas V, et al. The t(8;9)(p22;p24) translocation in atypical chronic myeloid leukaemia yields a new PCM1-JAK2 fusion gene. Oncogene. 2005;24:7248–7252.

39. Murati A, Adelaide J, Gelsi-Boyer V, et al. t(5;12)(q23-31;p13) with ETV6-ACSL6 gene fusion in polycythemia vera. Leukemia. 2006;20:1175–1178.

40. Reiter A, Walz C, Watmore A, et al. The t(8;9)(p22;p24) is a recurrent abnormality in chronic and acute leukemia that fuses PCM1 to JAK2. Cancer Res. 2005;65:2662–2667.

41. Mullighan CG, Morin R, Zhang J, et al. Next generation transcriptomic resequencing identifies novel genetic alterations in High-Risk (HR) childhood acute lymphoblastic leukemia (ALL): a report from the Children's Oncology Group (COG) HR ALL TARGET Project. Blood. 2009;114(22):704 (abstract).

42. Pardanani AD, Levine RL, Lasho T, et al. MPL515 mutations in myeloproliferative and other myeloid disorders: a study of 1182 patients. Blood. 2006;108:3472–3476.

43. Beer PA, Jones AV, Bench AJ, et al. Clonal diversity in the myeloproliferative neoplasms: independent origins of genetically distinct clones. Br J Haematol. 2009;144:904–908.

44. Kralovics R, Stockton DW, Prchal JT. Clonal hematopoiesis in familial polycythemia vera suggests the involvement of multiple mutational events in the early pathogenesis of the disease. Blood. 2003;102:3793–3796.

45. Campbell PJ, Baxter EJ, Beer PA, et al. Mutation of JAK2 in the myeloproliferative disorders: timing, clonality studies, cytogenetic associations, and role in leukemic transformation. Blood. 2006;108:3548–3555.

46. Theocharides A, Boissinot M, Girodon F, et al. Leukemic blasts in transformed JAK2-V617F-positive myeloproliferative disorders are frequently negative for the JAK2-V617F mutation. Blood. 2007;110:375–379.

47. Ding J, Komatsu H, Wakita A, et al. Familial essential thrombocythemia associated with a dominant-positive activating mutation of the c-MPL gene, which encodes for the receptor for thrombopoietin. Blood. 2004;103:4198–4200.

48. Viguie F, Aboura A, Bouscary D, et al. Common 4q24 deletion in four cases of hematopoietic malignancy: early stem cell involvement? Leukemia. 2005;19:1411–1415.

49. Couronné L, Lippert E, Andrieux J, Kosmider O, Radford-Weiss I, Penther D, Dastugue N, Mugneret F, Lafage M, Gachard N, Nadal N, Bernard OA, Nguyen-Khac F. Analyses of TET2 mutations in post-myeloproliferative neoplasm acute myeloid leukemias. Leukemia. 2010 Jan;24(1):201–3. Epub 2009 Aug 27.

50. Jankowska AM, Szpurka H, Tiu RV, et al. Loss of heterozygosity 4q24 and TET2 mutations associated with myelodysplastic/myeloproliferative neoplasms. Blood. 2009;113:6403–6410.

51. Tefferi A, Levine RL, Lim KH, et al. Frequent TET2 mutations in systemic mastocytosis: clinical, KITD816V and FIP1L1-PDGFRA correlates. Leukemia. 2009;23:900–904.

52. Tefferi A, Lim KH, Abdel-Wahab O, et al. Detection of mutant TET2 in myeloid malignancies other than myeloproliferative neoplasms: CMML, MDS, MDS/MPN and AML. Leukemia. 2009;23:1343–1345.

53. Tefferi A, Pardanani A, Lim KH, et al. TET2 mutations and their clinical correlates in polycythemia vera, essential thrombocythemia and myelofibrosis. Leukemia. 2009;23:905–911.

54. Lorsbach RB, Moore J, Mathew S, Raimondi SC, Mukatira ST, Downing JR. TET1, a member of a novel protein family, is fused to MLL in acute myeloid leukemia containing the t(10;11)(q22;q23). Leukemia. 2003;17:637–641.

55. Tahiliani M, Koh KP, Shen Y, et al. Conversion of 5-methylcytosine to 5-hydroxymethylcytosine in mammalian DNA by MLL partner TET1. Science. 2009;324:930–935.

56. Iyer LM, Tahiliani M, Rao A, Aravind L. Prediction of novel families of enzymes involved in oxidative and other complex modifications of bases in nucleic acids. Cell Cycle. 2009;8:1698–1710.

57. Nibourel O, Kosmider O, Cheok M, Boissel N, Renneville A, Philippe N, Dombret H, Dreyfus F, Quesnel B, Geffroy S, Quentin S, Roche-Lestienne C, Cayuela J-M, Roumier C, Fenaux P, Vainchenker W, Bernard OA, Soulier J, Fontenay M, Preudhomme C. Association of TET2 alterations with NPM1 mutations and prognostic value in de novo acute myeloid leukemia (AML). Blood. 2009;114 (22).

58. Hussein K, Abdel-Wahab O, Lasho TL, et al. Cytogenetic correlates of TET2 mutations in 199 patients with myeloproliferative neoplasms. Am J Hematol. 2009;85:81–83.

59. Kosmider O, Gelsi-Boyer V, Cheok M, et al. TET2 mutation is an independent favorable prognostic factor in myelodysplastic syndromes (MDSs). Blood. 2009;114:3285–3291.

60. Carbuccia N, Trouplin V, Gelsi-Boyer V, Murati A, Rocquain J, Adélaïde J, Olschwang S, Xerri L, Vey N, Chaffanet M, Birnbaum D, Mozziconacci MJ. Mutual exclusion of ASXL1 and NPM1 mutations in a series of acute myeloid leukemias. Leukemia. 2010 Feb;24(2):469–473. Epub 2009 Oct 29.

61. Cho YS, Kim EJ, Park UH, Sin HS, Um SJ. Additional sex comb-like 1 (ASXL1), in cooperation with SRC-1, acts as a ligand-dependent coactivator for retinoic acid receptor. J Biol Chem. 2006;281:17588–17598.

62. Fisher CL, Lee I, Bloyer S, Bozza S, Chevalier J, Dahl A, Bodner C, Helgason CD, Hess JL, Humphries RK, Brock HW. Additional sex combs-like 1 belongs to the enhancer of trithorax and polycomb group and genetically interacts with Cbx2 in mice. Dev Biol. 2010 Jan 1;337(1):9–15. Epub 2009 Oct 13.

63. Fisher CL, Pineault N, Brookes C, Helgason CD, Ohta H, Bodner C, Hess JL, Humphries RK, Brock HW. Loss-of-function Additional sex combs like 1 mutations disrupt hematopoiesis but do not cause severe myelodysplasia or leukemia. Blood. 2010 Jan 7;115(1):38–46. Epub 2009 Oct 27.

64. Beer PA, Delhommeau F, LeCouédic JP, Dawson MA, Chen E, Bareford D, Kusec R, McMullin MF, Harrison CN, Vannucchi AM, Vainchenker W, Green AR. Two routes to leukemic transformation after a JAK2 mutation-positive myeloproliferative neoplasm. Blood. 2010 Apr 8;115(14):2891–2900.

65. Abdel-Wahab O, Manshouri T, Patel J, Harris K, Yao J, Hedvat C, Heguy A, Bueso-Ramos C, Kantarjian H, Levine RL, Verstovsek S. Genetic analysis of transforming events that convert chronic myeloproliferative neoplasms to leukemias. Cancer Res. 2010 Jan 15;70(2):447–452. Epub 2009 Jan 12.

66. Jäger R, Gisslinger H, Berg T, Passamonti F, Cazzola M, Rumi E, Pietra D, Gisslinger B, Klampfl T, Harutyunyan A, Olcaydu D, and Kralovics R. Deletions of the Transcription Factor Ikaros in Myeloproliferative Neoplasms at Transformation to Acute Myeloid Leukemia. Blood (ASH Annual Meeting Abstracts), Nov 2009;114:435.

67. Mullighan CG, Miller CB, Radtke I, et al. BCR-ABL1 lymphoblastic leukaemia is characterized by the deletion of Ikaros. Nature. 2008;453:110–114.

68. Bench AJ, Nacheva EP, Hood TL, et al. Chromosome 20 deletions in myeloid malignancies: reduction of the common deleted region, generation of a PAC/BAC contig and identification of candidate genes. UK Cancer Cytogenetics Group (UKCCG). Oncogene. 2000;19:3902–3913.

69. Ebert BL, Pretz J, Bosco J, et al. Identification of RPS14 as a 5q- syndrome gene by RNA interference screen. Nature. 2008;451:335–339.

70. Starczynowski DT, Kuchenbauer F, Argiropoulos B, Sung S, Morin R, Muranyi A, Hirst M, Hogge D, Marra M, Wells RA, Buckstein R, Lam W, Humphries RK, Karsan A. Identification of miR-145 and miR-146a as mediators of the 5q- syndrome phenotype. Nat Med. 2010 Jan;16(1):49–58. Epub 2009 Nov 8.

71. van Haaften G, Dalgliesh GL, Davies H, et al. Somatic mutations of the histone H3K27 demethylase gene UTX in human cancer. Nat Genet. 2009;41:521–523.

72. Grand FH, Hidalgo-Curtis CE, Ernst T, et al. Frequent CBL mutations associated with 11q acquired uniparental disomy in myeloproliferative neoplasms. Blood. 2009;113:6182–6192.

73. Makishima H, Jankowska AM, Cazzolli H, Przychodzen BP, Prince C, Harish S, Rogers HJ, His ED, McDevitt MA, Advani A, Paquette R, Maciejewski JP. Cbl and TET2 Mutations Are Present in Refractory Ph+ Disorders Including Accelerated and Blast Crisis CML and ALL. Blood (ASH Annual Meeting Abstracts), Nov 2009;114:2173.

74. Muramatsu H, Makishima H, Jankowska AM, Cazzolli H, O'Keefe C, Yoshida N, Xu Y, Nishio N, Hama A, Yagasaki H, Takahashi Y, Kato K, Manabe A, Kojima S, Maciejewski JP. Mutations of an E3 ubiquitin ligase c-Cbl but not TET2 mutations are pathogenic in juvenile myelomonocytic leukemia. Blood. 2010 Mar 11;115(10):1969–1975. Epub 2009 Dec 11.

75. Sanada M, Suzuki T, Shih LY, et al. Gain-of-function of mutated C-CBL tumour suppressor in myeloid neoplasms. Nature. 2009;460:904–908.

76. Mardis ER, Ding L, Dooling DJ, et al. Recurring mutations found by sequencing an acute myeloid leukemia genome. N Engl J Med. 2009;361:1058–1066.

77. Pardanani A, Lasho T, McClure R, Lacy M, Tefferi A. Discordant distribution of JAK2V617F mutation in siblings with familial myeloproliferative disorders. Blood. 2006;107:4572–4573.

78. Pietra D, Li S, Brisci A, et al. Somatic mutations of JAK2 exon 12 in patients with JAK2 (V617F)-negative myeloproliferative disorders. Blood. 2008;111:1686–1689.

79. Rumi E, Passamonti F, Della Porta MG, et al. Familial chronic myeloproliferative disorders: clinical phenotype and evidence of disease anticipation. J Clin Oncol. 2007;25:5630–5635.

80. Rumi E, Passamonti F, Pietra D, et al. JAK2 (V617F) as an acquired somatic mutation and a secondary genetic event associated with disease progression in familial myeloproliferative disorders. Cancer. 2006;107:2206–2211.

81. Landgren O, Goldin LR, Kristinsson SY, Helgadottir EA, Samuelsson J, Bjorkholm M. Increased risks of polycythemia vera, essential thrombocythemia, and myelofibrosis among 24,577 first-degree relatives of 11,039 patients with myeloproliferative neoplasms in Sweden. Blood. 2008;112:2199–2204.

82. Pardanani A, Lasho TL, Finke CM, Gangat N, Wolanskyj AP, Hanson CA, Tefferi A. The JAK2 46/1 haplotype confers susceptibility to essential thrombocythemia regardless of JAK2V617F mutational status-clinical correlates in a study of 226 consecutive patients. Leukemia. 2010 Jan;24(1):110–114. Epub 2009 Oct 22.

83. Tefferi A, Lasho TL, Patnaik MM, Finke CM, Hussein K, Hogan WJ, Elliott MA, Litzow MR, Hanson CA, Pardanani A. JAK2 germline genetic variation affects disease susceptibility in primary myelofibrosis regardless of V617F mutational status:

nullizygosity for the JAK2 46/1 haplotype is associated with inferior survival. Leukemia. 2010 Jan;24(1):105–109. Epub 2009 Oct 22.

84. Olcaydu D, Skoda RC, Looser R, et al. The 'GGCC' haplotype of JAK2 confers susceptibility to JAK2 exon 12 mutation-positive polycythemia vera. Leukemia. 2009;23:1924–1926.

85. Cross NCP, Campbell P, Beer PA, Schnittger S, Vannucchi AM, Zoi K, Percy M, McMullin MF, Scott L, Silver RT, Oscier D, Harrison C, Green AR, and Chase A. The JAK2 46/1 Haplotype Predisposes to Myeloproliferative Neoplasms Characterized by Diverse Mutations. Blood (ASH Annual Meeting Abstracts), Nov 2009;114:433.

86. Seaman V, Jumaan A, Yanni E, et al. Use of molecular testing to identify a cluster of patients with polycythemia vera in eastern Pennsylvania. Cancer Epidemiol Biomarkers Prev. 2009;18:534–540.

87. Classen AK, Bunker BD, Harvey KF, Vaccari T, Bilder D. A tumor suppressor activity of Drosophila Polycomb genes mediated by JAK-STAT signaling. Nat Genet. 2009;41:1150–1155.

88. Capello D, Deambrogi C, Rossi D, et al. Epigenetic inactivation of suppressors of cytokine signalling in Philadelphia-negative chronic myeloproliferative disorders. Br J Haematol. 2008;141:504–511.

89. Fourouclas N, Li J, Gilby DC, et al. Methylation of the suppressor of cytokine signaling 3 gene (SOCS3) in myeloproliferative disorders. Haematologica. 2008;93:1635–1644.

90. Shi S, Calhoun HC, Xia F, Li J, Le L, Li WX. JAK signaling globally counteracts heterochromatic gene silencing. Nat Genet. 2006;38:1071–1076.

91. Dawson MA, Bannister AJ, Gottgens B, et al. JAK2 phosphorylates histone H3Y41 and excludes HP1alpha from chromatin. Nature. 2009;461:819–822.

92. O'Connell RM, Rao DS, Chaudhuri AA, et al. Sustained expression of micro-RNA-155 in hematopoietic stem cells causes a myeloproliferative disorder. J Exp Med. 2008;205:585–594.

93. Bruchova H, Merkerova M, Prchal JT. Aberrant expression of microRNA in poly-cythemia vera. Haematologica. 2008;93:1009–1016.

94. Bruchova H, Yoon D, Agarwal AM, Mendell J, Prchal JT. Regulated expression of microRNAs in normal and polycythemia vera erythropoiesis. Exp Hematol. 2007;35:1657–1667.

95. Guglielmelli P, Tozzi L, Pancrazzi A, et al. MicroRNA expression profile in granu-locytes from primary myelofibrosis patients. Exp Hematol. 2007;35:1708–1718.

96. Slezak S, Jin P, Caruccio L, et al. Gene and microRNA analysis of neutrophils from patients with polycythemia vera and essential thrombocytosis: down-regu-lation of micro RNA-1 and -133a. J Transl Med. 2009;7:39.

97. Lu J, Guo S, Ebert BL, et al. MicroRNA-mediated control of cell fate in meg-akaryocyte-erythrocyte progenitors. Dev Cell. 2008;14:843–853.

98. Zhao R, Follows GA, Beer PA, et al. Inhibition of the Bcl-xL deamidation path-way in myeloproliferative disorders. N Engl J Med. 2008;359:2778–2789.

99. Bellanne-Chantelot C, Chaumarel I, Labopin M, et al. Genetic and clinical impli-cations of the Val617Phe JAK2 mutation in 72 families with myeloproliferative disorders. Blood. 2006;108:346–352.

100. Saint-Martin C, Leroy G, Delhommeau F, et al. Analysis of the ten-eleven translocation 2 (TET2) gene in familial myeloproliferative neoplasms. Blood. 2009;114:1628–1632.

101. Rumi E. Familial chronic myeloproliferative disorders: the state of the art. Hematol Oncol. 2008;26:131–138.

Chapter 3

Cytogenetic Findings in Classical MPNs

John T. Reilly

Keywords: Cytogenetics • Pathogenesis • Prognosis • Primary myelofibrosis • Polycythemia vera • Essential thrombocythemia

Introduction

The myeloproliferative neoplasms (MPNs), as defined by the latest World Health Organisation's (WHO) revision, include a range of clonal haematopoietic disorders that are characterised by an increase in the number of one or more mature blood cell progeny. Classical cytogenetic analysis has played a crucial role in the identification of important oncogenes in many haematological malignancies, the paradigm being the identification of the t(9;22) in chronic myeloid leukaemia. This discovery led not only to the elucidation of the pathogenetic role of the *bcr-abl* fusion gene, but also to the development of effective targeted therapy. Other oncogenic events, involving the activation of different tyrosine kinases, were subsequently identified by the study of rare translocations. In contrast, the pathogenesis of the Philadelphia-negative MPNs namely, essential thrombocythemia (ET), polycythemia vera (PV), primary myelofibrosis (PMF), as well as chronic neutrophilic leukeamia (CNL), has not been greatly advanced by karyotypic analysis. Nevertheless, cytogenetic analysis still has a role in the routine investigation of such patients, as an abnormal profile provides evidence of clonality: a factor recognised by the WHO diagnostic criteria (Table 3.1). In addition, cytogenetic analysis may also provide valuable prognostic information in PMF, assist in the selection of specific therapy and ensure the exclusion of related disorders that may be associated with marrow fibrosis (see review [1]). The aim of this chapter is to review the current knowledge of chromosomal abnormalities in the MPN and to highlight possible pathogenetic consequences of such changes.

Essential Thrombocythaemia

ET is an MPN characterised by a persistently elevated platelet count of greater than 450×10^9/L, a bone marrow showing proliferation of the megakaryocytic lineage and, if no evidence of clonality by cytogenetic or molecular

S. Verstovsek and A. Tefferi (eds.), *Myeloproliferative Neoplasms: Biology and Therapy*, Contemporary Hematology, DOI 10.1007/ 978-1-60761-266-7_3,
© Springer Science+Business Media, LLC 2011

Table 3.1 Chromosomal changes and their associations in myeloproliferative neoplasms.

Chromosome	Karyotype	Disease association	Comments
1	Total or partial trisomy	PV/PMF (10%)	Critical regions 1q21–1q32
		Post-PV-MF (70–90%)	?Over-expression of protein tyrosine phosphatase
		ET (rare)	
	– der(1:7)(q10:p10)	ET	Poor prognosis
	– der(1)t(1:9)	PV/PMF	Poor prognosis
4	Normal	ET/PV/PMF	LOH at TET2 locus
5	del(5q)	ET/PV/PMF	?haplo-insufficiencyRPS14/consider lenalidamide
	monosomy 5	ET/PV/PMF	Poor prognosis/lack of response to therapy
6	der(6)t(1:6)(q23–25:p21–22)	PMF	?marker for PMF. ?involves *FKBP51*
	t(6;10)(q27;q11)	PMF	Poor prognosis related to acute transformation
7	del(7q)/monosomy 7	ET/PV/PMF	Poor prognosis/lack of response to therapy
8	Trisomy 8	PV (5%)/PMF (5%)	Poor prognosis PMF. Over-expression of microRNAs (miR-124a and miR-30d)
		ET (rare)	
9	Unbalanced translocations	PV	Critical region (p13-pter)
	– der(9;18)(p10;q10)	PV	Propensity to transformation
	LOH 9p	PV	JAK2 locus/results in homozygous JAK2-V617F
	Trisomy 9	ET/PV/PMF	
	Partial trisomy 9p	PV	
11	Complex	PMF	Lack committed erythroid progenitors
12	del(12q)	PMF	Poor prognosis/acute transformation
13	del(13q)	PV (3%)/PMF(6%)	Interstitial (13q12–13q22)/good prognosis
	Translocations involving 13q14	PMF (<1%)	Involve submicroscopic deletions
	Trisomy 13	PMF (rare)	?response to lenalidamide
20	Del(20q)	PV (10%)	Critical deleted regions (CDR) 20q11.2-q13.1
		PMF (10%)	Candidate gene ?*L3MBTL*
		ET (rare)	
21	Trisomy	PMF/CNL (uncommon)	

analyses, the absence of a reactive cause. Interestingly, cytogenetic analysis of haematopoietic colonies suggests that, at least in some patients, the disease can arise at the multi-potent stem cell level. Karyotypic abnormalities in ET are uncommon and occur in less than 5% of cases [2]. They are heterogeneous, including numerical gains, typically trisomy 8 and trisomy 9, or losses, classically del(13q) and del(20q), as well as unbalanced translocations. Recently, Steensma and Tefferi [3], in a review of the literature, have emphasised that abnormalities of most chromosomes have been reported in individual patients, a finding that might indicate a bystander effect. Interphase fluorescence in situ hybridisation (I-FISH) studies have been employed by a number of groups to determine the frequency of such abnormalities in ET, and the findings suggest a higher incidence than that reported by standard cytogenetics. However, not all studies have confirmed this observation and possible reasons include the different length of patient follow up, the concomitant use of cytoreductive therapy, as well as the source material analysed. Furthermore, an investigation using oligonucleotide array comparative genomic hybridization (aCGH) concluded that neither micro-deletions nor micro-duplications play a significant role in the pathogenesis of the disease [4].

A recent study by Gangat and colleagues [2] focused on the clinical and prognostic significance of an abnormal karyotypic at diagnosis in 402 cases of ET. For the first time, an association was noted between abnormal cytogenetics and palpable splenomegaly, current tobacco use, venous thrombosis and reduced haemoglobin levels (defined as less than 10 g/dL). In contrast, it was noted that such patients did not have a shorter survival, or an increased transformation to acute leukaemia or myelofibrosis. Rare cytogenetic abnormalities, however, may have an adverse prognosis, for example the de novo appearance of der(1;7(q10;p10)) in ET, unrelated to therapy. A total of eight cases have been reported, of which six were associated with leukaemic and one with a myelofibrotic transformation (reviewed in [1]). However, cytogenetic abnormalities are clearly more frequent at the time of leukaemic transformation, as is the case for all MPNs, with frequencies around 90%. This observation is consistent with the multi-step process of leukaemogenesis. Leukaemic transformations are commonly associated with poor prognostic changes, including -5/5q- and -7/-7q, and consequently respond poorly to intensive chemotherapy. Finally, it has been proposed that the Philadelphia-chromosome should be excluded in all cases of ET, as rarely CML may present with an identical phenotype. Although such presentations are rare, the success of targeted therapy in CML makes it important that such a diagnosis is not missed.

Polycythaemia Vera

The frequency of karyotypic changes has been documented in a limited number of patients, both at diagnosis and during follow-up, including both treated and untreated patients (see review [1]). Approximately, 15% of patients have chromosomal abnormalities at the time of diagnosis [5, 6], although like other MPNs, no specific abnormality has been reported. The use of either I-FISH or aCGH does not appear to significantly increase the detection rate in untreated patients [4]. The most frequent findings at presentation are trisomy 1q, trisomy 8, trisomy 9, as well as del(20q) [5], although many different changes have been noted [5, 6]. It is possible that del(13q) and abnormalities of chromosome 1 correlate with disease transformation to myelofibrosis [5]. The only clinical parameter that has been associated with an abnormal karyotype appears to be age, in contrast to thrombosis, haemorrhage, leukaemic or myelofibrotic transformation, *JAK2 V617F* allele burden or survival [6]. However, rare karyotypic abnormalities may be associated with a greater risk of undergoing myelofibrotic or leukaemic transformation. For example, on reviewing the literature, Larsen et al. [7] concluded that *JAK2 V617F*-positive cases with a der(9;18)(p10;q10) may have a high intrinsic propensity for such transformations. The molecular basis for this observation remains unclear, although the possibility of *JAK2* amplification requires further study.

Finally, specific therapies have been associated with a much higher frequency of abnormality. In one of the largest reported studies, for example, only 13% of untreated patients possessed a chromosomal change, when compared with more than half of those who had received 32P, or chemotherapy, especially the alkylating agent busulfan [5]. A further study demonstrated abnormalities in 18% treated with venesection alone, which increased to 60% in those receiving cytotoxic therapy.

Primary Myelofibrosis

In 1975, Kahn and colleagues, using G6PD isoenzyme analysis, were the first to demonstrate convincingly that erythrocytes, leucocytes and platelets were monoclonal in PMF. In contrast, the same technique was subsequently used to show that the fibroblast proliferation is polyclonal and not part of the underlying neoplastic process. Karyotypic studies have provided support for these conclusions, since circulating haematopoietic precursors, including pluripotent (CFU-GEMM) and lineage-restricted progenitor cells (BFU-E, CFU-GM and CFU-MK), are clonally involved. Such findings have contributed to the current pathogenetic model, in which a plethora of cytokines are thought to be released from intra-medullary, clonal megakaryocytes and monocytes, which in turn leads to the stimulation of a polyclonal or secondary stromal proliferation [8].

PMF has the highest aberration rate of the Philadelphia-negative MPNs, with one third of patients having an abnormal karyotype at presentation [9]. It should be noted that although most patients' bone marrow is a "dry tap", satisfactory results can usually be obtained from peripheral blood analysis. It has been proposed that many of the observed cytogenetic changes may represent secondary sub-clones, resultant upon the genetic instability of the original clone. Over the last two decades, the publication of a number of large studies has helped clarify the cytogenetic findings in this disorder [9–13]. Tefferi and colleagues [12], for example, in a retrospective single institution study of 165 cases, reported that the frequency of cytogenetic abnormalities increased with time from diagnosis, even in patients not previously exposed to cytoreductive therapy. All five studies suggest that deletions of 13q and 20q, trisomy 8 and abnormalities of chromosomes 1, 7 and 9 constitute more than 80% of all chromosomal changes. Abnormalities of chromosome 5 appeared to be more frequent in chemotherapy exposed cases [12]. Deletion of the long arm of chromosome 13 is the most common abnormality, occurring in approximately a quarter of those cases with an abnormal karyotype [10–12]. The next most frequently observed abnormalities are del(20q) and partial duplication of the long arm of chromosome 1 [10–12]. However, none of these lesions is specific for PMF, and they have all been reported in a wide range of myeloid malignancies, including the newly recognised category, myelodysplastic/ myeloproliferative neoplasms (MDS/MPN). Indeed, such findings indicate the likelihood of common pathways in the aetiology of both disorders. The only exception may be the scarce finding, der(6)t(1;6)(q23–25;p21–22), which has recently been proposed as a possible marker for PMF [14]. Interestingly, the gene coding the FK-506 binding protein 5 (*FKBP51*) is located in the involved region (6p21), and the protein has been shown to be over-expressed in CD34+ cell-derived megakaryocytes from PMF patients. The relevance of this observation is that the FK506 binding protein may confer anti-apoptotic effects through inhibition of calcineurin. In addition, abnormalities of chromosome 1, 5, 7 or 9 were noted to be almost always associated with additional karyotypic changes [12]. Finally, cytogenetic analysis has also suggested that tyrosine kinase activations other than *JAK2* and *MPL* mutations may be responsible for the pathogenesis of rare cases of PMF. For example, a patient with PMF and a t(5;12)(q22;q13) that was associated with a novel TEL-PDGFRβ fusion transcript has been reported to have responded to imatinib therapy.

In contrast to ET and PV, recent studies, using oligonucleotide micro-arrays on purified CD34+ cells, have highlighted a complexity in PMF far greater than suggested by standard cytogenetics. For example, one group reported a total of 95 highly differentially expressed genes, of which 75 could be used to accurately discriminate PMF stem cells from controls by using hierarchical clustering. Furthermore, it has been found that by using a set of only 8 out of a total of 174 differentially expressed genes, it was possible to separate not only PMF CD34 cells from controls, but also PMF granulocytes from those of PV and ET. Finally, *RARbeta2* has been shown to be a candidate tumour suppressor gene in PMF, by loss of heterozygosity (LOH) studies, although for most patients epigenetic changes may be the major determinant of reduced activity (see review [1]).

Cytogenetic evaluation is recommended in all cases of PMF for a number of clinical reasons. Not only can it confirm clonality, thereby excluding secondary causes of myelofibrosis, but also it can provide prognostic information. Occasionally, it may enable cases of *BCR-ABL1*-positive, or *PDGFRβ*-rearranged disease, which is present with an associated bone marrow fibrosis, to be excluded. Furthermore, it is important to identify patients with del(5q), which although rare, is more frequent in PMF than in other MPNs. Interestingly, the breakpoints are similar to those reported in myelodysplastic syndromes and patients with PMF-associated del(5q) show significant responses to the immuno-modulatory drug lenalidomide (CC-5013, Revlimid), in contrast to the limited response in those lacking such an abnormality. The mechanism of lenalidomide's action remains unclear but it may relate to the induction of G0-G1 growth arrest in malignant rather than normal cells. More recently, acute myeloid leukaemia-associated trisomy 13, a cytogenetic abnormality that also occurs rarely in PMF, has also been shown to respond to lenalidamide. Data from future clinical studies relating lenalidamide response to cytogenetic findings are awaited with interest.

A number of early studies suggested that an abnormal karyotype per se carries a poor prognosis for PMF patients. The first evidence, albeit indirect, was the observation that the response to androgen therapy was dependent on karyotype. Direct evidence was first provided by a French study, involving 47 cases, in which the adverse prognosis of an abnormal karyotype retained its significance on both univariate and multivariate analysis [10]. The same group subsequently confirmed these findings in a larger cohort of PMF patients [15] and demonstrated that an abnormal karyotype carried a greater risk of acute transformation. Similar prognostic results were reported by a British study [11] and led to the incorporation of karyotypic findings, together with haemoglobin levels and age, into a prognostic score. Patients younger than 69 years of age who did not have either anaemia (haemoglobin <10 g/dL) or an abnormal karyotype had a median survival of 180 months, compared with 22 months for the age-matched cohort, with both anaemia and abnormal cytogenetics. Interestingly, the outcome from allogeneic bone marrow transplantation may also be dependent on chromosomal findings. In a study of 56 patients, for example, it was concluded that an abnormal karyotype had the strongest negative effect on post-transplant mortality, other than the Lille score [15]. Interestingly, the frequency of chromosomal abnormalities appears to be age dependent, with significantly lower rates in younger patients, a fact that may account for their better prognosis [16]. This observation, and their clearly better outcome, suggests both a different pathogenesis and the need for a more conservative therapeutic approach.

Two recent reports from the Mayo Clinic, one retrospective [12] and the other prospective [17], suggest that not all cytogenetic abnormalities carry equal prognostic weight. For example, it was noted that the commonest abnormalities, namely del(13q) and del(20q), may have little impact on survival, in contrast to trisomy 8 and del(12q). Leukaemic transformation rates for patients with –7/del(7p), –5/del(5q), del(12p), abnormalities of chromosome 1, trisomy 8 and trisomy 9 (50%, 30%, 25%, 19%, 20%, 17%, respectively) were significantly higher for those with del(20q) and del(13q) (10% and 0%, respectively). Such a conclusion has been strengthened by similar results from a recent Japanese study [13], which found that not one of 28 patients with isolated del(13q) or del(20q) transformed to acute leukaemia, in contrast to approximately 17% for those with other cytogenetic abnormalities. Studies of post-polycythemia myelofibrosis (Post-PV-MF) and post-ET myelofibrosis (post-ET-MF) also support the above conclusions [18]. Recently, the International Working Group for Myelofibrosis Research and Treatment (IWG-MRT) has published the most robust prognostic scoring system to date [19]. This landmark study was based on the evaluation of presentation characteristics in 1,054 patients from seven centres, of whom 409 had available cytogenetic data. The presence of one or more karyotypic abnormalities was associated with reduced survival, but only in the intermediate risk I and II groups. Unfortunately, incomplete data sets did not enable the prognostic effects of different abnormalities to be determined. Finally, a retrospective analysis of 256 patients by the MD Anderson group has added further support for the differential prognostic effects of specific chromosomal defects [20]. Favourable cytogenetic abnormalities, namely isolated del(13q) and del(20q), or trisomy 9 with, or without, one other abnormality, had survival rates similar to those with normal karyotypes. In contrast, patients with unfavourable abnormalities, defined as rearrangements of chromosomes 5 or 7, or those with greater than 3 abnormalities, had an inferior median survival of 15 months. The worst outcome was for patients with abnormalities of chromosome 17, who only survived for a median of 5 months. Finally, although del(13q) has been associated with a poor prognosis in myeloma, this may result from the involvement of different gene(s).

A number of specific abnormalities have long been associated with prognosis in PMF, including der(1)t(1;9) (149) and t(6;10)(q27;q11). Structural abnormalities of the long arm of chromosome 12 in PMF confer a poor prognosis because of early leukaemic transformation. Chromosome 7 deletions ($-7/7q-$) have a poor prognosis, although somewhat surprisingly this does not appear to be due to blast transformation [21]. In addition, an association between a deficiency of committed erythroid progenitor cells and chromosome 11 abnormalities in PMF has been noted, a finding that suggests the existence of genes on this chromosome, which plays a key role during erythropoeisis.

Finally, detailed molecular profiling may provide additional prognostic information. For example, it has been reported that expression levels of both CD9 and DLK1 are associated with platelet count, whereas high WT1 expression identifies PMF cases with more active disease, as evidenced by elevated CD34+ cell count and a higher severity score.

Chronic Neutrophilic Leukaemia

CNL is a rare, but distinct, MPN that is recognised by the WHO and characterised by a persistent neutrophilia, hepato-splenomegaly, absence of bcr-abl transcripts and low G-CSF levels (reviewed in [22]). The diagnosis remains difficult, however, and an abnormal karyotype is of value in differentiating it from the more common leukemoid reaction, because of an underlying infection or malignancy. Furthermore, the diagnosis can only be made with certainty once chronic myeloid leukaemia has been excluded, especially as a similar phenotype that has been associated with the rare p230 bcr-abl transcript. The later situation, termed neutrophilic-chronic myeloid leukaemia (CML-N), may have a superior clinical outcome when compared with patients with the standard p210 transcript, a fact thought to be related to low p230 mRNA and protein expression levels.

Cytogenetic abnormalities occur in approximately one third of CNL cases, with del(20q) being the most frequent finding. Other reported abnormalities include trisomy 8, trisomy 21 and t(1;20), although as for all the MPN, none is disease specific. However, a normal karyotype is the usual finding, suggesting that the initial genetic event is submicroscopic and not visible by conventional cytogenetic analysis. Indeed, it has been postulated that the observed chromosomal changes may reflect cytogenetic evolution and be secondary events in the pathogenesis of the disease. Finally, karyotypic studies indicate that the neoplastic clone in CNL may originate at the committed stem cell level, although this conclusion has not been supported by X-linked clonality studies.

Specific Chromosomal Abnormalities

Chromosome 1

Structural changes leading to partial or total trisomy 1q are characteristic findings in Philadelphia-negative MPN. They account for approximately 10% of abnormal karyotypes in PV and PMF [11,12], a figure that increases to between 70 and 90% in patients with post-PV MF [23]. Trisomy 1q is likely to be an secondary event in post-PV MF, since it frequently coexists with other abnormalities known to be present at diagnosis, such as del(20q) [23]. The rearrangements of 1q follow a definite non-random pattern and may be caused by many mechanisms, including unbalanced translocations with many variable chromosome partners that results in trisomy 1q, as well as partial duplications of 1q that involve a critical region between 1q21 and 1q32 [23].

The underlying mechanisms for these changes are unclear, although the methylation status of the centromeric DNA of chromosome 1 could be relevant in MPN. For example, it is known that hypo- or demethylation of heterochromatin of chromosome 1 is associated with DNA de-condensation, making it more prone to breakage and subsequent rearrangements. Another study reported trisomy 1q in a case of dic(1;15)(p11;p11), in which the heterochromatic sequences were thought to play a role in the juxtaposition of the long arm of chromosome 1 and the peri-centromeric region of the acrocentric chromosome. Furthermore, it is likely that the heterochromatin juxtapositioning of the satellite II family of 1q and satellite III of 9q, because of their structural homologies, may favour heterochromatin recombination. The variable breakpoints and lack of a preferential translocation site indicates that an increase in gene(s) copy number could also be important. In support of this concept is the association of amplification and over-expression of a haematopoietic protein tyrosine phosphatase in such cases. However, a number of alternative hypotheses have been proposed, including the silencing of genes closely located to heterochromatin that have been moved as a result of the chromosome abnormality and/or the interference of proteins that normally associate with heterochromatin [24].

Chromosome 8

Trisomy 8 is commonly associated with myeloid malignancies, especially PV and PMF [11, 12], and is principally found as an isolated finding, although found occasionally in association with trisomy 9 [23]. The result of conventional cytogenetic analysis, however, can be uncertain; including situations where only a single abnormal metaphase is identified since, according to the ISCN definition (ISCN), clonality requires the observation of two or more abnormal cells to be present. Interestingly, it appears that the incorporation of FISH studies, with centromeric probes for chromosome 8, can be of value in such cases as its sensitivity appears greater than standard cytogenetics. The genetic consequences of chromosome 8 duplication remain unclear, although a recent study has suggested a role for microRNAs (miRNAs). The latter are small, non-coding, RNAs of between 19 and 25 nucleotides that act as regulators of gene expression by inducing translational inhibition and cleavage of target mRNAs. Recently, their expression has been linked to haematopoiesis and cancer. Interestingly, in cases of trisomy 8, *miR-124a* and *miR-30d* located on 8p21 and 8q23, respectively, are over-expressed suggesting that a gene dosage effect may be contributing to this finding. It may be relevant that *miR-124a* targets the myeloid transcription factor CEBPalpha [25], although pathogenetic studies in CMPDs are awaited.

Chromosome 9

Studies incorporating I-FISH and comparative genomic hybridisation (CGH) have provided evidence for the pathogenetic involvement of 9p in PV.

Such techniques can be applied to non-dividing cells and, as a result, have a greater sensitivity than conventional cytogenetics. For example, Amiel and colleagues [26] provided preliminary data to suggest that trisomy 9, as well as trisomy 8, were more common in PV than had previously been appreciated. Subsequent studies have reported partial trisomy of 9p, as well as an additional i(9)(p10), to be new and recurrent primary chromosomal abnormalities in PV and suggest that amplification of a gene, or genes, on 9p may be pathogenetically important. Such an interpretation has been supported by data from several other groups. For example, gain of 9p, either as a trisomy or tetrasomy, resulting from an unbalanced translocation, or as a sole abnormality, has been reported in PV patients, with the critical region appearing to lie between p13 and pter. A gain of 9p due to an unbalanced rearrangement der(9;18) has been reported, while Al-Assar and colleagues [27], in a study incorporating CGH, reported gains of 9p in 50% of PMF cases, involving 9p13 and 9p23. A similar amplified region 9p22–p24.3 has been identified in a case of PV that transformed to acute myeloid leukaemia with resultant amplification of *MLLT3*, *JMJD2C*, *JAK2* and *SMARCA2* genes [28]. Although amplification of such genes has been implicated in solid tumours, their role in MPN remains unclear. Nevertheless, these findings suggest that gene(s) on 9p, rather than 9q, are relevant to the pathogenesis of PV.

In an attempt to clarify further the genomic regions that cause the PV phenotype, genome-wide micro-satellite screen for LOH has been undertaken. Three genomic regions were identified on chromosomes 9p, 10q and 11q, with LOH of the 9p being found in a third of cases, making it the most frequent chromosomal lesion described at the time. It has been concluded that mitotic recombination accounted for the 9pLOH, as there are no cytogenetic losses in affected subjects and that the involved region extends to the telomere. Interestingly, this finding of uniparental disomy, which involves the entire short arm of chromosome 9, is not detectable by cytogenetic analysis, FISH or CGH. Subsequently, markers from the 9pLOH region were reported not to co-segregate with the phenotype in familial PV, suggesting that a somatic event caused the 9pLOH. Ultimately, fine mapping of the region identified JAK2, located at 9p24.1, as a likely candidate gene and led to the group detecting the JAK2 V617F activating mutation in the majority of PV patients. Three other teams, using different methodological approaches, reported identical findings at around the same time (reviewed in [1]).

Chromosome 13

Del(13q) is a common abnormality in MPN, especially PMF, although to a lesser extent in Post-PV-MF [11, 12, 23]. It is usually interstitial with proximal and distal breakpoints in 13q12 and 13q14-q22, respectively. Since the retinoblastoma susceptibility gene (*RB-1*) is located in the critically deleted region, it is possible that its inactivation could be of pathogenetic importance. However, no structural changes in *Rb-1*, even in cases with obvious LOH at the locus, have been reported. Karyotypic analysis of these cases failed to detect a del(13q), suggesting the presence of cryptic deletions [Gaidano, pers. commun]. However, FISH studies to detect *Rb-1* deletions have documented hemizygous gene deletion only in those cases with del(13q) on standard metaphase analysis. Similarly, *Rb-1* allelic loss, in addition to the micro-satellite loci D13S319 and D13S25, occurs in cases of myeloid malignancy with deletion/translocation at 13q14.

Additional studies have confirmed these findings and indicate that del(13q), like del(20q), is associated with considerable genetic loss [29] and that cryptic deletions are rare.

Rare translocations involving 13q14 have been studied [29] in the hope that such cases would assist the identification of pathogenetically relevant genes. Unfortunately, large submicroscopic deletions involving the same CDR as present in del(13q) are a feature of these apparently balanced translocations [29]. This suggests that 13q14 translocations may have the same underlying pathogenetic mechanism and that study of further cases is unlikely to reduce the CDR. Finally, it is possible that more than one gene is involved on chromosome 13, as a study of a case of PMF and t(4;13)(q25;q12) suggested the involvement of a novel gene on 13q12.

Trisomy 13, although a well-described abnormality in acute leukaemia, has occasionally been reported in Philadelphia-negative MPNs. A few cases have been diagnosed as PMF, although the majority appear to have a "CML-like" disorder. As previously discussed, such cases may respond to lenalidamide and further emphasise the clinical importance of cytogenetic data in MPNs.

Chromosome 20

Deletion of the long arm of chromosome 20 (del20q), although first described in 1966 as an F-group chromosomal deletion in PV, is now known to occur in a wide range of myeloproliferative disorders. It has been reported not only in PV [5], but also in PMF, ET, CNL, myelodysplastic syndromes and acute myeloid leukaemia, although rarely in lymphoid neoplasms [1, 10–12]. Del(20q) is usually an isolated finding, although can occur in association with other abnormalities, most commonly del(5q), monosomy 7, trisomy 8, deletions and translocations of 13q and trisomy 21 [30].

The 20q breakpoints are heterogeneous, as evidenced by the variable size of the deletion by standard cytogenetics, FISH analysis and by early molecular studies, which revealed the variable retention of *SRC*. Nacheva and colleagues [31] confirmed this finding, by using high-resolution banding, and identified a commonly deleted region (CDR) spanning 20q11.2–q13.1. Furthermore, Roulston and colleagues [32] defined a CDR flanked by D20S17 (MLRG) distally and *RPN2* (20q11.2) proximally, while a further group [33] narrowed it to 8 Mb, flanked by a proximal boundary between markers D20S206 and D20S107 and a distal boundary between D20S119 and D20S424. The Cambridge group [34] further refined the CDR to a 2.7-Mb region spanning from D20S108 to D20S481 and identified six genes and ten unique expressed sequence tags (ESTs). Importantly, five of these are expressed in both normal bone marrow and purified CD34+ cells and are therefore likely candidates for the 20q target. One of the most promising genes is *L3MBTL* (also known as h-l(3)mbt), a conclusion also supported by the findings of MacGrogan et al. [35].

L3MBTL was identified as a candidate suppressor gene by virtue of its homology to the *Drosophila* tumour suppressor gene *lethal* [3] *malignant brain tumour* [36]. It appears that tightly controlled levels of L3MBT, a member of the Polycomb group of proteins, are required for normal mitosis, as both over-expression and loss of activity can affect cell division. Recently, Boccuni et al. [37] have suggested that the protein functions as a histone deacetylase (HDAC) independent transcription repressor, which can be recruited by direct binding to TEL (ETV6). Despite these findings, the pathogenetic relevance of *L3MBT* in the context of del(20q) myeloid disorders is uncertain, since sequence alterations have not been identified [38], although the demonstration that *L3MBTL* is monoallelically methylated and transcribed only from the paternally derived allele might be pathogenetically relevant [39].

Studies of patients with del(20q) have provided some valuable insights into the biology of the MPNs. They suggest that the lymphoid lineage may be clonally involved in some patients. For example, a patient with ET and del(20q) was shown to exhibit the cytogenetic abnormality in the myeloid, erythroid and CD34+ progenitor cells, as well as CD10+ lymphoid cells [40]. Furthermore, a lymphoblastoid cell line derived from a patient with *bcr-abl*-positive ALL possessed the del(20q), as did the CFU-GM, CFU-GEMM and BFU-E [41]. Both studies suggest that MPN may arise from an early progenitor cell that possesses both myeloid and lymphoid potential. This conclusion is strengthened by studies in PMF, in which the involvement of B and T cells has also been documented [42]. Intriguingly, a case of myelodysplasia has been reported in which the del(20q) was present in the pluripotential cells, in contrast to the circulating lymphocytes [43]. Explanations for such a finding are either that the clonal B cells have a reduced lifespan, or that the involved progenitor cells have an impaired ability to produce mature B lymphocytes. A further insight from cytogenetic studies is the paradoxical observation that del(20q) may be associated with severe impairment of granulocyte release from bone marrow. Asimakopoulos et al. [44], for example, have documented that some patients, with del(20q) in all bone marrow metaphases, can possess cytogenetically normal circulating granulocytes. The likely explanation is that the del(20q) cells are preferentially retained and/or destroyed in the bone marrow.

Karyotype, Haplotype and *JAK2-V617F*

A number of studies have correlated the karyotypic abnormality in patients with MPN with their *JAK2* mutational status. Campbell and colleagues, for example, reported that del(20q) occurred preferentially together with the *JAK2-V617F* in 28 of 29 MPN cases studied [45]. Similar findings were also reported for patients with trisomy 9/+9p, while a recent FISH study has confirmed these findings in a cohort of PV patients [46]. It may be relevant that most cases in the later study possessed multiple copies of *JAK2*, in addition to the *JAK2-V617F* mutation, suggesting that *JAK2* amplification may be important. These results imply a role for co-operating mutations in the pathogenesis of *JAK2-V617F* MPNs and support the hypothesis that dosage of JAK2 contributes to the disease phenotype in which an increased constitutive activation of JAK2 provides a proliferative advantage [46]. In studies of acute transformation of MPN, cytogenetics combined with *JAK2* mutational screening has also provided evidence that *JAK2* mutations may not be the initiating event. Theocharides and colleagues [47], for example, reported a single case *of JAK2-V617F* PMF in which the *JAK2-V617F* was absent from the blasts at the time of transformation. However, the karyotypic abnormality, del(11q), was present in all metaphases by cytogenetic analysis and by I-FISH, suggesting that the *JAK2-V617F*-negative blasts and the *JAK2-V617F*-positive bone marrow cells carried the same deletion. Intriguingly, the same region on chromosome 11 had been reported in a genome-wide screening for LOH. This cytogenetic finding implies the presence of sub-clones from a common clonal ancestor in the development of PMF and AML and that an initial clonal event may precede the acquisition of *JAK2-V617F* in the pathogenesis of MPNs [48].

Recently, a detailed analysis of two patients, with del(20q) and *JAK2-V617F*, revealed that the size of the clone carrying the del(20q) greatly exceeded the size of the *JAK2-V617F* clone, implying that the del(20q) event occurred first [49]. Subsequently, a European group explored the temporal order of acquisitions further by screening single burst-forming units-erythroid (BFU-E) and colony-forming units-granulocytes (CFU-G) colonies, from 14 patients positive for both del(20q) and *JAK2-V617F*. Each individual colony from a given patient was genotyped for both del(20q) and *JAK2-V617F*. Intriguingly, two patients possessed colonies in which del(20q) was noted in association with both wild type *JAK2* and *JAK2-V617F*, while other cases possessed colonies that were *JAK2-V617F*-positive but with normal chromosomes 20. It was concluded that the failure to find a consistent temporal order of abnormalities makes it unlikely that del(20q) represents a predisposing event for *JAK2* mutations. Furthermore, using micro-satellite analysis, Schaub and colleagues [50] reported that somatic events, such as del(20q) and 9pLOH, can occur more than once in the same patient, since sub-clones were identified in which the abnormality affected both paternal and maternal chromosomes. These finding imply that the MPN clone carries a predisposition to acquiring such genetic alterations, as *JAK2-V617F* and del(20q). The multiple genetic hits could be linked to environmental factors, including radiation or toxins. However, the concept for an underlying genetic predisposition has received support from three recent studies that report a significant association between the risk of developing a *JAK2-V617F* MPN and a specific germline haplotype that includes the 3′ portion of *JAK2*. This association is strong, with the odds of developing a MPN being three- to-fourfold for those carrying the specific haplotype, which has been termed 46/1. At least two hypotheses have been proposed: first, the haplotype confers a hypermutability property on the *JAK2* locus; second, *JAK2* mutations occur at the same rate but those that develop in association with the "46/1" haplotype produce a stronger selective advantage. Future studies exploring these two possibilities will undoubtedly have implications beyond the MPN field and could help unravel the complicated interactions between germline and somatic genetics that almost certainly exist in many neoplasms.

References

1. Reilly JT. Pathogenetic insight and prognostic information from standard and molecular cytogenetic studies in the BCR-ABL-negative myeloproliferative neoplasms (MPNs). Leukemia. 2008; 22: 1818–1827.
2. Gangat N, Tefferi A, Thanarajasingam G, et al. Cytogenetic abnormalities in essential thrombocythemia: prevalence and prognostic significance. Eur J Haematol. 2009; 83: 17–21.
3. Steensma DP, Tefferi A. Cytogenetic and molecular genetic aspects of essential thrombocthemia. Acta Haematol. 2003; 108: 55–65.
4. Borze I, Mustjoki S, Juvonen E, Knuutila S. Oligoarray comparative genomic hybridization in polycythemia vera and essential thrombocythemia. Haematologica. 2008; 93: 1098–1100.
5. Diez-Martin JL, Graham DL, Petitt RM, Dewald GW. Chromosome studies in 104 patients with polycythemia vera. Mayo Clin Proc. 1991; 66: 287–299.

6. Gangat N, Strand J, Lasho TL, et al. Cytogenetic studies at diagnosis in polycythemia vera: clinical and JAK2 V617F allele burden correlates. Eur J Haematol. 2008; 80: 197–200.

7. Larsen TS, Hasselbalch HC, Pallisgaard N, Kerndrup GB. A der(18)t(9;18) (p13;p11) and a der(9;18)(p10;q10) in polycythemia vera associated with a hyper-proliferative phenotype in transformation to postpolycythemia myelofibrosis. Cancer Genet Cytogenet. 2007; 172: 107–112.

8. Reilly JT. Pathogenesis and management of idiopathic myelofibrosis. Bailliere's Clin Haematol. 1998; 11: 751–767.

9. Hussein K, Huang J, Lasho T, et al. Karyotype complements the International Prognostic Scoring System for primary myelofibrosis. Eur J Haematol. 2009; 82: 255–259.

10. Demory JL, Dupriez B, Fenaux P, et al. Cytogenetic studies and their prognostic significance in agnogenic myeloid metaplasia: a report on 47 cases. Blood. 1988; 72: 855–859.

11. Reilly JT, Snowden JA, Spearing RL. et al. Cytogenetic abnormalities and their prognostic significance in idiopathic myelofibrosis: a study of 106 cases. Br J Haematol. 1997; 98: 96–102.

12. Tefferi A, Mesa RA, Schroeder G, Hanson CA, Li CY, Dewald GW. Cytogenetic findings and their clinical relevance in myelofibrosis with myeloid metaplasia. Br J Haematol. 2001; 113: 763–771.

13. Hidaka T, Shide K, Shimoda H, et al. The impact of cytogenetic abnormalities on the prognosis of primary myelofibrosis: a prospective survey of 202 cases in Japan. Eur J Haematol. 2009; 83: 328–333.

14. Dingli D, Grand FH, Mahaffey V, et al. Der(6)t(1;6)(q21-23;p21.3): the first specific cytogenetic abnormality in myelofibrosis with myeloid metaplasia. Br J Haematol. 2005; 130: 229–232.

15. Dupriez B, Morel P, Demory JL, et al. Prognostic factors in agnogenic myeloid metaplasia: a report on 195 cases with a new scoring system. Blood. 1996; 88: 1013–1018.

16. Cervantes F, Barosi G, Hernandez-Boluda J-C, Marchetti M, Montserrat E. Myelofibrosis with myeloid metaplasia in adult individuals 30 years old or younger: presenting features, evolution and survival. Eur J Haematol. 2001; 66: 324–327.

17. Tefferi A, Dingli D, Li C-Y, Dewald GW. Prognostic diversity among cytogenetic abnormalities in myelofibrosis with myeloid metaplasia. Cancer. 2005; 104: 1656–1660.

18. Dingli D, Schwager SM, Mesa RA, Li C-Y, Dewald GW, Tefferi A. Presence of unfavourable cytogenetic abnormalities is the strongest predictor of poor survival in secondary myelofibrosis. Cancer. 2006; 106: 1985–1989.

19. Cervantes F, Dupriez B, Pereira A. et al. New prognostic scoring system for primary myelofibrosis based on a study of the International Working Group for Myelofibrosis Research and Treatment. Blood. 2009; 113: 2895–2901.

20. Tam CS, Abruzzo LV, Lin KI, et al. The role of cytogenetic abnormalities as a prognostic marker in primary myelofibrosis: applicability at the time of diagnosis and later during disease course. Blood. 2009; 113: 4171–4178.

21. Strasser-Weippl K, Steurer M, Kees M, et al. Chromosome 7 deletions are associated with unfavourable prognosis in myelofibrosis with myeloid metaplasia. Blood. 2005; 105: 4146.

22. Reilly JT. Chronic neutrophilic leukaemia: a distinct clinical entity? Br J Haematol. 2002; 116: 10–18.

23. Andrieux J, Demory JL, Caulier MT, et al. Karyotypic abnormalities in myelofibrosis following polycythemia vera. Cancer Genet Cytogenet. 2003; 140: 118–123.

24. Busson-Le Coniat M, Salomon-Nguven F, Dastugue N. et al. Fluorescence in situ hybridization analysis of chromosome 1 abnormalities in hematopoietic disorders: rearrangements of DNA satellite II and new recurrent translocations. Leukemia. 1999; 13: 1975–1981.

25. Lim LP, Lau LC, Garrett-Engele P, et al. Microarray analysis shows that some micro-RNAs downregulate large numbers of target mRNAs. Nature. 2005; 433: 769–773.

26. Amiel A, Gaber E, Manor Y, et al. Fluorescence in situ hybridization for the detection of trisomies 8 and 9 in polycythemia vera. Cancer Genetic Cytogenet. 1995; 79: 153–156.

27. Al-Assar O, Ul-Hassan A, Brown A, Wilson GA, Hammond DW, Reilly JT. Gains of 9p are common genomic aberrations in idiopathic myelofibrosis: a comparative genomic hydridization study. Br J Haematol. 2005; 129: 66–71.

28. Helias C, Struski S, Gervais C, et al. Polycythaemia vera transforming to acute myeloid leukemia and complex abnormalities of *MLLT3, JMJD2C, JAK2*, and *SMARCA2*. Cancer Genetic Cytogenetic. 2008; 180: 51–55.

29. Sinclair EJ, Forrest EC, Reilly JT, Watemore AE, Potter AM. Fluorescence in situ hybridization analysis of 25 cases of idiopathic myelofibrosis and two cases of secondary myelofibrosis. Monoallelic loss of RB1, D13S319 and D13S25 loci associated with cytogenetic deletion and translocation involving 13q14. Br J Haematol. 2001; 113: 365–368.

30. Kurtin PJ, Dewald GW, Shields DJ, Hanson CA. Hematologic disorders associated with deletion of chromosome 20q: a clinicopathologic study of 107 patients. Am J Clin Path. 1996; 106: 680–688.

31. Nacheva E, Holloway T, Carter N, Grace C, White N, Green AR. Characterization of 20q deletions in patients with myeloproliferative disorders or myelodysplastic syndromes. Cancer Genet Cytogenet. 1995; 80: 87–94.

32. Roulston S, Espinosa R III, Stoffel M, Bell GI, Le Beau MM. Molecular genetics of myeloid leukaemia:identification of the commonly deleted segment of chromosome 20. Blood. 1993; 82: 3424–3429.

33. Wang PW, Eisenbart JD, Espinosa R, Davis EM, Larson RA, Le Beau MM. Refinement of the smallest commonly deleted segment of chromosome 20 in malignant myeloid diseases and development of a PAC-based physical and transcription map. Genomics. 2000; 67: 28–39.

34. Bench AJ, Nacheva EP, Hood TL, et al. Chromosome 20 deletions in myeloid malignancies: reduction of the common deleted region, generation of a PAC/BAC contig and identification of candidate genes. UK Cancer Cytogenetic Group (UKCCG). Oncogene. 2000; 20: 4150–4160.

35. MacGrogan D, Alvarez S, DeBlasio T, Jhanwar SC, Nimer SD. Identification of candidate genes on chromosome band 20q12 by physical mapping of translocation breakpoints found in myeloid leukaemia cell lines. Oncogene. 2001; 20: 4150–4160.

36. Koga H, Matsui S, Hirota T, Takebayashi S, Okumura K, Saya H. A human homolog of Drosophila lethal (3) malignant brain tumor (1(3)mbt) protein associates with condensed mitotic chromosomes. Oncogene. 1999; 18: 3799–3809.

37. Boccuni P, MacGrogan D, Scandura JM, Nimer SD. The human L(3)MBT polycomb group protein is a transcriptional repressor and interacts physically and functionally with TEL (ETV6). J Bio Chem. 2003; 278: 15412–15420.

38. Bench AJ, Li J, Huntly BJP, Delabesse E, et al. Characterization of the imprinted polycomb gene *L3MBTL*, a candidate 20q tumour suppressor gene, in patients with myeloid malignancies. Br J Haematol. 2004; 127: 509–518.

39. Li J, Bench AJ, Vassiliou GS, Fourouclas N, Ferguson-Smith AC, Green AC. Imprinting of the human L3MBTL gene, a polycomb family member located in a region of chromosome 20 deleted in human myeloid malignancies. Proc Natl Acad Sci USA. 2004; 101: 7341–7346.

40. Knuutila S, Teerenhovi L, Larramendy ML, et al. Cell lineage involvement of recurrent chromosomal abnormalities in hematologic neoplasms. Genes Chromsomes Cancer. 1994; 10: 95–102.

41. Hollings PE, Beard MEJ, Rosman I. A 20q deletion originating in a pluripotential stem cell. Blood. 1994; 83: 306–307.

42. Reeder TL, Bailey RJ, Dewald GW. Tefferi A Both B and T lymphocytes may be clonally involved in myelofibrosis with myeloid metaplasia. Blood. 2003; 101: 1981–1983.

43. White NJ, Nacheva E, Asimakopoulos FA, Paul B, Green AR. Deletion of chromosome 20q in myelodysplasia can occur in a multipotent precursor of both myeloid cells and B cells. Blood. 1994; 83: 2809–2816.

44. Asimakopoulos FA, Holloway TL, Nacheva EP, Scott MA, Fenaux P, Green AR. Detection of chromosome 20q deletions in bone marrow metaphases but not peripheral blood granulocytes in patients with myeloproliferative disorders or myelodysplastic syndromes. Blood. 1996; 87: 1561–1570.

45. Campbell PJ, Baxter EJ, Beer PA, et al. Mutation of JAK2 in the myeloproliferative disorders: timing, clonality studies, cytogenetic associations, and role in leukemic transformation. Blood. 2006; 108: 3548–3555.

46. Najfeld V, Cozza A, Berkofsy-Fessler W, Prchal J, Scalise A. Numerical gain and structural rearrangements of JAK2, identified by FISH, characterize both JAK2617V>F-positive and -negative patients with Ph-negative MPD, myelodysplasia, and B-lymphoid neoplasms. Exp Hematol. 2007; 35: 1668–1676.

47. Theocharides A, Boissinot M, Girodon F, et al. Leukemic blasts in transformed JAK2-V617F-positive myeloproliferative disorders are frequently negative for the JAK2-V617F mutation. Blood. 2007; 110: 375–379.

48. Hsiao HH, Yang WC, Liu YC, Lee CP, Lin SF. Disappearance of JAK2 V617F mutation in a rapid leukemic transformed essential thrombocythemia patient. Leuk Res. 2008; 32: 1323–1324.

49. Kralovics R, Teo SS, Li S, et al. Acquisition of the V617F mutation of JAK2 is a late genetic event in a subset of patients with myeloproliferative disorders. Blood. 2006; 108: 1377–1380.

50. Schaub FX, Jager R, Looser R, Hao-Shen H, Hermouet S, Girodon F, Tichelli A, Gisslinger H, Kralovics R, Skoda RC. Clonal analysis of deletions on chromosome 20q and JAK2-V617F in MPD suggests that del20q acts independently and is not one of the predisposing mutations for JAK2-VI6F. Blood. 2009; 113: 2022–2027.

Chapter 4

Prognostic Factors in Classic Myeloproliferative Neoplasms

Francisco Cervantes and Juan-Carlos Hernández-Boluda

Keywords: Myeloproliferative neoplasms • Prognosis • Thrombosis • *JAK2* mutation

Introduction

The term "classic" BCR/ABL-negative chronic myeloproliferative neoplasms (MPNs) includes three clonal diseases arising in a pluripotent hemopoietic stem cell that share clinical, hematological, and biological features: polycythemia vera (PV), essential thrombocythemia (ET), and primary myelofibrosis (PMF). The recent discovery of mutations in the *JAK2* gene in a high proportion of these patients has given biological support to the early notion by Dameshek placing the three disorders within a same group. With regard to survival, PMF is associated with a substantial reduction in life expectancy [1–7], ET affects more the patients' quality of life than their survival, whereas PV is associated with both a substantial morbidity but also a certain reduction in the patients' life expectancy [8–10]. Because of this, prognostic studies in the MPNs have been carried out primarily in PMF. In the last years, however, attention is increasingly being paid to the identification of prognostic factors in ET and PV, primarily focused on the risk of thrombosis. The recent progress in the knowledge of the biology of the MPNs has prompted the study of the possible correlations between the biological features and prognosis of the disease.

The present chapter summarizes the current status of survival and prognosis in patients with MPNs. Since these diseases are infrequent in children, this subpopulation will not be considered in this review.

Prognosis of PMF

PMF, also known as idiopathic myelofibrosis or myelofibrosis with myeloid metaplasia, is a rare disease usually affecting elderly people. Median survival ranges from 4 to 5.5 years in modern series [1–7] (Fig. 4.1). When the survival of PMF patients has been compared with that of age- and sex-matched individuals

S. Verstovsek and A. Tefferi (eds.), *Myeloproliferative Neoplasms: Biology and Therapy*, Contemporary Hematology, DOI 10.1007/ 978-1-60761-266-7_4,
© Springer Science+Business Media, LLC 2011

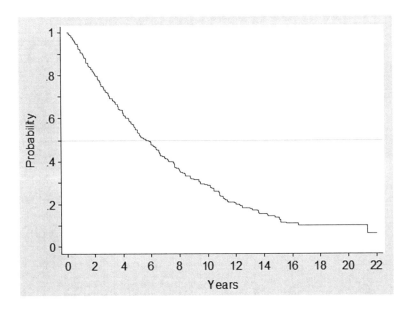

Fig. 4.1 Actuarial survival curve of the 1,054 patients with primary myelofibrosis of the International Working Group for Myelofibrosis Research and Treatment

from the general population, a substantial reduction in life expectancy has been observed [7, 8]. Main causes of death in PMF are evolution to acute leukemia (observed in 20% of cases at 10 years of diagnosis), infection and bleeding secondary to bone marrow failure, portal hypertension or hepatic failure secondary to hepatic/splenoportal vein thrombosis or myeloid metaplasia of the liver, thromboses in other territories, and heart failure [4, 5].

With regard to young individuals with PMF, as more intensive therapeutic options for the disease are available (notably, allogeneic stem cell transplantation), there is an increasing interest for a better knowledge of their prognosis [11, 12]. Thus, in a survey of 121 patients 55-year-old or younger from four European institutions [11] found that their prognosis was substantially better than that of the general PMF patients, with a median survival of 128 months, i.e., more than twice that of the overall PMF patients. PMF seldom affects persons younger than 30 years. In a survey of 323 PMF cases collected in two European institutions, nine patients younger than 30 years were identified, representing less than 3% of the total [12]. In all the cases the disease presented without adverse prognostic factors and remained stable for years, with only two patients having died, at 10.7 and 9.9 years from diagnosis, while the remaining five being asymptomatic and without need for treatment.

Survival of patients with post-ET or post-PV myelofibrosis does not seem to differ from that of those with PMF [13, 14].

Prognostic Factors and Prognostic Classifications of PMF

The wide variability in the survival of PMF patients has stimulated the interest for the identification of variables predicting for survival. Among the clinical factors assessed for prognostic significance in PMF, an association between the presence of hypermetabolic or constitutional symptoms (i.e., fever, night sweats, and weight loss) and shorter survival has been found in all the studies in which it has been analyzed [3–5, 7, 15]. Age at presentation is another variable linked to the prognosis of PMF [1–3, 5–7], with younger subjects surviving longer. Male sex was associated with worse prognosis at univariate study in the Lille series, but lost significance at multivariate level [4].

The initial hemoglobin (Hb) concentration is the parameter most consistently associated with the prognosis of PMF, with the 10 g/dL value being the cut-off level usually determining a more unfavorable course of the disease [1, 2, 4–6, 7, 13, 14]. Low leukocyte count was a poor prognostic indicator in the Lille and Mayo series [4, 15], whereas high leukocyte counts had poor prognostic weight in the latter and other studies [4, 6, 7, 15]. According to Hb level and leukocyte count, Dupriez et al. based on the analysis of the Lille series [4], proposed a score (the so-called Lille scoring system), which was able to identify three distinct prognostic groups. In the low-risk group (Hb > 10 g/dL and WBC > 4 × 10^9/L and <30 × 10^9/L) patients had a median survival of 93 months, whereas those in the intermediate (Hb < 10 g/dL or WBC < 4 × 10^9/L or >30 × 10^9/L) and high (Hb < 10 g/dL and WBC < 4 × 10^9/L or >30 × 10^9/L) risk groups had median survivals of 26 and 13 months, respectively. This prognostic score has been widely used in stratifying patients in clinical trials. More recently, Tefferi et al. from the analysis of 334 patients, improved the Dupriez's score by adding thrombocytopenia (<100 × 10^9/L) and monocyte count ≥1 × 10^9/L to Hb and leukocyte count [15]. According to the number of the latter four factors, the Mayo prognostic scoring system was able to identify three subpopulations of patients with median survivals of 134, 50, and 29 months, respectively.

The presence of thrombocytopenia [6, 15], immature myeloid precursors [1, 2], or (≥1%) circulating blasts in peripheral blood [4, 5, 7, 15] at diagnosis has been associated with poorer prognosis. In contrast, bone marrow histologic findings did not have prognostic relevance [5].

An increased number of CD34+ cells is typically observed in the peripheral blood of patients with PMF, and this parameter is also considered as a marker of the disease progression, since it has been found to be correlated with disease duration, splenomegaly size, and evolution to a leukemic phase [16]. With regard to prognosis, in two studies a correlation was found between circulating CD34+ cell counts and PMF risk groups, the higher the number of such cells the more unfavorable the patient′s risk group [16, 17]. Besides, a strong correlation was found between CD34+ cell counts and the probability of acute transformation, with patients presenting with more than 300 × 10^6/L CD34+ cells in blood having a 50% probability of developing acute leukemia by 11 months from diagnosis [16]. However, the adverse prognostic influence of circulating CD34+ cells could not be demonstrated in another series [18].

An abnormal karyotype can be observed in about a third of PMF patients at diagnosis, and its detection has generally been linked to shorter survival. Dupriez et al. [4] demonstrated the independent prognostic value of cytogenetic abnormalities, as this feature retained its unfavorable influence even in the low-risk PMF subgroup. Karyotypic abnormalities had also an adverse prognostic weight in the series by Reilly et al. [6], whereas they had not in the study by Tefferi et al. [19] when the abnormalities were considered as a whole. In this latter study, however, the negative influence of chromosome changes was restricted to trisomy 8 and deletion of 12p, while deletions of 13q and 20q did not involve shorter survival. Similarly, a study from the MD Anderson showed the impact on survival of a set of cytogenetic abnormalities detected at baseline or during the disease evolution [20]. Thus, the sole detection of deletions of 13q and 20q was associated with a survival comparable with that of patients with a normal dyploid karyotype, whereas patients with abnormalities in chromosome 5, 7, and 17 or with complex aberrations had a significantly worse outcome.

Recently, a new prognostic scoring system was proposed by the International Working Group for Myelofibrosis Research and Treatment based on data from 1,054 patients consecutively diagnosed with PMF at seven institutions, representing the largest prognostic study ever performed in this disease [7]. Multivariate analysis of parameters obtained at diagnosis identified age >65 years, presence of constitutional symptoms, Hb < 10 g/dL, WBC > 25 × 10⁹/L, and circulating blast cells ≥1% as predictors of shortened survival. Based on the presence of 0 (low risk), 1 (intermediate risk-1), 2 (intermediate risk-2), or ≥3 (high risk) of these variables four risk groups with no overlapping in their survival curves could be identified, with their respective median survivals being 135, 95, 48, and 27 months (Fig. 4.2). Of note, cytogenetic abnormalities were associated with shorter survival, but their independent contribution to prognosis was restricted to patients in the intermediate-risk groups.

In individuals with PMF younger than 55 years, the factors associated with poor prognosis are anemia (Hb value <10 g/dL), constitutional symptoms, and presence of blast cells in peripheral blood [11]. It is worth noting that in these younger patients no association was found between the presence of cytogenetic abnormalities and survival, although only 17% of them displayed such a finding [11]. On the basis of the above-mentioned three variables, two prognostic groups could be clearly identified: a "low-risk" group, including patients with none or one of the bad prognostic factors, and a "high-risk" group, integrated by patients with two or the three unfavorable factors. The "low-risk" group encompassed three quarters of the overall patients and its median survival approached 15 years, whereas the "high-risk" group included a quarter of the patients, with a median survival of less than 3 years. This prognostic scoring system is of help at the time of making treatment decisions in young patients with PMF.

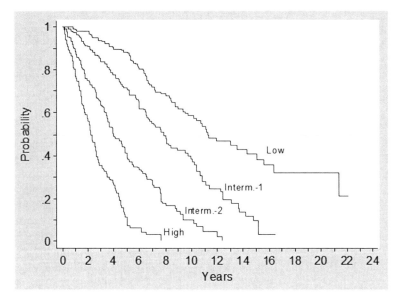

Fig. 4.2 Actuarial survival curves of the four risk groups of patients defined according to the new PMF International Prognostic Scoring System

Several studies have evaluated the prognostic relevance of the *JAK2* V617F mutation in PMF, with somewhat divergent results. Campbell et al. [21] found that the presence of the *JAK2* V617F mutation in PMF patients was associated with higher leukocyte counts and inferior survival. In a longitudinal prospective study, Barosi et al. [22] found that the *JAK2* mutation predicted the evolution towards large splenomegaly, need of splenectomy, and leukemic transformation. The strongest influence of the mutated genotype was exerted on the risk of leukemic transformation, which was 5.2 times higher than in nonmutated patients. In contrast, a more recent study from the Mayo Clinic [23] did not find any significant difference in the probability of leukemic transformation or survival among patients with or without the *JAK2* mutation. In fact, patients with a high *JAK2* V617F allele burden had a similar outcome to that of the nonmutated cases, whereas those with a low *JAK2* V617F allele burden had a shortened overall- and leukemia-free survival that could not be accounted for by other relevant risk factors.

Finally, prognostic factors for acute transformation of PMF include severe anemia or thrombocytopenia, a high proportion of immature myeloid cells in blood, and a high number of circulating CD34+ cells [16, 24]. In one series, an increased risk of acute leukemia was registered in patients submitted to splenectomy [25], but this was not confirmed in a study from the Mayo Clinic [26].

Prognosis of PV and ET

Survival studies in PV and ET are relatively scarce. A study on 831 patients with PV and ET followed for a median time about 10 years provided evidence that life expectancy of PV patients is reduced when compared with that of the general population, while the survival of patients with ET is not significantly shortened [9]. Other study from the Mayo Clinic including 322 patients with ET followed for a median time of 13.6 years confirmed that the survival in the first decade of the disease is not shortened, but became significantly worse thereafter [10]. In the Pavia study, the standardized mortality ratio (SMR), which is the ratio of the observed number of deaths in the patients' population to the number of deaths expected in the reference population, was 1.6 in PV and 1.0 in ET [9], which means that PV patients have a 1.6-fold higher mortality than the general population, while ET patients do not have an increased mortality. When the SMR was analyzed according to the patient's age at diagnosis, mortality was 3.3-fold higher in PV patients younger than 50 years and 1.6-fold higher in those over 50 years, while it was not increased in ET patients from each age category with regard to the reference population. ET is therefore the more indolent of the MPNs, and young patients with PV would accumulate time-dependent disease-related complications.

The World Health Organization (WHO) recognized in 2001 [27] a new entity within the MPNs, the so-called "prefibrotic" stage of PMF, which would include patients that would have been classified as ET using the Polycythemia Vera Study Group (PVSG) criteria. Although it has been claimed that patients with "prefibrotic" PMF had a loss in life-expectancy when compared to those with ET [28], no differences in clinical outcome were observed in a recent study focused on the pathological and clinical distinction between ET and "prefibrotic" PMF [29]. Moreover, from the biological point of view, neither circulating CD34+ cell count, as an expression of stem cell mobilization, nor granulocyte *JAK2* V617F allele burden differs between the two conditions [30]. The recently proposed revision of the WHO classification for chronic MPNs [31] allows to diagnose this condition only if the typical histopathological findings are present with, at least, two of the following criteria: leukoerythroblastosis, increase in serum lactate dehydrogenase level, anemia, and palpable splenomegaly.

Life-expectancy of patients with PV or ET is mainly affected by disease-related complications, such as vascular disease (thrombosis and hemorrhage) and transformation to either myelofibrosis or leukemia. The incidence of disease-related complications varies significantly between the two diseases. Indeed, PV patients would have a higher incidence of thrombosis and evolution to myelofibrosis and leukemia than ET patients [9]. Conversely, the incidence of solid cancers does not differ between the two conditions, indicating that disease and disease-specific treatments do not directly influence the occurrence of extra-hematological malignancies. In PV, the incidence of thrombosis was 18 per 1,000 person-years, being about 5 per 1,000 person-years for myelofibrosis and leukemia, whereas in ET, the incidence of thrombosis was 12 per 1,000 person-years, being 1.6 per 1,000 person-years for myelofibrosis and 1.2 per 1,000 person-years for leukemia. The results of the European Collaboration on Low-dose Aspirin in Polycythemia Vera (ECLAP) study [32] showed that cardiovascular mortality in PV patients accounted for 45% of all deaths, whereas hematologic transformation was the cause of death in 13% of cases. Therefore, given that thrombosis is, by far, the more frequent complication of PV and ET, there is a clear rationale for stratifying patients at diagnosis according to their thrombosis risk.

Prognostic Factors in PV and ET

Prognostic Factors for Thrombosis
Age at diagnosis and a previous history of thrombosis are the two most important prognostic factors for thrombosis in PV and ET and represent the state-of-the-art for risk stratification in treatment decision-making for these patients (Table 4.1). The relationship of age at presentation and prior history of thrombosis with the subsequent risk of thrombosis has been demonstrated in several large studies in both PV [32, 33] and ET [34–36]. Thus, patients with any of the two risk factors at diagnosis are considered at high risk for thrombosis, while those with none of them are considered at low risk and require a different treatment approach.

Table 4.1 Initial risk factors in patients with polycythemia vera and essential thrombocythemia according to their current role in treatment decision-making.

Events	Risk factors considered in treatment decision-making
Thrombosis	• Age ≥60 years
	• Prior thrombosis
Hemorrhage	• Platelet count ≥1,500 × 10^9/L
	Risk factors not currently considered in treatment decision-making
Thrombosis	• Arterial hypertension
	• Smoking
	• Hypercholesterolemia
	• Diabetes mellitus
	• Leukocyte count
Leukemia	• Age at diagnosis
	• Leukocyte count at diagnosis
Pregnancy	• *JAK2* (V617F) mutation

No evidence is available for the link between the initial platelet count and the risk of subsequent thrombosis in either PV or ET. On the other hand, there is a more evident correlation between extreme thrombocytosis and bleeding risk, which would be attributed to an acquired von Willebrand disease [37]. Therefore, in treatment decision-making, platelet counts over $1,500 \times 10^9/L$ should be considered as a risk factor for hemorrhage.

Increased leukocyte count has been identified as an independent risk factor for thrombosis in both PV and ET [10, 38, 39]. In the ECLAP study on PV, patients with a leukocyte count exceeding $15 \times 10^9/L$ had a significant increase in the risk of myocardial infarction as compared with those with leukocyte counts below $10 \times 10^9/L$ [38]. In ET, a significant correlation has been found between the initial leukocyte count and the subsequent risk of thrombosis in two studies. In both, a cut-off value for the leukocyte count was identified, being $15 \times 10^9/L$ in a study including 322 patients [10] and $8.7 \times 10^9/L$ in other study analyzing 439 patients [39]. However, no correlation between initial leukocyte count and subsequent thrombosis was observed in a study from the Mayo Clinic including 605 ET patients [40]. Therefore, for the time being, the burden of evidence would not be sufficient to consider leukocyte count as a risk factor at time of treatment decision-making, given the fact that the relationship between the initial leukocyte count and the subsequent thrombosis may be affected by treatment. From a functional point of view, a role for leukocytes, platelets, and leukocyte–platelet aggregates as cooperating mechanisms for the thrombosis in PV and ET has been shown. Thus, their activation [41] as well as the correlation with the *JAK2* mutational status might be more important than the number of leukocytes per se. In this sense, a correlation has also been found recently between the *JAK2* status and hemostasis activation parameters [41], leukocyte activation (by means of leukocyte alkaline phosphatase) [30], and platelet activation [42].

Several studies have been published on the possible contribution of well-defined cardiovascular risk factors, such as arterial hypertension, smoking habit, hypercholesterolemia, and diabetes mellitus, to the risk of thrombosis, but the results have been conflicting [10, 35, 36]. Taking into account that these cardiovascular risk factors may have additional influence on the expected risk of thrombosis in PV and ET, patients with such risk factors are usually considered to belong to an intermediate-risk category. Nevertheless, the use of cytoreductive treatment is not recommended in these patients, but an appropriate management of the reversible risk factors is mandatory.

Despite the value of risk stratification based on clinical parameters to guide the treatment of patients with MPNs, a better molecular understanding of these diseases may improve our ability to identify those patients destined to develop thrombosis. In this sense, several studies have recently analyzed the possible association between the V617F mutation of the *JAK2* gene and the occurrence of thrombosis in the MPNs (Table 4.2). Thus, a post hoc genetic analysis of the high-risk ET cohort in the Medical Research Council Primary Thrombocythemia-1 study demonstrated that the mutation was associated with higher Hb and white blood counts, and that such patients had higher rates of venous thromboses [43]. In another study of 179 ET patients, the frequency of thrombosis in *JAK2* mutants was significantly increased (33 vs. 17%) and comparable to that of PV patients [44]. Conversely, other retrospective concurrent studies with more than 100 patients each [10, 39] reported that the

Table 4.2 *JAK2* V617F mutation and the risk of thrombosis in ET.

Author	Study	No. of patients	Type of analysis	*JAK2* V617F prognostic value
Wolanskyj et al. 2006 [10]	Retrospective/ prospective	150	Univariate	Mutation not associated with thrombohemorrhagic events
Campbell et al. 2005 [43]	Prospective	806	Multivariate	Mutation associated with venous but not arterial thrombotic events
Carobbio et al. 2007 [39]	Retrospective	277	Multivariate	Mutation not an independent predictor of thrombosis occurring in the course of the disease
Finazzi et al. 2007 [44]	Retrospective	179	Univariate	Mutation associated with thrombotic events
Vannucchi et al. 2007 [45]	Retrospective	639	Multivariate	Homozygous mutation associated with thrombotic events
Kittur et al. 2007 [46]	Retrospective	176	Multivariate	Mutation and allele burden associated with venous thrombosis during follow-up, but not with arterial or venous thrombosis at diagnosis
Antonioli et al. 2008 [47]	Retrospective	260	Multivariate	Mutation and allele burden associated with arterial thrombosis at diagnosis. No difference between patients with mutant and wild-type alleles in rate of venous thrombosis

mutation status was not associated with the incidence of thrombohemorrhagic events. Reasons for these conflicting results might be the inadequacy of clinical criteria for distinguishing ET from PV, different patient selection and study design, and reliance solely on qualitative *JAK2* V617F expression and not quantitative allele burden measure.

About a third of PV patients and 2–4% of patients with ET harbor the mutation in the so-called homozygous state, a condition in which at least 51% of *JAK2* alleles in the granulocytes are mutated as a result of the mitotic recombination process. In a multicenter retrospective study including ET and PV patients, thrombotic events were significantly more frequent in homozygous patients with ET than in wild-type or heterozygous patients [45]. Employing quantitative assays for V617F allele, two retrospective series of ET patients demonstrated that *JAK2* mutation and its allele burden were associated with thrombosis [46, 47]. However, while one series provided evidence that only venous thrombosis occurring during follow-up was correlated with allele burden [46], the other showed that only arterial thrombosis at diagnosis proved associated with allele burden [47]. Of note, the independent predictive role of *JAK2* mutant allele burden was maintained after elimination of potential confounders at multivariate analysis, in which well-established risk factors for thrombosis, such as age, previous thrombosis, and leukocytosis, were included [45–47].

Given the extremely high incidence of the *JAK2* mutation in PV, the utility of the presence of the mutated allele itself is not likely to be of prognostic value in this disease. Indeed, in a large multicenter retrospective study no significant differences were observed in the overall rate and the type of major thrombosis between heterozygous and homozygous PV patients [45]. However, in a subsequent prospective study from the same group employing quantitative assays for V617F allele at diagnosis in PV patients, the occurrence of cardiovascular events (either at diagnosis or during follow-up) progressively increased from 10%, 14%, and 24% to 37% in the different groups according to categorized *JAK2* V617F allele burden [48]. Accordingly, the risk ratio of total thrombosis was 3.6-fold higher in patients with greater than 75% mutant allele as compared to a reference population.

In conclusion, findings of large studies indicate that identification of the *JAK2* V617F mutation might be a prognostic marker for thrombosis in ET. However, accurate determination of *JAK2* V617F allele burden using quantitative assay, rather than merely defining heterozygosity versus homozygosity, seems to be important for the assessment of the prognostic role of *JAK2* V617F allele in ET and PV. If these findings are corroborated in future prospective trials, a high V617F allele burden might represent a novel risk factor for thrombosis in ET and PV, in addition to age, previous thrombosis, and leukocytosis.

Prognostic Factors for Transformation to Myelofibrosis and Leukemia

Since the incidence of leukemia is low and this complication occurs late in the evolution of PV and ET, large and long-term studies are required to identify the risk factors at diagnosis for developing such a complication. A French study showed that the incidence of leukemia did not reach a plateau over time [49]. Patient's age [34, 49] and leukocyte count [50, 51] influenced the risk of leukemia in both ET and PV. No clear association has been demonstrated between leukemia and a specific drug exposure history [9, 34, 49, 52], with the exception of ^{32}P and chlorambucil [33], while the use of more than one cytoreductive therapy clearly increased the risk of leukemia [9, 33]. In PV, the ECLAP study failed to show significant differences in terms of leukemic evolution between patients treated with hydroxyurea and those managed with phlebotomy only [53]. Recently, no correlation between specific therapies and the occurrence of leukemia in ET was observed in a study from the Mayo Clinic, whereas a leukocyte count exceeding 15×10^9/L was the more relevant adverse prognostic factor [51].

Concerning the evolution of PV to myelofibrosis, recent studies identified that patients with homozygous *JAK2* V617F mutation or with a leukocyte count $>15 \times 10^9$/L at PV diagnosis had a higher risk of developing post-PV myelofibrosis [14]. With regard to ET, factors associated with a higher risk of myelofibrotic transformation were the presence of anemia [34] and increased reticulin accumulation in bone marrow [54] at ET diagnosis. In addition, it has been found that the longer the duration of PV or ET the higher the risk of developing myelofibrosis [14, 32, 34].

Concluding Remarks

The prognosis of PMF patients mainly relies on the degree of anemia at diagnosis. Although it is quite likely that this parameter will remain the basic tool for predicting the patients' outcome, international collaborative efforts are currently in progress to help refining the prognostic assessment of this disease by considering time-dependent factors. With regard to PV and ET, the prognostic parameters currently considered for the patients' clinical management are age >60 years, a history of thrombosis or bleeding, and platelet counts $>1,500 \times 10^9$/L, since they have a proven value to distinguish patients with low or high risk of vascular complications. However, in the setting of future prospective clinical trials, other factors such as leukocyte count, and *JAK2* V617F mutational status and allele burden should be tested for prognostic influence.

References

1. Barosi G, Berzuini C, Liberato LN, Costa A, Polino G, Ascari E. A prognostic classification of myelofibrosis with myeloid metaplasia. Br J Haematol 1988; 70:397–401.
2. Visani G, Finelli C, Castelli U, et al. Myelofibrosis with myeloid metaplasia: Clinical and haematological parameters predicting survival in a series of 133 patients. Br J Haematol 1990; 75:4–9.
3. Rupoli S, Da Lio L, Sisti, et al. Primary myelofibrosis: A detailed statistical analysis of the clinicopathological variables influencing survival. Ann Hematol 1994; 68:205–212.
4. Dupriez B, Morel P, Demory JL, et al. Prognostic factors in agnogenic myeloid metaplasia: A report on 195 cases with a new scoring system. Blood 1996; 88:1013–1018.
5. Cervantes F, Pereira A, Esteve J, Cobo F, Rozman C, Montserrat E. Identification of "short-lived" and "long-lived" patients at presentation of idiopathic myelofibrosis. Br J Haematol 1997; 97:635–640.
6. Reilly JT, Snowden JA, Spearing RL, et al. Cytogenetic abnormalities and their prognostic significance in idiopathic myelofibrosis: A study of 106 cases. Br J Haematol 1997; 98:96–102.
7. Cervantes F, Dupriez B, Pereira A, et al. New prognostic scoring system for primary myelofibrosis based on a study of the International Working Group for Myelofibrosis Research and Treatment. Blood 2009; 113:2895–2901.
8. Rozman C, Giralt M, Feliu E, Rubio D, Cortes MT. Life expectancy of patients with chronic nonleukemic myeloproliferative disorders. Cancer 1991; 67:2658–2663.
9. Passamonti F, Rumi E, Pungolino E, et al. Life expectancy and prognostic factors for survival in patients with polycythemia vera and essential thrombocythemia. Am J Med 2004; 117:755–761.
10. Wolanskyj AP, Schwager SM, McClure RF, Larson DR, Tefferi A. Essential thrombocythemia beyond the first decade: Life expectancy, long-term complication rates, and prognostic factors. Mayo Clin Proc 2006; 81:159–166.
11. Cervantes F, Barosi G, Demory JL, et al. Myelofibrosis with myeloid metaplasia in young individuals: Disease characteristics, prognostic factors and identification of risk groups. Br J Haematol 1998; 102:684–690.
12. Cervantes F, Barosi G, Hernández-Boluda JC, Marchetti M, Montserrat E. Myelofibrosis with myeloid metaplasia in adult individuals 30 years old or younger: Presenting features, evolution and survival. Eur J Haematol 2001; 66:324–327.
13. Cervantes F, Alvarez-Larrán A, Talarn C, Gómez M, Montserrat E. Myelofibrosis with myeloid metaplasia following essential thrombocythemia: Actuarial probability, presenting characteristics and evolution in a series of 195 patients. Br J Haematol 2002; 118:786–790.
14. Passamonti F, Rumi E, Caranella M, et al. A dynamic prognostic model to predict survival in post-polycythemia vera myelofibrosis. Blood 2008; 111:3383–3387.
15. Tefferi A, Huang J, Schwager S, et al. Validation and comparison of contemporary prognostic models in primary myelofibrosis. Analysis based on 334 patients from a single institution. Cancer 2007; 109:2083–2088.
16. Barosi G, Viarengo G, Pecci A, et al. Diagnostic and clinical relevance of the number of circulating CD34+ cells in myelofibrosis with myeloid metaplasia. Blood 2001; 98:3249–3255.
17. Sagaster V, Jager E, Weltermann A, et al. Circulating hematopoietic progenitor cells predict survival in patients with myelofibrosis with myeloid metaplasia. Haematologica 2003; 88:1204–1212.

18. Arora B, Sirhan S, Hover JD, Mesa RA, Tefferi A. Peripheral blood CD34 count in myelofibrosis with myeloid metaplasia: A prospective evaluation of prognostic value in 94 patients. Br J Haematol 2004; 128:42–48.

19. Tefferi A, Mesa RA, Schroeder G, Hanson CA, Li Ch-Y, Dewald GW. Cytogenetic findings and their clinical relevance in myelofibrosis with myeloid metaplasia. Br J Haematol 2001; 113:763–771.

20. Tam CS, Abruzzo LV, Lin KI, et al. The role of cytogenetic abnormalities as a prognostic marker in primary myelofibrosis: Applicability at the time of diagnosis and later during disease course. Blood 2009; 113:4171–4178.

21. Campbell PJ, Griesshammer M, Döhner K, et al. V617F mutation in JAK2 is associated with poorer survival in idiopathic myelofibrosis. Blood 2006; 107:2098–2100.

22. Barosi G, Bergamaschi G, Marchetti M, et al. JAK2 V617F mutational status predicts progression to large splenomegaly and leukemic transformation in primary myelofibrosis. Blood 2007; 110:430–436.

23. Tefferi A, Lasho TL, Huang J, et al. Low JAK2V617F allele burden in primary myelofibrosis, compared to either a higher allele burden or unmutated status, is associated with inferior overall and leukemia-free survival. Leukemia 2008; 22:756–761.

24. Huang J, Chin-Yang L, Mesa RA, et al. Risk factors for leukemic transformation in patients with primary myelofibrosis. Cancer 2008; 112:2726–2732.

25. Barosi G, Ambrosetti A, Centra A, et al. Splenectomy and risk of blast transformation in myelofibrosis with myeloid metaplasia. Blood 1998; 91:3630–3636.

26. Tefferi A, Mesa RA, Nagorney DN, Schroeder G, Silverstein MN. Splenectomy in myelofibrosis with myeloid metaplasia: A single-institution experience with 223 patients. Blood 2000; 95:2226–2233.

27. Vardiman JW, Harris NL, Brunning RD. The World Health Organization (WHO) classification of the myeloid neoplasms. Blood 2002; 100:2292–2302.

28. Thiele J, Kvasnicka HM. Chronic myeloproliferative disorders with thrombocythemia: A comparative study of two classification systems (PVSG, WHO) on 839 patients. Ann Hematol 2003; 82:148–152.

29. Wilkins BS, Erber WN, Bareford D, et al. Bone marrow pathology in essential thrombocythemia: Inter-observer reliability and utility for identifying disease subtypes. Blood 2008; 111:60–70.

30. Passamonti F, Rumi E, Pietra D, et al. Relation between JAK2 (V617F) mutation status, granulocyte activation, and constitutive mobilization of CD34+ cells into peripheral blood in myeloproliferative disorders. Blood 2006; 107:3676–3682.

31. Tefferi A, Thiele J, Orazi A, et al. Proposals and rationale for revision of the World Health Organization diagnostic criteria for polycythemia vera, essential thrombocythemia, and primary myelofibrosis: Recommendations from an ad hoc international expert panel. Blood 2007; 110:1092–1097.

32. Marchioli R, Finazzi G, Landolfi R, et al. Vascular and neoplastic risk in a large cohort of patients with polycythemia vera. J Clin Oncol 2005; 23:2224–2232.

33. Berk PD, Goldberg JD, Donovan PB, Fruchtman SM, Berlin NI, Wasserman LR. Therapeutic recommendations in polycythemia vera based on Polycythemia Vera Study Group protocols. Semin Hematol 1986; 23:132–143.

34. Passamonti F, Rumi E, Arcaini L, et al. Prognostic factors for thrombosis, myelofibrosis, and leukemia in essential thrombocythemia: A study of 605 patients. Haematologica 2008; 93:1645–1651.

35. Cortelazzo S, Viero P, Finazzi G, D'Emilio A, Rodeghiero F, Barbui T. Incidence and risk factors for thrombotic complications in a historical cohort of 100 patients with essential thrombocythemia. J Clin Oncol 1990; 8:556–562.

36. Besses C, Cervantes F, Pereira A, et al. Major vascular complications in essential thrombocythemia: A study of the predictive factors in a series of 148 patients. Leukemia 1999; 13:150–154.

37. Michiels JJ. Acquired von Willebrand disease due to increasing platelet count can readily explain the paradox of thrombosis and bleeding in thrombocythemia. Clin Appl Thromb Hemost 1999; 5:147–151.

38. Landolfi R, Di Gennaro L, Barbui T, et al. Leukocytosis as a major thrombotic risk factor in patients with polycythemia vera. Blood 2007; 109:2446–2452.

39. Carobbio A, Finazzi G, Guerini V, et al. Leukocytosis is a risk factor for thrombosis in essential thrombocythemia: Interaction with treatment, standard risk factors, and Jak2 mutation status. Blood 2007; 109:2310–2313.

40. Tefferi A, Gangat N, Wolanskyj A. The interaction between leukocytosis and other risk factors for thrombosis in essential thrombocythemia. Blood 2007; 109:4105.

41. Falanga A, Marchetti M, Evangelista V, et al. Polymorphonuclear leukocyte activation and hemostasis in patients with essential thrombocythemia and polycythemia vera. Blood 2000; 96:4261–4266.

42. Arellano-Rodrigo E, Alvarez-Larrán A, Reverter JC, Villamor N, Colomer D, Cervantes F. Increased platelet and leukocyte activation as contributing mechanisms for thrombosis in essential thrombocythemia and correlation with the JAK2 mutational status. Haematologica 2006; 91:169–175.

43. Campbell PJ, Scott LM, Buck G, et al. Definition of subtypes of essential thrombocythaemia and relation to polycythaemia vera based on JAK2 V617F mutation status: A prospective study. Lancet 2005; 366:1945–1953.

44. Finazzi G, Rambaldi A, Guerini V, Carobbo A, Barbui T. Risk of thrombosis in patients with essential thrombocythemia and polycythemia vera according to JAK2 V617F mutation status. Haematologica 2007; 92:135–136.

45. Vannucchi AM, Antonioli E, Guglielmelli P, et al. Clinical profile of homozygous JAK2 617V>F mutation in patients with polycythemia vera or essential thrombocythemia. Blood 2007; 110:840–846.

46. Kittur J, Knudson RA, Lasho TL, et al. Clinical correlates of JAK2V617F allele burden in essential thrombocythemia. Cancer 2007; 109:2279–2284.

47. Antonioli E, Guglielmelli P, Poli G, et al. Influence of JAK2V617F allele burden on phenotype in essential thrombocythemia. Haematologica 2008; 93:41–48.

48. Vannucchi AM, Antonioli E, Guglielmelli P, et al. Prospective identification of high-risk polycythemia vera patients based on $JAK2^{V617F}$ allele burden. Leukemia 2007; 21:1952–1959.

49. Kiladjian JJ, Rain JD, Bernard JF, Brière J, Chomienne C, Fenaux P. Long-term incidence of hematological evolution in three French prospective studies of hydroxyurea and pipobroman in polycythemia vera and essential thrombocythemia. Semin Thromb Hemost 2006; 32:417–421.

50. Gangat N, Strand J, Chin-Yang L, Wu W, Pardanani A, Tefferi A. Leucocytosis in polycythemia vera predicts both inferior survival and leukaemic transformation. Br J Haematol 2007; 138:354–358.

51. Gangat N, Wolanskyj AP, McClure RF, et al. Risk stratification for survival and leukemic transformation in essential thrombocythemia: A single institutional study of 605 patients. Leukemia 2007; 21:270–276.

52. Finazzi G, Caruso V, Marchioli R, et al. Acute leukemia in polycythemia vera: An analysis of 1638 patients enrolled in a prospective observational study. Blood 2005; 105:2664–2670.

53. Landolfi R, Marchioli R, Kutti J, et al. Efficacy and safety of low-dose aspirin in polycythemia vera. N Engl J Med 2004; 350:114–124.

54. Campbell PJ, Bareford D, Erber WN, et al. Reticulin accumulation in essential thrombocythemia: Prognostic significance and relationship to therapy. J Clin Oncol 2009; 27:2991–2999.

Chapter 5

Therapy of Polycythemia Vera and Essential Thrombocythemia

Guido Finazzi and Tiziano Barbui

Keywords: Chronic myeloproliferative neoplasms • Polycythemia vera • Essential thrombocythemia

Introduction

Understanding of the pathophysiology of polycythemia vera (PV) and essential thrombocythemia (ET) dramatically improved following the description, in the last years, of recurrent molecular abnormalities represented by: the V617F mutation in *JAK2* exon 14, that is the most frequent and involves >95% of PV and ≅60–70% of ET patients; a number of molecular alterations located in *JAK2* exon 12, that have been described in 50–80% of the *JAK2*-wild-type PV patients; mutations in *MPL*, mostly represented by the W515L or W515K allele, that are presented by ≅7% of ET patients; and mutations of the TET2 (10–11 translocation 2) gene reported in 20% of MDS and MPN/MDS and 8–15% of Myeloproliferative Neoplasm (MPN) (see Chap. 2 of this book). Genotyping for such molecular abnormalities has already become a standard tool in the diagnostic work-up of patients suspected to have a MPN and constitutes a major criterion for diagnosis, according to the new WHO classification of myeloid neoplasms (Chap. 1 of this book). As a consequence of an early diagnosis, it is very likely that the frequency and clinical presentation of these disorders will change in the next future.

Recommendations for management of PV and ET are adapted to the risk of thrombosis based on a limited number of randomized clinical trials performed within national or international collaborative groups. In addition, several observational studies described the clinical course of the diseases and indirectly evaluated the role of different treatments. Remarkably, criteria of inclusion and evaluation of responses in these studies did not consider the new molecular and histopathological findings (Chaps. 2 and 4 of this book). Thus, sound methodological evidence is limited and its application to currently diagnosed patients may be questionable. In practice, therapeutic recommendations are largely based on consensus of experts [1, 2]. The first step is to identify

S. Verstovsek and A. Tefferi (eds.), *Myeloproliferative Neoplasms: Biology and Therapy,* Contemporary Hematology, DOI 10.1007/ 978-1-60761-266-7_5, © Springer Science+Business Media, LLC 2011

the potential risk to develop major thrombotic or hemorrhagic complications. Then, patients should be stratified with the aim to focus chemotherapy only on high-risk cases, since the concern of increased rate of leukemia transformation limits the use of potentially leukemogenic cytotoxic drugs.

Incidence and Type of Thrombosis

Thrombosis is the most frequent clinical complications in ET and PV. In two randomized clinical trials in ET, the cumulative rates for major vascular complications during follow-up was 2.7 and 6.2 per 100 persons per year, respectively [3, 4]. In the prospective European Collaboration on Low-dose Aspirin in Polycythemia (ECLAP) study, cardiovascular mortality accounted for 1.5 deaths per 100 persons per year and the cumulative rate of nonfatal thrombosis was 3.8 events per 100 persons per year [5].

The most frequent types of major thrombosis include stroke, transient ischemic attack, myocardial infarction, peripheral arterial thrombosis, and deep venous thrombosis often occurring in unusual sites, such as hepatic, portal, and mesenteric veins. In addition to large vessel occlusions, ET and PV patients may suffer from microcirculatory symptoms, including vascular headaches, dizziness, visual disturbances, distal paresthesia, and acrocyanosis. The most characteristic of these disturbances is erythromelalgia, consisting of congestion, redness, and burning pain involving the extremities.

Risk Stratification

The largest prospective study evaluating risk factors for survival and thrombosis in PV is the ECLAP [5]. In this study, 1,638 PV patients were monitored prospectively to provide the profile of the disease as it is determined by the current clinical practice of a sample of specialized clinical centers across several European countries and to characterize the presently unmet therapeutic need of polycythemic patients. The incidence of cardiovascular complications was higher in those aged more than 65 years (5.0% pt-yr, hazard ratio (HR) 2.0, 95% confidence interval (CI) 1.22–3.29, $P < 0.006$) or with a history of thrombosis (4.93% pt-yr, HR 1.96, 95% CI 1.29–2.97, $P = 0.0017$) than in younger subjects with no history of thrombosis (2.5% pt-yr, reference category). These two variables, age and previous thrombotic history, were associated with an increased rate of vascular complications also in other large studies in ET (reviewed in ref. [6]). Other potential determinants of thrombotic risk, including cardiovascular risk factors (i.e. smoking, hypertension, hypercholesterolemia, diabetes mellitus) or the presence of thrombophilic conditions, are more contentious. However, it is wise to assume that patients with MPN presenting common cardiovascular risk factors have the same relative risk (RR) as those estimated in the general population and deserve to be treated accordingly.

The ECLAP and several prospective studies in ET [6] failed to show a clear association between platelet count and thrombotic events. Actually, the theory that elevated platelet count increases thrombosis risk in ET has been challenged. In a cohort study of 1,063 patients Carobbio et al. [7] found that a platelet count at diagnosis greater than $1,000 \times 10^9/L$ was associated with significantly lower rate of thrombosis in multivariable analysis. If this is combined with leukocytes less than 11×10^9/L, a "low-risk" category with a rate of thrombosis of 1.59% of patients/year was identified. On the contrary, the highest risk category (thrombosis rate, 2.95% of patients/year) was constituted of patients with leukocytosis, lower platelet count, and a JAK2V617F mutated genotype (77 vs. 26% in the low-risk group).

At variance of thrombocytosis, leukocytosis was found to be an independent risk factor for thrombosis and survival in most studies both in PV and ET (reviewed in ref. [8]). In PV, time-dependent multivariate analysis, adjusted for potential confounders including cytoreductive and antithrombotic treatment, showed that patients participating in the ECLAP study with a leukocyte count greater than 15×10^9/L had a significant increase in the risk of thrombosis when compared to patients with leukocyte lower than 10×10^9/L (HR, 1.71, 95% CI 1.1–2.6), mainly due to an higher rate of myocardial infarction (HR 2.84; 95% CI 1.25–6.46, $P = 0.01$). In another study in PV, leukocyte count $>15 \times 10^9$/L was an independent predictor of inferior survival, leukemic transformation, and venous thrombosis. In ET, three large cohort studies reported that an increased baseline leukocyte count was an independent risk factor for both thrombosis and inferior survival. In "low-risk" ET patients (i.e. below 60 years and without previous thrombosis), leukocytosis confers a thrombotic risk comparable to that of treated "high-risk" patients without leukocytosis. In a study of 53 ET patients carried out in Taiwan, thrombotic events were significantly correlated with leukocytosis, older age, and JAK2 V617F mutation. White blood cells (WBC) count above 9.5×10^9/L at diagnosis were independently associated with thrombosis during follow-up (RR = 1.8, $P = 0.03$) in 187 patients with ET and PV evaluated in Italy. More recently, the association of leukocytosis and JAK2 V617F mutation with thrombotic events has been confirmed in a retrospective study of 108 patients with ET and PV [9]. These findings have been confuted by the Mayo Clinic investigators in a retrospective study of 407 low-risk patients with ET [10]. Leukocytosis at the time of diagnosis, defined by a cut-off level of either 15 or 9.4×10^9/L, did not appear to be predictive of either arterial or venous thrombosis during follow-up. However, in an analysis by Passamonti et al. [11] of 194 low-risk ET patients, the increase in leukocyte count within 2 years of diagnosis (observed in 9% of patients), rather than leukocytosis at diagnosis, was associated with an higher risk of vascular complications during follow-up.

In ET and PV, an in vivo leukocyte activation has been consistently documented, in association with signs of activation of both platelets and endothelial cells, particularly in patients carrying the V617F JAK2 mutation [8]. Thus, leukocyte and platelet activation may play a role in the generation of the prethrombotic state that characterizes these disorders. However, whether leukocytosis should be simply considered a marker for vascular disease or whether elevated WBC levels actually contribute directly to causing such disorders should be a matter of prospective studies.

The influence of the JAK2 V617F mutational status and allele burden on the thrombotic risk has been evaluated in several studies (reviewed in ref. [12]). In 173 patients with PV, those harboring greater than 75% JAK2 V617F allele were at higher relative risk to develop major cardiovascular events during follow-up than those with less than 25% mutant allele (RR 7.1; $P = 0.003$). A trend towards more thrombotic events in 105 PV patients having greater than 80% mutant allele has also been reported. On the other hand, Tefferi et al. measured V617F allele burden in bone marrow-derived DNA obtained from 103 PV patients at variable times after diagnosis, and found that it was not correlated with major cardiovascular events. In ET, the presence of the V617F JAK2 mutation in about 60% of patients raised the question whether mutated and nonmutated patients differ in terms of thrombotic risk. The largest prospective study on 806 patients suggested that JAK2 mutation in ET was associated with anamnestic venous but not arterial events. An increased risk of thrombosis in JAK2 mutated patients was retrospectively observed by other investigators. However, the rate of vascular complications was not affected by the presence of the mutation in two relatively large retrospective studies, including 150 and 130 ET patients, respectively. A systematic literature review was carried out to compare the frequency of thrombosis between JAK2 V617F-positive and wild-type patients with ET [13]. This study showed that JAK2 V617F patients have a twofold risk of developing thrombosis (odds ratio 1.92, 95% CI 1.45–2.53) but a significant heterogeneity between studies should be pointed out. In addition to the prognostic role of JAK2 mutation for the first thrombotic episode, recent data would indicate that the mutation has also a role to predict recurrent thrombotic episodes in patients with ET [14].

As to the presence of an *MPL* mutation, higher rates of arterial thrombosis were found in the Italian study [15] but not in the Primary Thrombocythemia-1 (PT-1) trial cohort [16]. Interestingly, data derived from the PT-1 have identified increased bone marrow reticulin fibrosis at diagnosis as an independent predictor of subsequent thrombotic and hemorrhagic complications [17].

In conclusion, by incorporating this body of knowledge in a clinically oriented scheme (Table 5.1), we have now consistent information to stratify the patients with either PV or ET in a "high-risk" or "low-risk" category according to their age and previous history of thrombosis; an "intermediate-risk" category, that would include younger patients with coexisting generic cardiovascular risk factors in the absence of previous thrombosis, is also defined, but formal proof of its relevance to stratify patients is still lacking. Putative novel variables, such as leukocytosis and *JAK2*V617F mutational status and allele burden and bone marrow reticulin, might be incorporated in the risk classification, possibly allowing better definition of the low-risk group, once more information is available and when they have been eventually validated in prospective studies.

Table 5.1 Risk stratification in PV and ET based on thrombotic risk.

Risk category	Age ≥60 years or history of thrombosis	Cardiovascular risk factors[a]
Low	No	No
Intermediate	No	Yes
High	Yes	

Extreme thrombocytosis (platelet count >1,500 × 10^9/L) is a potential risk factor for bleeding in ET
Increasing leukocyte count and JAK2 V617F mutation have been identified as novel risk factors for thrombosis, but confirmation in prospective studies is required
[a]Hypertension, hypercholesterolemia, diabetes, and smoking

Treatment of "Low-Risk" Patients

Phlebotomy

The only randomized study comparing phlebotomy with myelosuppressive therapy was published by the Polycythemia Vera Study Group (PVSG) more than 20 years ago (01 trial) [18]. Patients treated in the phlebotomy arm had a better overall median survival (13.9 years) than the other two arms (chlorambucil 8.9 years, radiophosphorus 11.8 years) due to a reduced incidence of acute leukemia and other malignancies. In contrast, an excess of thrombosis was observed in phlebotomized patients during the first 3 years. The difficulty to maintain PV patients on phlebotomy only was underlined by Najean et al. [19] who reported that of the 104 patients entered by the French group into the phlebotomy arm of the PVSG study, more than 50% were excluded by the 5th year and 90% by the 10th year. The patient's poor compliance was one of the most frequent causes of treatment changes.

In the PVSG-01 trial, the target hematocrit (HCT) was set at 45% and this was based on a small, retrospective study of PV that showed in univariate analysis a progressive increase in the incidence of vascular occlusive episodes at HCT levels higher than 44% [20]. However, no controlled study confirmed such findings. In the ECLAP study, despite the recommendation of maintaining the HCT values at less than 0.45, only 48% of patients had values below this threshold, while 39% and 13% of patients remained between 0.45 and 0.50 and greater than 0.50, respectively. Multivariate models considering all the confounders failed to show any correlation between these HCT values and thrombosis. A total of 164 deaths (10%), 145 (8.85%) major thrombosis, and 226 (13.8%) total thrombosis were encountered during 4,393 person-years of follow-up (median 2.8 years). An association between relevant outcome events (thrombotic events, mortality, and hematological progression) and HCT in the evaluable range of 40–55% was found neither in the multivariate analysis at baseline nor in the time-dependent multivariate model [21]. For the time being, the recommended hematocrit target is below 45%, according to the phlebotomy management described in Table 5.2, but the uncertainty described above prompted Italian Investigators to launch a prospective, randomized clinical study (CYTO-PV) addressing the issue of the optimal target of cytoreduction in PV (EudraCT 2007-006694-91).

Low-Dose Aspirin

The efficacy and safety of low-dose aspirin (100 mg daily) in PV has been assessed in the ECLAP double-blind, placebo-controlled, and randomized clinical trial [22]. In this study, 532 PV patients were randomized to receive 100 mg aspirin or placebo. After a follow-up of about 3 years, data analysis showed a significant reduction of a primary combined end-point including cardiovascular death, nonfatal myocardial infarction, nonfatal stroke, and major venous thromboembolism (RR 0.4, 95% CI 0.18–0.91, $P = 0.0277$). The estimated benefit of low-dose aspirin in terms of reduction of major cardiovascular end-points is shown in Fig. 5.1. Major bleeding was not significantly increased by aspirin (RR 1.6, 95% CI 0.27–9.71). It is important to underline that the ECLAP trial was conducted in a relatively low-risk population since it recruited only patients in whom the benefit/risk ratio of ASA use was

Table 5.2 Management and dosing of cytoreductive therapy in PV and ET.

Phlebotomy

Phlebotomy should be started withdrawing 250–500 cc of blood daily or every other day until a hematocrit between 40 and 45% is obtained. In the elderly or those with a cardiovascular disease, smaller amount of blood (200–300 cc) should be withdrawn twice weekly. Once normalization of the hematocrit has been obtained, blood counts at regular intervals (every 4–8 weeks) will establish the frequency of future phlebotomies. Sufficient blood should be removed to maintain the hematocrit below 45%. Supplemental iron therapy should not be given.

Hydroxyurea

The starting dose of HU is 15–20 mg/kg/day until response is obtained (for response criteria, see ref. [39]). Thereafter, a maintenance dose should be administered to keep the response without reducing WBC count values below $2,500 \times 10^9$/L. Supplemental phlebotomy should be performed if needed in PV patients. Complete hemogram should be recorded every 2 weeks during the first 2 months, then every month, and, in steady state in responding patients, every 3 months.

Interferon

IFN is contraindicated in patients with thyroid and/or mental disorders: for this reason an accurate evaluation of thyroid function and inquiry of previous or present mental disorders in candidate patients are recommended. IFN should be administered at the dose of 3 MU daily until a response is reached [39]; then, therapy has to be adjusted at the lowest weekly doses which maintain the response. Complete hemogram must be recorded every week during the first month of therapy, every 2 weeks during the second month, then every month and, in steady state in responding patients, every 3–4 months. Peg-IFN is given at a starting dose of 0.5 μg/kg once weekly. In patients who failed to achieve a response after 12 weeks, the dose is increased up to 1.0 μg/kg/week. Then, therapy has to be adjusted at the lowest dose that maintain the response and monitored as above.

Anagrelide

The recommended starting dosage of oral anagrelide for adults is 0.5 mg twice daily; this dosage should be maintained for at least 1 week and thereafter titrated individually to achieve a platelet count $<600 \times 10^9$/L and ideally $150–400 \times 10^9$/L. Dosages should be increased by no more than 0.5 mg/day in a single week, and should not exceed 10 mg/day. The recommended maximum single dose is 2.5 mg. Patients with cardiovascular disease or hepatic dysfunction should be monitored closely. The drug is contraindicated in patients with severe cardiac insufficiency as well as hepatic (Child–Pugh classification C) or renal (creatinine clearance <30 mL/min) impairment.

judged to be uncertain by the responsible physicians. As a consequence, most high-risk patients were excluded from randomization for having a clear indication to ASA use. Patients with a history of previous thrombotic event had an annual risk approximately equal to 8% events and at low to moderate bleeding risk. In comparison to aspirin only, the combination of aspirin plus clopidogrel could reduce thrombotic complications. Thus, a phase II, randomized, double-blind, placebo-controlled international study of clopidogrel and aspirin for the treatment of PV (ISCLAP) is currently underway.

In ET, aspirin, 100 mg daily, has been found to control microvascular symptoms, such as erythromelalgia, and transient neurological and ocular disturbances including dysarthria, hemiparesis, scintillating scotomas, amaurosis fugax, migraine, and seizures. Higher doses, up to 500 mg daily, may be necessary in the acute phase of erythromelalgia. Translating evidence from the ECLAP randomized study in PV, the use of low-dose aspirin as primary prophylaxis of vascular events can be considered. However, formal

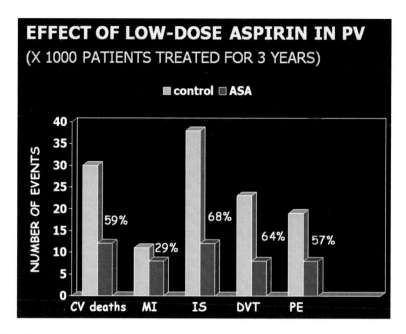

Fig. 5.1 Expected benefit of aspirin, 100 mg daily, on major cardiovascular (CV) end-points in PV patients, according to ECLAP study [22]. *MI* myocardial infarction, *IS* ischemic stroke, *DVT* deep vein thrombosis, and *PE* pulmonary embolism

clinical trials addressing this issue in ET have not been produced so far. In a randomized study comparing hydroxyurea vs. anagrelide in high-risk patients with ET discussed in detail below [3], low-dose aspirin was given to both groups. An increased rate of major bleeding was registered in the anagrelide plus aspirin arm and this may be due to a synergistic effect of the two drugs on platelet function inhibition.

Treatment of High-Risk Patients

The cytoreductive drugs most commonly used for the treatment of high-risk ET and PV patients, nowadays, include hydroxyurea, interferon-alpha (IFN-alpha), and anagrelide. Early studies on these drugs are quoted in ref. [6]. Practical recommendations for their management and dosing are reported in Table 5.2.

Hydroxyurea

The first group of investigators who studied HU in the management of PV was the PVSG. Hydroxyurea (HU) is an antimetabolite that prevents DNA synthesis and, at that time, it was assumed to be not leukemogenic. In a paper summarizing their long-term experience with HU in 51 patients followed for a median of 8.6 years, the PVSG reported an incidence of leukemia of 9.8% (vs. 3.7% in the historical phlebotomized controls) but less myelofibrosis (7.8 vs. 12.7%) and fewer total deaths (39.2 vs. 55.2%). In the ECLAP study, HU alone was not found to enhance the risk of leukemia in comparison with patients treated with phlebotomy only (HR 0.86, 95% CI 0.26–2.88, $P = 0.8$). However, the risk was significantly increased by exposure to radiophosphorus, busulphan, or pipobroman (HR 5.46, 95% CI 1.84–16.25, $P = 0.002$). The use of HU in patients already treated with alkylating agents or radiophosphorus also enhanced the leukemic risk (HR 7.58, 95% CI 1.85–31, $P = 0.0048$) [23]. Two studies did not find significant differences in the rate of leukemic transformation in PV patients treated with HU or pipobroman, an alkylating agent with a mechanism of action that also involves metabolic competition with pyrimidine basis. However, different results were observed by prolonging the observation time. In a recent long-term analysis of a randomized clinical trial comparing HU to Pipobroman in 292 PV patients (median follow-up 16.3 years), median survival was 20.3 years in HU arm and 15.4% in Pipobroman arm. Cumulative incidence of AML/MDS at 10, 15, and 20 years was 6.6%, 16.5%, and 24% in the HU and 13%, 34%, and 52% in the Pipobroman arm, respectively ($P = 0.004$) [24].

HU has emerged as the treatment of choice also in high-risk patients with ET because of its efficacy and only rare acute toxicity. The efficacy of HU in preventing thrombosis in high-risk ET patients was demonstrated in a seminal randomized clinical trial [4]. One hundred and fourteen patients were randomized to long-term treatment with HU ($n = 56$) or to no cytoreductive treatment ($n = 58$). During a median follow-up of 27 months, 2 thromboses were recorded in the HU-treated group (1.6%/pt-yr) compared with 14 in the control group (10.7% pt-yr; $P = 0.003$). Notably, the antithrombotic effect of HU may recognize additional mechanisms of action besides panmyelosuppression, including qualitative changes in leukocytes, decreased expression of endothelial adhesion molecules, and enhanced nitric oxide generation [25]. Some long-term follow-up studies revealed that a proportion of ET patients treated with HU developed acute leukemia, particularly when given before or after alkylating agents or radiophosphorus. In other studies, however, the use of this drug as the only cytotoxic treatment was rarely associated with secondary malignancies: in an analysis of 25 ET patients younger than 50 years and treated with HU alone for a high risk of thrombosis, no case of leukemic or neoplastic transformation occurred after a median follow-up of 8 years (range 5–14 years). Interestingly, in a recent, large population-based nested case-control study in Sweden, the risk of AML/MDS in MPNs was strongly associated with P32 (RR 3.39, 95% CI 1.28–8.99, $P = 0.01$) and alkylator treatments (RR 4.46, 95% CI 1.22–16.31, $P = 0.03$). In contrast, in this survey HU (>1,000 mg) did not significantly increase the risk for transformation to AML/MDS (RR 1.01, 0.28–3.6) [26]. Further support to the low, if any, leukemogenic potential of HU comes from a systematic review of the efficacy and safety of this drug in sickle cell disease. This study analyzed HU toxicities not only in patients with sickle cell disease but also in patients with other diseases, including MPNs, and concluded that, albeit limited, current evidence suggests that hydroxyurea treatment in adults does not increase the risk for leukemia [27].

Major side effects of hydroxyurea include hematopoietic impairment, leading to neutropenia and macrocytic anemia, and mucocutaneous toxicity, most frequently presenting as oral and leg ulcers and skin lesions. In addition, it is estimated that about 10% of patients receiving HU do not achieve the desired reduction in blood cell counts using recommended doses. Recently, an international working group (WG) in the frame of the European Leukemia Net was convened to develop a consensus formulation of clinically significant criteria for defining resistance/intolerance to HU in ET. The WG proposed that the definition of resistance/intolerance should require the fulfillment of at least one of the following criteria: platelet count greater than 600,000/μL after 3 months of at least 2 g/day of HU (2.5 g/day in patients with a body weight over 80 kg); platelet count greater than 400,000/μL and WBC less than 2,500/μL or Hb less than 10 g/dL at any dose of HU; presence of leg ulcers or other unacceptable mucocutaneous manifestations at any dose of HU; and HU-related fever [28].

Interferon Alpha

IFN-alpha was considered for the treatment of patients with MPDs since this agent suppresses the proliferation of hematopoietic progenitors, has a direct inhibiting effect on bone marrow fibroblast progenitor cells, and antagonizes the action of platelet-derived growth factor, transforming growth factor-beta and other cytokines, which may be involved in the development of myelofibrosis. Published reports concern small consecutive series of patients in whom hematological response and side effects were evaluated. One review analyzed the cumulative experience with IFN-alpha in 279 patients with PV from 16 studies [29]. Overall responses were 50% for reduction of HCT to less than 0.45% without concomitant phlebotomies, 77% for reduction in spleen size, and 75% for reduction of pruritus. In a review article, Silver updated his experience on the long-term use (median 13 years) of IFN-alpha in 55 patients with PV [30]. Complete responses, defined by phlebotomy free, HCT less than 45%, and platelet number below 600×10^9/L, were reached in the great majority of cases after 1–2 years of treatment, and the maintenance dose could be decreased in half of the patients. Noteworthy is the absence of thrombohemorrhagic events during this long follow-up.

IFN-alpha has also been used in ET patients. The results of several cohort studies, reviewed in Lengfelder et al. [31], indicate that reduction of platelet count below 600×10^9/L can be obtained in about 90% of cases after about 3 months with an average dose of three million IU daily. IFN-alpha is not known to be teratogenic and does not cross the placenta. Thus, it has been used successfully throughout pregnancy in some ET patients with no adverse fetal or maternal outcome. The main problem with IFN-alpha therapy, apart from its costs and parental route of administration, is the incidence of side effects. Fever and flu-like symptoms are experienced by most patients and usually require treatment with paracetamol. Signs of chronic IFN-alpha toxicity, such as weakness, myalgia, weight and hair loss, severe depression, and gastrointestinal and cardiovascular symptoms, make it necessary to discontinue the drug in about one third of the patients.

Pegylated forms of IFN-alpha allow weekly administration, potentially improving compliance and possibly providing more effective therapy. A phase 2 study has shown that following pegylated IFN alpha-2a therapy the malignant clone as quantitated by the percentage of the mutated allele JAK2V617F was reduced [32]. More limited effects on JAK2 mutational status have been reported after therapy with pegylated IFN-alpha-2b in a small group of patients with PV and ET [33]. Kiladjian et al. performed a prospective sequential quantitative evaluation of the percentage of mutated JAK2 allele (%V617F) by real-time polymerase chain reaction (PCR) in patients treated with pegylated IFN-alpha-2a [34]. The % JAK2V617F was decreased in 26 (89.6%) of 29 treated patients, from a mean of 45% to a mean of 22.5% after 12 months of treatment (median decrease of 50%; $P < 0.001$), with no evidence for a plateau being achieved. In two patients, JAK2V617F was no longer detectable after 12 months, such complete molecular response being observed in a total of seven patients (24%) at the time of last analysis after a median follow-up of 31.4 months. These impressive results have been confirmed by the M.D. Anderson Cancer Center investigators [35]. In a phase II study of pegylated IFN-alpha-2a in 79 patients with PV and ET, an overall hematologic response rate was observed in 80% of PV and 81% of ET (complete in 70% and 76% of patients, respectively). The molecular response rate was 38% in ET and 54% in PV, being complete (undetectable JAK2 V617F) in 6% and 14%, respectively. The JAK2 V617F mutant allele burden continued to decrease with no clear evidence for a plateau. The tolerability of PEG-IFN-alpha-2a at 90 μg weekly was excellent. Thus, this agent may have an important role in the treatment of PV and other clonal MPN.

Anagrelide

Anagrelide, a member of the imidazoquinazolin compounds, has a potent platelet reducing activity devoid of leukemogenic potential and appeared to be the option to HU for reducing platelet counts in younger ET patients at high risk for thrombosis. The largest analysis reported so far comprised 3,660 patients (2,251 with ET) [36]. With maximum follow-up of 7 years, anagrelide achieved platelet control in over 75% of patients and did not increase the conversion to AL. However, other complications of the drug include palpitations, congestive heart failure, headache, and depression.

HU and anagrelide (plus aspirin in both groups) have been compared head to head in a randomized clinical trial (PT-1) including 809 ET patients [3]. Patients in the Anagrelide arm showed an increased rate of arterial thrombosis (OR 2.16, 95% CI 1.04–2.37, $P = 0.03$), major bleeding (OR 2.61, 95% CI 1.27–5.33, $P = 0.008$), and myelofibrotic transformation (OR 2.92, 95% CI 1.24–6.86, $P = 0.01$) but a decreased incidence of venous thrombosis (OR 0.27, 95% CI 0.11–0.71, $P = 0.006$) compared to HU. In addition, Anagrelide was more poorly tolerated than HU and presented significantly greater rates of cardiovascular ($P < 0.001$), gastrointestinal ($P < 0.02$), neurological ($P < 0.001$), and constitutional ($P < 0.001$) side effects. Transformation to AL was comparable between the two arms (4 anagrelide vs. 6 HU) although the small number of transformations and short follow-up prevented firm conclusions about leukemogenicity.

Responses to the treatment in the PT-1 trial were influenced by JAK2 status [37]. Patients who were V617F-positive randomized to anagrelide had higher rates of arterial thrombosis than those randomized to hydroxyurea (19 vs. 5 patients; $P = 0.003$), whereas for V617F-negative patients there were equal numbers of arterial thromboses in the two groups (10 patients in each group; $P = 0.9$). In addition, V617F-positive patients required substantially lower doses of hydroxyurea and yet had greater reductions in platelet counts, white cell counts, and hemoglobin concentration than did V617F-negative patients. No such effect was seen in patients receiving anagrelide. These findings suggest that V617F-positive patients gain particular benefit from hydroxyurea compared with anagrelide. Anagrelide does appear to provide partial protection from thrombosis, particularly in JAK2 V617F neg. ET patients, and may therefore be suitable as second line therapy for patients in whom hydroxyurea is inadequate or not tolerated, according to the criteria described above.

Therapy with anagrelide, but not with hydroxyurea, was also associated with progressive anemia and an increase in bone marrow fibrosis [17]. The increased fibrosis was reversible in a small number of patients upon withdrawal of anagrelide, and follow-up trephine biopsies are therefore recommended for patients receiving this agent, perhaps every 2–3 years. It is important to note that the diagnosis of ET in the PT1-trial was made according to the PVSG classification and it remains questionable if these recommendations can be applied to ET patients diagnosed according to the WHO classification.

In this connection, useful information is expected from the Anahydret trial [38]. The Anahydret was a randomized single blind international multicenter phase III study designed to evaluate the noninferiority of anagrelide vs. hydroxyurea in 258 high-risk ET patients diagnosed according to the 2008 WHO diagnostic criteria. This classification, at variance of PVSG criteria required in the PT-1 trial, included a more homogenous category of patients excluding those with early myelofibrosis. During the whole study period, 11 major ET-related complications occurred in the anagrelide group (5 arterial events, 2 venous thrombotic complications, and 4 bleedings) and 12 major events were seen in the hydroxyurea arm (5 arterial events, 5 venous thrombositic events, and 2 bleedings). Transformations to myelofibrosis were not reported. This study provides preliminary evidence for noninferiority of anagrelide compared to hydroxyurea in the treatment of ET diagnosed according to the WHO classification. However, compared to PT-1, the number of patients enrolled was small, duration of follow-up relatively short, and considerably fewer end-point events were recorded. It is therefore questionable whether this study has the statistical power to detect the differences observed in the PT-1 study.

Summary

Our practice recommendations for the treatment of patients with ET and PV are summarized in Table 5.3. Several areas of uncertainties still remain and call for further appropriate clinical trials. In order to uniform the response criteria from new drugs to be used in clinical trials, European experts were convened to develop a definition of response to treatment in PV and ET [39]. Clinico-hematologic, molecular, and histologic response were selected and are expected to provide a means to compare the results from different patient cohorts and to facilitate communication within the scientific community.

Table 5.3 Risk-adapted therapy in PV and ET.

Risk stratification
  At least one of the following defines high-risk patients
    Age above 60 years
    Previous major thrombotic or hemorrhagic complication

Therapy
  Low-risk patients
    PV: Target hematocrit below 45% plus aspirin 100 mg/day
    ET: aspirin 100 mg/day if microcirculatory symptoms (i.e. erythromelalgia)

  High-risk patients
  As above, plus myelosuppressive therapy:
    Hydroxyurea as first choice
    PEG-interferon in special situations (young patients, pregnancy)
    Anagrelide in ET patients intolerant or refractory to hydroxyurea

Special Treatment Issues

Management of Pregnancy

Normal pregnant women are at an increased risk of thrombosis, calculated to be approximately six times higher than in nonpregnant women, and the risk is compounded if they also have MPD. As a consequence, women with MPD may present a high incidence not only of pregnancy-related venous thromboembolism, but also of other vascular complications of pregnancy involving occlusion of the placental circulation. The paucity of published data, however, makes it difficult to obtain a clear view of the overall risk of these events.

Clinical Epidemiology and Risk Factors

In the Italian guidelines for the therapy of ET [1], the outcomes of 461 pregnancies reported in retrospective and prospective cohort studies were pooled. The mean age at pregnancy was 29 years, with a mean platelet count at the beginning of pregnancy of $1,000 \times 10^9/L$. During the second trimester, a spontaneous decline was registered to a nadir of $599 \times 10^9/L$. This decrease seems larger than the reduction seen in normal pregnancies, which is attributed to an increase in plasma volume. The mechanism is not known, but could involve placental or fetal production of a factor that down-regulates platelet production. In the postpartum period the platelet counts rise back up to their earlier levels and rebound thrombocytosis may occur in some patients. This increases the probability of vascular complications at this time, which is a period of high thrombotic risk, like in other conditions of thrombophilia as well as in normal women.

Overall, 50–70% of ET women had successful live births; first-trimester loss occurred in about 25–40% and late pregnancy loss in 10% of cases. This is in agreement with a recent Mayo Clinic study of 63 pregnancies, 60% ended in live births and 32% in first trimester miscarriages [40]. Abruptio placentae was reported in 3.6% of cases, higher than in the general population (1%). Pre-eclampsia rates were similar to the normal population (1.7%), and intrauterine growth retardation (IUGR) was reported in 4–5%. Maternal thrombosis or hemorrhage is uncommon. In the pooled analysis cited above [1], postpartum thrombotic episodes were reported in 13 patients, occurring in 5.2% of pregnancies, and minor or major, pre- or postpartum bleeding events in other 13 cases. The maternal vascular risk may be higher in women with previous venous or arterial events or hemorrhages attributed to MPD, independent of whether they occurred in a previous pregnancy or not. Similarly, severe complications in a previous pregnancy, such as ≥3 first-trimester or ≥1 second or third-trimester losses, birth weight <5th centile of gestation, pre-eclampsia, intrauterine death, or stillbirth, are considered to raise the risk of subsequent events for the mother and the fetus. Other vascular risk factors in pregnant women are age, obesity, immobilization, and other causes of genetic and acquired thrombophilia including antiphospholipid antibodies. A recent paper analyzed risk factors associated with pregnancy complications in 103 pregnancies occurring in 62 women with ET [41]. The live birth rate was 64% and a full-term normal delivery was seen in 51% of cases. Fetal complications occurred in 40% and maternal complications in 9% of pregnancies (5% pre-eclampsia, 4% arterial hypertension), respectively. Fetal loss in women with ET was 3.4-fold higher compared with the general population. Most interestingly, the presence of the JAK2 V617F mutation occurring in half of the patients was an independent predictor of pregnancy complications. However, other studies are needed to confirm this preliminary information.

In comparison with the situation in ET, pregnancy in PV is a rare event since only 15% of PV patients are <40 years at presentation. In a review of this issue, a total of 36 pregnancies have been reported in 18 PV patients [42]. There was a live birth rate of 58% (21 of 36 pregnancies). However, three babies out of these 21 live births subsequently had an early neonatal death, and thus the surviving neonatal rate was 50% (18 of 36 pregnancies). Similarly to ET, spontaneous abortion during the first trimester was the most frequent complication occurring in 22% (8 of 36 pregnancies). Late pregnancy loss and IUGR occurred in 19.4% (7 of 36 pregnancies) and preterm delivery in 13.8% (5 of 36 pregnancies). In contrast to ET, maternal morbidity was significant. Eight of the reported 18 patients (44.4%) had significant complications: 1 death, 4 pre-eclampsia, 2 postpartum pulmonary emboli, and 1 large postpartum hemorrhage.

Treatment

A detailed personal and family history should be taken and a woman with MPD who plans a pregnancy should be put under the joint care of a hematologist and an obstetrician experienced in the care of patients with high-risk pregnancies in order to assess the risks and agree on the most appropriate therapy. It is recommended that the patient stop any possibly teratogenic drugs at least 3 months before conception. Depending on the risk of maternal vascular events and pregnancy morbidity, the various treatment options range from no therapy, aspirin alone, low molecular weight heparin (LMWH) to cytoreductive therapy (Table 5.4).

In the absence of clear contraindications, all patients with ET and PV should be given aspirin (100 mg daily) throughout pregnancy, although not all studies agree on the value of aspirin therapy in reducing miscarriages rates. Low-dose aspirin

Table 5.4 Practice recommendations for management of pregnancy in ET and PV.

Risk stratification
At least one of the following defines high-risk pregnancy
Previous major thrombotic or bleeding complication
Previous severe pregnancy complications[a]
Platelet count >1,500 × 10^9/L
Therapy
Low-risk pregnancy
Target hematocrit should be kept below 45%
Aspirin 100 mg/day
LMWH 4,000 U/day after delivery until 6 weeks postpartum
High-risk pregnancy
As above, plus
If previous major thrombosis or severe pregnancy complications: LMWH throughout pregnancy (stop aspirin if bleeding complications)
If platelet count >1,500 × 10^9/L: consider IFN-alpha
If previous major bleeding: avoid aspirin and consider IFN-alpha to reduce thrombocytosis

[a]Severe pregnancy complications: ≥3 first-trimester or ≥1 second or third-trimester losses, birth weight <5th centile of gestation, pre-eclampsia, intrauterine death or stillbirth

is considered safe in pregnancy and should preferably be started before conception to facilitate placental and fetal development. Bleeding complications are rare but particular attention should be paid to patients with platelet count above $1,000-1,500 \times 10^9$/L since the risk of bleeding may increase significantly.

LMWH in pregnancy is indicated for prophylaxis and treatment of deep venous thrombosis in selected high-risk ET women, and to reduce fetal morbidity. The suggested dose of enoxaparin is 4,000 U (40 mg) once daily increasing to 4,000 U twice daily from 16 weeks, dropping to 4,000 U daily for 6 weeks postpartum, preterm delivery, and IUGR. To increase the antithrombotic efficacy in very high-risk situations LMWH was used in combination with low-dose aspirin.

Cytoreductive therapy in pregnant women with ET and PV is a very controversial area. During pregnancy, hematocrit (Hct) and platelet count may undergo a natural fall and this could reduce the need of phlebotomy or cytoreductive drugs. The target Hct in PV is not yet well established. The recommendation is to reduce Hct to below 0.45 by venesection, since currently no evidence to support a different level in males and females is available. Platelet-lowering therapy in pregnancy is also controversial, since the available data did not indicate a relation between platelet count and adverse pregnancy outcome. In any case, drugs should be avoided in the first trimester. According to the Italian guidelines [1] and expert judgement [42, 43], candidates for platelet-lowering drugs are high-risk women, such as those with a previous history of major thrombosis or major bleeding, particularly when platelet count is greater than $1,000-1,500 \times 10^9$/L, or when familial thrombophilia or cardiovascular risk factors are documented. If cytoreduction has to be given, IFN-alpha is probably the safest option. Generally, patients should not be receiving hydroxyurea when they conceive or in the first trimester. Anagrelide may cause fetal harm by crossing the placenta and results in severe thrombocytopenia. It is therefore not recommended in pregnancy.

Management of Venous Thrombosis in Unusual Sites

Venous thrombosis occurring in unusual sites calls for particular comments, as recently reviewed [44] and summarized in Table 5.5.

Cerebral vein thrombosis requires anticoagulant therapy even in the presence of radiological signs of intracranial hemorrhage because these are considered secondary to the obstruction of the venous outflow. However, in a recent review, Martinelli et al. [45] suggested that, in the absence of clear data on efficacy and safety of early anticoagulation in these patients, anticoagulation should be delayed until a stabilization or reduction of hemorrhage is documented. The duration of oral anticoagulant depends on whether the thrombotic episode was unprovoked or secondary to a transient risk factors. In case of recurrent thrombosis, lifelong oral anticoagulation is recommended.

Abdominal vein thrombosis, including extrahepatic portal vein occlusion, Budd–Chiari Syndrome, and mesenteric vein thrombosis, is frequently encountered in MPNs. Diagnosis may be difficult because the most frequent symptom, i.e. abdominal pain, is aspecific. Doppler ultrasonography, CT scan, and MRI are usually required to achieve a diagnosis. Full-dose anticoagulation is recommended despite the high risk of gastrointestinal bleeding. In a survey of the current outcome of portal vein thrombosis in 136 patients, 42 (31%) with an MPN, anticoagulant therapy reduced the risk of recurrence

Table 5.5 Management of thrombosis in unusual sites.

Cerebral vein thrombosis
Common presenting symptoms
Severe headache (>90% of cases)
Paresis, aphasia
Seizures, mental status disorder
Recommended diagnostic procedures
Magnetic resonance imaging
Angiography
Treatment
Standard anticoagulant therapy[a]
Abdominal vein thrombosis (hepatic, portal, and mesenteric)
Common presenting symptoms
Abdominal pain
Hepatomegaly and ascites (in hepatic thrombosis)
Recommended diagnostic procedures
CT scan
Hepatic ultrasonography (in hepatic thrombosis)
Angiography
Treatment
Standard anticoagulant therapy[a]
Invasive procedures if needed (in hepatic thrombosis)
Liver transplantation if needed (in hepatic thrombosis)

[a]*Standard anticoagulant therapy*: full heparinization followed by oral anticoagulation with PT INR range 2.0–3.0 (long-life?)

or extension of thrombosis by two thirds without any real increase in the incidence or severity of bleeding [46]. In the Budd–Chiari syndrome, MPN may not be clinically obvious because concurrent hypersplenism, occult gastrointestinal bleeding, and hemodilution can mask blood count abnormality. Of significant diagnostic help is the determination of JAK2 V617F mutation found in 45% of Budd–Chiari syndrome and 34% of portal vein thrombosis [47]. Intensive medical management including anticoagulation is mandatory but more aggressive procedures, such as trans-jugular intrahepatic portosystemic shunt, angioplasty with or without stenting, surgical shunts, up to liver transplantation should be considered in the most severe cases.

Management of Bleeding
Hemorrhage is both a less frequent and generally less severe clinical complication than thrombosis in patients with MPD. Untreated low-risk PV patients in the control arm of the ECLAP trial showed a rate of major and minor bleeding of 0.3 and 1.5 events per 100 persons per year, respectively [22]. Recent large prospective studies enrolling high-risk patients, mostly treated with HU plus aspirin, reported rates of major bleeding of, respectively, 0.8 and 0.9 events per 100 persons per year in PV and ET [3, 5]. The main sites affected are skin, mucous membranes, and gastrointestinal tract. Intracranial bleeding occurs rarely but can be severe and potentially fatal, requiring hospital admission. Intra-articular, retroperitoneal, and deep intramuscular hematomas, like those seen in hemophilia, are distinctly unusual.

Hemorrhagic symptoms are more frequent in patients with platelet counts in excess of $1,000–1,500 \times 10^9$/L, and this may be related to an acquired deficiency of von Willebrand factor (vWF) [48]. This is not restricted to MPD and has also been described in patients with reactive thrombocytosis, suggesting a primary effect of absolute platelet number as opposed to dysfunctional clonal platelets. Normalization of the platelet count was accompanied by restoration of a normal plasma vWF multimeric distribution and regression of the hemorrhagic tendency. A practical consequence of these observations is the recommendation to give prophylactic cytoreductive therapy to all ET patients whose platelet count is over $1,500 \times 10^9$/L [1]. Serious bleeding may be triggered by simultaneous antithrombotic therapy with anticoagulants or antiplatelet agents. These drugs should be avoided in patients with previous hemorrhagic events, or with anatomical conditions with a high bleeding risk (e.g. gastric ulcers or esophageal varices secondary to abdominal vein thrombosis and portal hypertension). The combination of aspirin with anagrelide can increase the risk of bleeding, as shown in the PT1 clinical trial [3].

Treatment of bleeding events in MPDs should start with withdrawal of any concomitant antithrombotic therapy and correction of extreme thrombocytosis if associated with vWF deficiency [48]. This latter situation is usually treated with HU but platelet apheresis may be indicated in an emergency. Other potential measures include antifibrinolytic agents, such as tranexamic acid, but desmopressin or vWF-containing therapeutic products are of limited value. Platelet transfusions have been rarely used although the defective platelet function in MPDs may represent a rationale for their indication. The utility of recombinant factor VII has not been reported on in MPD patients with uncontrolled life-threatening bleeding and merits further study. Occasional patients may present with a simultaneous occurrence of both bleeding and thrombosis: in this difficult cases, treatment should be based on the prevalent clinical symptoms and tailored on individual basis.

Management of Surgery

Patients with MPDs have an increased risk of morbidity and mortality when they require surgical procedures. In a retrospective survey on the outcome of 311 surgical interventions in 105 patients with PV and 150 with ET, Italian investigators recorded 12 cases (3.8%) with postsurgery arterial thrombosis, 12 (3.8%) with venous thromboembolism, 23 (7.4%) with major hemorrhagic complications requiring transfusions, and 5 (1.6%) surgery-related deaths within 3 months from the procedure [49]. Although it is conceivable that different types of surgical interventions may carry different risks of bleeding and thrombosis, the data in literature are too scanty to allow some stratification of patients accordingly.

A high-risk intervention is splenectomy, particularly when it is needed for the management of symptomatic splenomegaly because of portal vein thrombosis or myelofibrosis. In one large series of patients with myelofibrosis [50], perioperative fatal and nonfatal bleeding occurred in 4.5% and 14.5% of patients, respectively; fatal and nonfatal major thrombotic events were reported in an additional 1.3% and 7.2% and overall operative mortality was as high as 9%. Thrombocytopenia (platelet count $<100 \times 10^9$/L) was the only preoperative variable that was significantly correlated with postoperative thrombosis. Severe thrombocytopenia (platelet count $<50 \times 10^9$/L) and bone marrow hypocellularity or normocellularity were significantly associated with a worse perioperative survival.

The optimal management of MPD during surgery is uncertain because of the lack of controlled trials. The appropriate control of erythrocytosis and thrombocytosis with phlebotomy and/or myelosuppression has been recommended [48]. Platelet count should be kept below 400×10^9/L, particularly when splenectomy is planned, because of the potential for postoperative extreme thrombocytosis. This may lead to the development or exacerbation of a vWF deficiency and associated hemorrhagic diathesis. Aspirin should be withheld for at least 1 week before elective surgery involving a high risk of bleeding or in which even minor bleeding could result in life-threatening complications, such as neurosurgery, or requiring heparin prophylaxis. The drug can be restarted 24 h after stopping heparin [1]. LMWH at a prophylactic dose (4,000 U s.c. starting 12 h before surgery) is probably indicated in all patients with MPD because of the high thrombotic risk, although there are no prospective studies in this setting. Finally, these patients must be followed carefully for the paradoxical predisposition to both bleeding and thrombotic perioperative complications.

References

1. Barbui T, Barosi G, Grossi A, et al. Practice guidelines for the therapy of essential thrombocythemia. A statement from the Italian Society of Hematology, the Italian Society of Experimental Hematology and the Italian Group for Bone Marrow Transplantation. Haematologica 2004; 89: 215–232
2. McMullin MF, Bareford D, Campbell P, et al. Guidelines for the diagnosis, investigation and management of polycythemia/erythrocytosis. Br J Haematol 2005; 130: 174–195
3. Harrison CN, Campbell PJ, Buck G, et al. Hydroxyurea compared with anagrelide in high-risk essential thrombocythemia. N Engl J Med 2005; 353: 33–45
4. Cortelazzo S, Finazzi G, Ruggeri M, et al. Hydroxyurea in the treatment of patients with essential thrombocythemia at high risk of thrombosis: a prospective randomized trial. N Engl J Med 1995; 332: 1132–1136
5. Marchioli R, Finazzi G, Landolfi R, et al. Vascular and neoplastic risk in a large cohort of patients with polycythemia vera. J Clin Oncol 2005; 23: 2224–2232
6. Finazzi G, Barbui T. Evidence and expertise in the management of polycythemia vera and essential thrombocythemia. Leukemia 2008; 22: 1494–1502
7. Carobbio A, Finazzi G, Antonioli A et al., Thrombocytosis and leukocytosis interaction in vascular complications of essential thrombocythemia. Blood 2008; 112: 3135–3137
8. Barbui T, Carobbio A, Rambaldi A, Finazzi G. Perspectives on thrombosis in essential thrombocythemia and polycythemia vera: is leukocytosis a causative factor? Blood 2009; 114: 759–763
9. Kundranda MN, Maiti B, Iqbal N et al., The association of leukocytosis, thrombocytosis and JAK2V617F mutation with thrombotic events in myeloproliferative disorders (MPD's). Blood 2008; 112: abstr. 2803
10. Gangat N, Wolanskyj AP, Schwager SM et al., Leukocytosis at diagnosis and the risk of subsequent thrombosis in patients with low-risk essential thrombocythemia and polycythemia vera. Cancer 2009; 115: 5740–5745
11. Passamonti F, Rumi E, Pascutto C, et al. Increase in leukocyte count over time predicts thrombosis in patients with low-risk essential thrombocythemia. J Thromb Haemost 2009; 7: 1587–1589
12. Vannucchi AM, Antonioli E, Guglielmelli P et al., Clinical correlates of JAK2V617F presence or allele burden in myeloproliferative neoplasms: a critical reappraisal. Leukemia 2008; 22: 1299–1307
13. Lussana F, Caberlon S, Pagani C et al., Association of V617F Jak2 mutation with the risk of thrombosis among patients with essential thrombocythemia or idiopathic myelofibrosis: a systematic review. Thromb Res 2009; 124: 409–417

14. De Stefano V, Za T, Rossi Eet al., Increased risk of recurrent thrombosis in patients with essential thrombocythemia carrying the homozygous JAK2 V617F mutation. Ann Hematol 2010; 89: 141–146

15. Vannucchi AM, Antonioli E, Guglielmelli Pet al., Characteristics and clinical correlates of MPL 515W>L/K mutation in essential thrombocythemia. Blood 2008; 112: 844–847

16. Beer PA, Campbell PJ, Scott LMet al., MPL mutations in myeloproliferative disorders: analysis of the PT-1 cohort. Blood 2008; 112: 141–149

17. Campbell PJ, Bareford D, Erber WNet al., Reticulin accumulation in essential thrombocythemia: prognostic significance and relationship to therapy. J Clin Oncol 2009; 27: 2991–2999

18. Berk PD, Goldberg JD, Donovan PB, et al. Therapeutic recommendations in polycythemia vera based on Polycythemia Vera Study Group protocols. Semin Hematol 1986; 23: 132–143

19. Najean Y, Rain J-D. The very long term evolution of polycythemia vera: an analysis of 318 patients initially treated by phlebotomy or ^{32}P between 1969 and 1981. Semin Hematol 1997; 34: 6–16

20. Pearson TC, Wetherley-Mein G. Vascular occlusive episodes and venous haematocrit in primary proliferative polycythaemia. Lancet 1978; 2: 1219–1222

21. Di Nisio M, Barbui T, Di Gennaro L, et al. The hematocrit and platelet target in polycythemia vera. Br J Haematol 2007; 136: 249–259

22. Landolfi R, Marchioli R, Kutti J, et al. Efficacy and safety of low-dose aspirin in polycythemia vera. N Engl J Med 2004; 350: 114–124

23. Finazzi G, Caruso V, Marchioli R, et al. Acute leukemia in polycythemia vera. An analysis of 1,638 patients enrolled in a prospective observational study. Blood 2005; 105: 2664–2670

24. Kiladjian JJ, Chevret S, Dosquet Cet al., Long-term outcome in polycythemia vera: final analysis of a randomized trial comparing hydroxyurea (HU) to pipobroman (Pi). Blood 2008; 112: abstr. 1746

25. Maugeri N, Giordano G, Petrilli MPet al., Inhibition of tissue factor expression by hydroxyurea in polimorphonuclear leukocytes from patients with myeloproliferative disorders: a new effect for an old drug? J Thromb Haemost 2006; 4: 2593–2598

26. Bjorkholm J, Derolf AR, Ekstrand Cet al., Clinical risk for AML/MDS transformation in Philadelphia negative chronic myeloproliferative neoplasms. A population-based nested case-control study in Sweden. 14th Congress European Hematology Association, Berlin June 4–7, 2009; abstr. 1085

27. Lanzkron S, Strouse JJ, Wilson Ret al., Systematic review: hydroxyurea for the treatment of adults with sickle cell disease. Ann Intern Med 2008; 148: 939–955

28. Barosi G, Besses C, Birgegard Get al., A unified definition of clinical resistance/intolerance to hydroxyurea in essential thrombocythemia: results of a consensus process by an international working group. Leukemia 2007; 21: 277–280

29. Lengfelder E, Berger U, Hehlmann R. Interferon alpha in the treatment of polycythemia vera. Ann Hematol 2000; 79: 103–109

30. Silver RT. Long-term effects of the treatment of polycythemia vera with recombinant interferon-alpha. Cancer 2006; 107: 451–458

31. Lengfelder E, Griesshammer M, Hehlmann R. Interferon-alpha in the treatment of essential thrombocythemia. Leuk Lymphoma 1996; 22 (Suppl.1): 135–142

32. Kiladjian JJ, Cassinat B, Turlure P, et al. High molecular response rate of polycythemia vera patients treated with pegylated interferon alpha-2a. Blood 2006; 108: 2037–2040

33. Samuelsson J, Mutschler M, Birgegard G, et al. Limited effects on JAK2 mutational status after pegylated interferon α-2b therapy in polycythemia vera and essential thrombocythemia. Haematologica 2006; 91: 1281–1282

34. Kiladjian JJ, Cassinat B, Chevret Set al., Pegylated interferon alpha-2a induces complete hematologic and molecular responses with low toxicity in polycythemia vera. Blood 2008; 112: 3065–3072

35. Quintas-Cardama A, Kantarjian H, Manshouri Tet al., Pegylated interferon alpha-2a yields high rates of hematologic and molecular response in patients with advanced essential thrombocythemia and polycythemia vera. J Clin Oncol 2009; 27: 5418–5424

36. Fruchtman SM, Petitt RM, Gilbert HS, et al. Anagrelide: analysis of long term efficacy, safety and leukemogenic potential in myeloproliferative diseases. Leuk Res 2005; 5: 481–491

37. Campbell PJ, Scott LM, Buck G, et al. Definition of subtypes of essential thrombocythaemia and relation to polycythemia vera based on JAK2 V617F mutation status: a prospective study. Lancet 2005; 366: 1945–1953

38. Gisslinger H, Gotic M, Holowiecki Jet al., Final results of the ANAHYDRET study: non-inferiority of anagrelide compared to hydroxyurea in newly diagnosed WHO essential thrombocythemia patients. Blood 2008; 112: abstr. 661

39. Barosi G, Birgegard G, Finazzi Get al., Response criteria for essential thrombocythemia and polycythemia vera: result of a European LeukemiaNet consensus conference. Blood 2009; 113: 4829–4833

40. Gangat N, Wolanskyj AP, Schwager S, Tefferi A. Predictors of pregnancy outcome in essential thrombocythemia: a single institution study of 63 pregnancies. Eur J Haematol 2009; 82: 350–353

41. Passamonti F, Randi ML, Rumi Eet al., Increased risk of pregnancy complications in patients with essential thrombocythemia carrying the JAK2 (617V>F) mutation. Blood 2007; 110: 485–489

42. Griesshammer M, Struve S, Harrison CM. Essential thrombocythemia/polycythemia vera and pregnancy: the need for an observational study in Europe. Semin Thromb Hemost 2006; 32: 422–429

43. Tefferi A, Passamonti F. Essential thrombocyythemia and pregnancy: observations from recent studies and management recommenadtions. Am J Hematol 2009; 84: 629–630

44. Barbui T, Finazzi G. Myeloproliferative disease in pregnancy and other management issues. Hematology Am Soc Hematol Educ Program 2006; 246–252

45. Martinelli I, Franchini M, Mannucci PM. How I treat rare venous thrombosis. Blood 2008; 112: 4818–4823

46. Condat B, Pessione F, Hillaire Set al., Current outcome of portal vein thrombosis in adults: risk and benefit of anticoagulant therapy. Gastroenterology 2001; 120: 490–497

47. Kiladjian JJ, Cervantes F, Leebek FWGet al., The impact of JAK2 and MPL mutations on diagnosis and prognosis of splanchnic vein thrombosis: a report on 241 cases. Blood 2008; 111: 4922–4929

48. Elliott MA, Tefferi A. Thrombosis and haemorrhage in polycythaemia vera and essential thrombocythaemia. Br J Haematol 2004; 128: 275–290

49. Ruggeri M, Rodeghiero F, Tosetto Aet al., Postsurgery outcomes in patients with polycythemia vera and essential thrombocythemia: a retrospective survey. Blood 2008; 111: 666–671

50. Tefferi A, Mesa RA, Nagorney DM, Schroeder G, Silverstein MN. Splenectomy in myelofibrosis with myeloid metaplasia: a single-institution experience with 223 patients. Blood 2000; 95: 226–233

Chapter 6

Conventional and Investigational Therapy for Primary Myelofibrosis

Giovanni Barosi

Keywords: Primary myelofibrosis • SDF-1 • CXCR4 • TGF-β (beta) • JAK2V617F • MPLW515L/K • Androgens • Nandrolone • Fluoxymesterolone • Methandrostenolone • Oxymetolone • Metenolone • Danazol • Erythropoietin • rHuEpo • Darbepoetin • Thalidomide • Anemia • Transfusion-dependent anemia • Symptomatic splenomegaly • Leukemic transformation • Pulmonary hypertension • Erythropoiesis-stimulating agents • EUMNET • IWG-MRT • Iron overload • Deferoxamine • Deferiprone • Deferasirox • Hydroxyurea • Busulphan • Interferon • Pegylated interferon • Splenic radiotherapy • Splenectomy • Portal vein thrombosis • Post-splenectomy hepatomegaly • 2-chlorodexoxyadenosine • Liver radiotherapy • Extramedullary hematopoiesis • Abdominal radiotherapy • Paraspinal extramedullary hematopoiesis • Lenalidomide • Pomalidomide • Tipifarnib • Bortezomib • Vascular Endothelial Growth Factor • Epigenetics • Azacitidine • Decitabine • Vorinostat • Givinostat

Background

Primary myelofibrosis (PMF), also known as myelofibrosis with myeloid metaplasia or agnogenic myeloid metaplasia, is a clonal myeloproliferative neoplasm that, in patients with fully expressed disease, is characterized by profound remodeling of bone marrow architecture and derangement of hematopoiesis. Bone marrow appears with almost constant expanded population of megakaryocytes and clusters of dystrophic and dysmature elements, deposition of excessive amounts of collagen, and other extracellular matrix proteins resulting in marrow reticulin or collagen fibrosis, increase in microvessel density, and osteosclerosis. Specific hallmarks of hematopoiesis derangement consist in the aberrantly decreased expression of disease-associated surface receptors on hematopoietic stem cell, such as SDF-1 receptor CXCR4, TGF-β (beta) receptor, and TPO receptor MPL, associated with high levels of stromal molecules, like SDF-1, elastase, and metalloproteinases. These stem cell and microenvironmental alterations bring to disruption of bone marrow niches with ensuing

S. Verstovsek and A. Tefferi (eds.), *Myeloproliferative Neoplasms: Biology and Therapy*,
Contemporary Hematology, DOI 10.1007/ 978-1-60761-266-7_6,
© Springer Science+Business Media, LLC 2011

mobilization and homing of neoplastic hematopoietic stem cells in new or reinitialized niches in the spleen and liver. These features result in extramedullary hematopoiesis (EMH) with splenomegaly, anemia with a leukoerythroblastic blood picture, and possible neutropenia and thrombocytopenia.

Recently, the definition of PMF has been extended to patients who do not express all the biological characteristics of the disease and who bear a disease phenotype referred to as prefibrotic PMF. This disease variant is characterized by morphological alterations of megakaryocytes in the absence of bone marrow fibrosis and an attenuated clinical profile that resembles that of essential thrombocythemia.

The discovery of recurrent mutations in janus kinase 2 (*JAK*2V617F) or MPL (*MPL*W515L/K) has rapidly improved the knowledge on the pathogenesis of the disease. The *JAK*2V617F mutation is located in the JH2 pseudo-kinase domain of JAK2 and likely results in the loss of auto-inhibitory control of JAK2. Expression of V617F-mutated allele in cytokine-dependent cell lines and experiments with mice transplanted with marrow cells transduced with a retrovirus expressing the mutated allele, or with transgenic mice, have all suggested that the *JAK*2V617F mutation is an integral component of the myeloproliferative process that underlies PMF and other myeloproliferative neoplasms (MPNs). The frequency of *JAK*2V617F mutation is estimated at approximately 60% in PMF.

PMF is an infrequent disease, with an estimated incidence in the Western countries that ranges from 0.4 to 1.46 new cases per 100,000 persons/year. It affects mainly elderly people, since the median age at presentation is about 65 years, but 22% of patients are 55 year old or younger at diagnosis. The major causes of death are represented by infections, bleeding, thrombotic events, portal hypertension, pulmonary hypertension, and leukemia transformation. Median survival of patients with MF ranges from 3.5 to 6 years in modern series. However, there is a wide variability, with some patients dying within 1 or 2 years from diagnosis, while others surviving for even decades.

Medical Needs

PMF can affect patients in a variety of ways. Approximately 25% of patients are entirely asymptomatic and come to medical attention because of an enlarged spleen detected during routine physical examination or because of an abnormal blood cell count or peripheral blood smear. However, in the majority of the patients, the disease interferes with the quality of life and social activities. Some of the symptoms and disease complications, such as hemorrhagic or thrombotic events, infections, and portal hypertension, need treatments that are not specific for PMF. On the contrary, relief of anemia or splenomegaly, treatment of extramedullary nonhepato-splenic hematopoiesis, treatment of pulmonary hypertension, and therapy for the accelerated phase and of blast transformation of the disease are PMF-specific medical needs (Table 6.1).

Severe anemia (hemoglobin less than 10 g/dL) affects 20% of patients at diagnosis or develops in 50% of patients after 3.5 years from the diagnosis. Anemia may be arigenerative or may be caused by ineffective red cell production and shortened red blood cell (RBC) survival. However, hypochromic microcytic anemia resulting from iron deficiency secondary to blood loss may develop in 5% of the PMF patients.

Table 6.1 Medical needs requiring specific disease-targeted therapies in PMF.

Common
Relief of severe anemia
Relief of transfusion-dependent anemia
Relief of symptomatic splenomegaly
Relentless of spleen enlargement in progressive splenomegaly
Reversion of accelerated phase or blast transformation of the disease
Rare
Treatment of extramedullary nonhepato-splenic hematopoiesis
Therapy of portal hypertension
Therapy of pulmonary hypertension
Undetermined
Treatment of transfusion-dependent iron overload

Transfusion-dependency is the fate of many PMF anemic patients who do not respond to treatment for anemia. In thalassemia, significant iron overload occurs after as few as 10–20 RBC units, and patients develop cardiac, hepatic, and endocrine dysfunction. In PMF, the role of iron overload in morbidity and mortality remains largely undefined. The only available evidence is that PMF patients who received at least 24 RBC units showed MRI T2*-detectable hepatic iron, and that only patients with severe hepatic iron overload showed cardiac T2* value indicative of dangerous myocardial iron deposition [1].

Symptomatic splenomegaly, i.e., spleen extending more than 10 cm from the left costal margin, affects 10% of patients at diagnosis, or develop in 50% of patients after approximately 4 years from the diagnosis. Increase of spleen volume in PMF is mostly acknowledged as the result of splenic EMH. Neoangiogenesis, however, gives a significant contribution to the spleen volume expansion as documented by the measurement of capillary vascular density in spleen sections. With enlargement of the spleen, abdominal discomfort ensues, characterized by pressure of the spleen on the stomach that may lead to delayed gastric emptying and early satiety. In addition, the bulk of the spleen can result in areas of ischemia and painful episodes of splenic infarction, simulating an acute abdominal emergency. Pressure of the spleen on the colon or small bowel may be responsible for severe disabling diarrhea. Finally, splenomegaly can result in the development or exacerbation of cytopenias from spleen sequestration.

Accelerated phase of the diseased and leukemic transformation of PMF are subsequent phases of blast accumulation that occur in approximately 10–15% of patients and bear a dramatic symptomatic burden of disease, and short life expectancy. In a recent series of 91 consecutive PMF patients who experienced leukemic transformation, the disease was fatal in 98% of patients after a median of 2.6 months [2].

On turn, patients with PMF may present medical needs that are oriented to contrast rare presentations or disease complications. Extramedullary nonhepato-splenic hematopoiesis might cause symptoms in various organs, particularly in advanced phases of the disease and after splenectomy. The most common sites are pulmonary, gastrointestinal, central nervous, and genitourinary systems.

PMF may be associated with the development of pulmonary hypertension. Several mechanisms for this complication have been proposed, including thromboembolic occlusion of the pulmonary vasculature, EMH diffusely involving the lung, and pulmonary fibrosis due to the elaboration

Table 6.2 International Working Group (IWG) consensus criteria for treatment response in PMF [3].

Complete remission (CR):

- Complete resolution of disease-related symptoms and signs including palpable hepatosplenomegaly.
- Peripheral blood count remission defined as hemoglobin level at least 11 g/dL, platelet count at least 100×10^9/L, and absolute neutrophil count at least 1.0×10^9/L. In addition, all the three blood counts should be no higher than the upper normal limit.
- Normal leukocyte differential including disappearance of nucleated red blood cells, blasts, and immature myeloid cells in the peripheral smear, in the absence of splenectomy.
- Bone marrow histological remission defined as the presence of age-adjusted normocellularity, no more than 5% myeloblasts, and an osteomyelofibrosis grade no higher than 1.

Partial remission (PR):

- Requires all of the above criteria for CR except the requirement for bone marrow histological remission. However, a repeat bone marrow biopsy is required in the assessment of PR and may or may not show favorable changes that do not, however, fulfill criteria for CR.

Clinical improvement (CI):

Requires one of the following in the absence of both disease progression and CR/PR assignment.

- A minimum 20 g/L increase in hemoglobin level or becoming transfusion-independent (applicable only for patients with baseline hemoglobin level less than 100 g/dL).
- Either a minimum 50% reduction in palpable splenomegaly of a spleen that is at least 10 cm at baseline or a spleen that is palpable at more than 5 cm at baseline becomes not palpable.
- A minimum 100% increase in platelet count and an absolute platelet count of at least $50,000 \times 10^9$/L (applicable only for patients with baseline platelet count below 50×10^9/L).
- A minimum 100% increase in ANC and an ANC of at least 0.5×10^9/L (applicable only for patients with baseline absolute neutrophil count below 1×10^9/L).

---

of fibrogenic cytokines from dysfunctional circulating megakaryocytes and platelets. Patients with PMF-associated pulmonary hypertension are present with progressive dyspnoea, signs of biventricular heart failure, and rapidly increasing hepato-splenomegaly. Many of these patients succumb to cardiopulmonary complications within less than 2 years of the documentation of pulmonary artery hypertension.

Besides these therapy-oriented medical needs, an operational medical need in PMF is that patients who receive a treatment for the disease should not be treated for an inappropriately long time when therapy fails. Accordingly, the development of a standardized definition for monitoring and assessing treatment responses, based on rigorous, consistent, and feasible criteria, has been exploited (Tables 6.2 and 6.3) [3,4].

Conventional Therapeutic Strategies

Except for the minority of patients who can receive an allogeneic stem cell transplantation, PMF remains an incurable disease, with its therapy being merely palliative and primarily aimed at alleviation of the symptoms and

Table 6.3 Clinico-hematologic response criteria for PMF proposed by the European Myelofibrosis Network (EUMNET) [4].

Complete response

Complete response in anemia, splenomegaly, constitutional symptoms, platelet, and leukocyte count. (Complete response in anemia: hemoglobin ≥12 g/dL for transfusion-independent patients or ≥11 g/dL for transfusion-dependent patients; complete response in splenomegaly: spleen not palpable; complete response in constitutional symptoms: absence of constitutional symptoms (fever, drenching night sweats, or ≥10% weight loss). Complete response in platelet count: platelet count 150–400 × 10^9/L; complete response in leukocyte count: leukocyte count 4–10 × 10^9/L).

Major response

- Any response in anemia and splenomegaly without progression in constitutional symptoms *OR*
- Complete response in anemia or partial response in anemia that is transfusion-dependent, and response in constitutional symptoms without progression in splenomegaly, *OR*
- Any response in splenomegaly and response in constitutional symptoms without progression in anemia. (Partial response in anemia: Either a ≥2 g/dL increase in hemoglobin level or >50% decrease in transfusion requirement; partial response in splenomegaly: either ≥50% decrease in spleen size if baseline ≤10 cm from LCM or ≥30% decrease if baseline ≥10 cm from LCM; partial response in platelet count: a ≥50% decrease in the platelet count if baseline >800 × 10^9/L or platelet count increase by ≥50 × 10^9/L if baseline <100 × 10^9/L; partial response in leukocyte count: a ≥50% decrease in leukocyte count if baseline >20 × 10^9/L or leukocyte count increase by ≥1 × 10^9/L if baseline <4 × 10^9/L. Progression in anemia: a hemoglobin decrease of ≥2 g/dL *or* a ≥50% increase in transfusion requirement *or* becoming transfusion-dependent; progression in splenomegaly: a ≥50% increase in spleen size if baseline ≤ 10 cm from LCM *or* a ≥30% increase if baseline >10 cm from LCM; progression in constitutional symptoms: appearance of constitutional symptoms).

Moderate response

- Complete response in anemia with progression in splenomegaly, *OR*
- Partial response in anemia without progression in splenomegaly, *OR*
- Any response in splenomegaly without progression in anemia and constitutional symptoms.

Minor response

Any response in WBC or platelet count without progression in anemia, splenomegaly, or constitutional symptoms.

No response

Any response that does not satisfy minor response

improvement in the patients' quality of life, but without having a real impact on survival. This is the reason why patients who are asymptomatic at diagnosis should be maintained untreated. A thorough communication with the patient is necessary to make him aware of the nature of the disease and of the disease's chronic course. Untreated patients should be followed up to underscore the appearance of therapy-requiring symptoms.

Treatment of Anemia

Androgens

Nandrolone, fluoxymesterolone, methandrostenolone, oxymetholone, and metenolone acetate have been reported to improve the anemia of PMF in 30–60% of cases. In 1982, Besa and coworkers reported that 57% of 23 patients with PMF who received androgen therapy exhibited sustained increase in the hematocrit of greater than 30% and elimination of the need for transfusion [5]. In that study, 92% of the patients with normal karyotypes and 22% of the patients with abnormal karyotypes responded to androgen therapy, suggesting that chromosomal analysis could predict a patient's response to androgen therapy. Good responses to androgen therapy have been confirmed recently by Shimoda and colleagues who reported 39 anemic patients treated with anabolic steroids, mostly metenolone acetate [6]. The authors defined a "good" response as a hemoglobin increase of ≥1.5 g/dL, cessation of transfusion dependence, and a hemoglobin concentration of >10 g/dL maintained for at least 8 weeks. Favorable responses were achieved in 17 patients (44%), with 20.5% good responses. None of the pretreatment variables, such as the lack of transfusion dependence, a higher hemoglobin concentration at the start of treatment, or the absence of cytogenetic abnormalities, were associated with the response.

Danazol, a synthetic attenuated androgen, has been proposed as a substitute of anabolic steroids due to the advantage of also being able to correct thrombocytopenia in some cases and producing a less virilising effect. Danazol has unique properties similar to those of corticosteroids, such as inhibition of both interleukin-1 and TNF-α (alpha) production, and decreases the number of the Fcγ (gamma) receptors. Cervantes and colleagues reported 33 anemic patients with PMF who received an initial dose of 600 mg/day of danazol, with a favorable response in 37%, with 27% having a complete response after a median time of 5 months [7]. A complete response was defined as the cessation of transfusion requirements with hemoglobin >11 g/dL. Variables associated with response were lack of transfusion requirement and higher hemoglobin level.

Danazol is usually well tolerated. The most frequent toxicity consists of a moderate increase in the liver enzymes during the first months of treatment that improves following a reduction in the danazol dose. Headache and a mild increase in the muscle mass have been occasionally observed. Screening for prostate cancer before using androgen therapy in males is recommended, and monitoring toxic effects on transaminases is a mandatory procedure.

Erythropoiesis-Stimulating Agents

Erythropoiesis-stimulating agents (ESAs) are widely used for the treatment of PMF-associated anemia, even though serum erythropoietin (s-Epo) levels in patients with PMF are appropriately elevated for the degree of anemia, suggesting that exogenous administration of ESA might have limited value in this disease. The experience with the use of recombinant human erythropoietin (rHuEpo) in PMF has been reported in a pool analysis by Cervantes and colleagues [8], and in two other studies [9,10] before 2009 for a total of 96 patients (Table 6.4). The response rates of these studies ranged from 16 to 60%. S-Epo levels <125 U/L, favorable cytogenetic abnormality (13q- or 20q-), absence of homozygous *JAK2* V617F mutation, low beta-2-microglobulin serum levels, and slight to moderate splenomegaly were variably found to be associated with a favorable response. The Mayo Clinic experience on use of rHuEpo has been recently reported by Huang and Tefferi [11]. A query from a master database of PMF patients identified 43 patients treated with r-Hu-Epo. Response was defined as a minimum 2.0 g/dL increase in hemoglobin level or becoming transfusion-independent over a minimum of 1-month period. The overall response rate to rHuEpo was 23%: 0% (0 of 16) among transfusion-dependent patients and 37% (10 of 27) among transfusion-independent patients. In the

Table 6.4 Results in studies using erythropoiesis-stimulating agents in PMF.

Drug	Study	No. of patients	Total response (%)	Major response (%)
RHuEpo	Cervantes et al. [8] (pooled analysis)	51	55	31
	Tefferi et al. [9]	25	16	NR
	Tsiara et al. [10]	20	60	NR
	Huang and Tefferi [11]	43	23	NR
Darbepoetin-α (alpha)	Cervantes et al. [12]	20	40	30

latter instance, response was seen only in the presence of <10 g/dL baseline hemoglobin level. Response was not correlated with baseline s-Epo level, PMF-specific treatment history, use of concurrent cytoreductive therapy, cytogenetic findings, or *JAK2*V617F presence.

Darbepoetin-α *(alpha) is* a novel hyperglycosylated erythropoiesis-stimulating protein, with greater *in vivo* activity and longer half-life than rHuEpo, allowing less frequent administration. Darbepoetin-α *(alpha)* was given to 20 PMF patients with hemoglobin £10 g/dL at a weekly subcutaneous dose of 150 μg, which was increased to 300 μg when no hemoglobin increase was noted at 4 weeks or a partial response had not been attained at 8 weeks [12]. Oral iron supplements were given whenever inadequate iron status was observed. By using the EUMNET response criteria (Table 6.3), eight patients (40%) showed a favorable response to treatment, including six complete and two partial responses. Median time to response was 2 months. In three patients the response followed a dose increase at 4 weeks. At univariate analysis, older age was the only factor associated with a favorable response. Treatment was well tolerated. One patient had a moderate increase in splenomegaly.

Thalidomide

Since the Food and Drug Administration (FDA) of the United States of America approved thalidomide as a therapeutic agent for erythema nodosum leprosum in 1998, a number of investigators have renewed interest in the clinical applications of the drug. The rationale for thalidomide therapy in PMF is based on the drug's anti-angiogenetic and immunomodulatory activity. It inhibits neoangiogenesis by downregulating VEGF, bFGF, and TNF-α (alpha) production.

Multiple trials have explored the use of thalidomide in the treatment of anemia in PMF (Table 6.5) [13–20]. The highest response rate was obtained by Mesa and coworkers combining low-dose thalidomide (50 mg per day) with prednisone [15]. With this regimen, 40% of patients with a RBC transfusion requirement became transfusion-independent. Recently, the response to thalidomide has been analyzed according to EUMNET criteria (Table 6.3) in a trial that enrolled 15 patients [20]. After low-dose thalidomide ± prednisolone, overall 40% of patients achieved major or moderate responses. All responses began within the first 12 weeks of treatment, suggesting that thalidomide could be stopped if there is no response by this time. Among responders, the median response duration was 16 weeks. The two patients not treated with prednisolone demonstrated a minor and no response, respectively. Five out of 13 patients (38%) were

Table 6.5 Results in studies using thalidomide in PMF.

Drug	Study	No. of pts.	Total response (%)
Thalidomide (standard-dose)	Merup et al. [13]	15	0
	Barosi et al. (pool analysis) [14]	49	29
	Strupp et al. [16]	10	60
	Abgrall et al. (randomized vs. placebo) [18]	18	5
	Thomas et al. [19]	35	20
Thalidomide (low-dose + prednisone)	Mesa et al. [15]	21	62
	Weinkove et al. [20]	15	40
Thalidomide (low-dose)	Marchetti et al. [17]	49	22

positive for the *JAK2*V617F mutation and were indistinguishable from negative patients.

The most common side effects of thalidomide are peripheral neuropathy, constipation, and somnolence. Thromboembolism is rarely reported in patients with PMF, however, assessment of thrombotic risk and thromboprophylaxis for high-risk patients is recommended.

Treatment Strategy for Anemia

Due to the possible side effects of treatments and the modest impact that moderate anemia has on quality of life and physical performance, it is commonly thought that in PMF a treatment for anemia should be established when hemoglobin reduces under 10 g/dL. In the absence of comparative trials between the treatment options, it is hard to provide evidence-based recommendations on how to approach PMF-associated anemia. Many centers prefer androgen, particularly danazol, as the first therapeutic option due to safety and low cost. In the case of a lack of response to androgen, thalidomide or ESA should be considered, being aware that the results of the trials suggest that ESA should be avoided in those patients who are transfusion-dependent. Other centers recommend that first-line therapy for PMF-associated anemia should include ESA if endogenous Epo level is below 100 mU/mL and a combination of either an androgen preparation or low-dose thalidomide with a tapering dose of prednisone.

Treatment of Transfusional Iron Overload

Direct evidence that treatment of iron overload in PMF results in reduction of morbidity or mortality is still lacking. In a retrospective review of the British Columbia provincial experience, transfusion dependence in PMF was associated with inferior survival, and within the transfusion-dependent group, the overall survival was superior in patients receiving iron-chelating therapy [21]. However, iron overload assessment was made by clinical criteria and serum ferritin levels rather than by imaging or biopsy. Thus, it remains difficult to be certain retrospectively whether individual deaths were related to toxicity from iron. In a study in 185 patients with PMF at the Mayo Clinic [22], 12% of the cases had serum ferritin >1,000 ng/mL and 17% were RBC transfusion-dependent at diagnosis. During median follow-up of 28 months, peak serum ferritin levels exceeded 1,000 ng/mL in 22% of the patients. On multivariable analysis, RBC transfusion need at diagnosis, but not increased serum ferritin or transfusion load, predicted shortened survival. This result was in favor of the hypothesis that the presence of a more severe erythropoietic defect, and not iron overload, has an adverse prognostic value.

Different options are currently available for chelation therapy, e.g., subcutaneous deferoxamine, oral once daily administration of the iron chelator deferasirox, or oral chelation with deferiprone. Adopting a precautionary principle, physicians sometimes use oral iron chelation, mostly deferasirox, for treating patients who attain high levels of serum ferritin after 10–20 units of blood transfusions and who have a long life expectancy. The appropriateness of such a therapy should be investigated prospectively.

In anecdotal reports in PMF, iron-chelation therapy resulted in the improvement in the hemoglobin level and reduction in the transfusion dependence [23–24]. These data open new insights regarding the benefit of iron-chelation therapy not only for transfusional iron overload of PMF patients but also for the increase in hemoglobin levels.

Treatment of Splenomegaly

Medical Therapies

Current medical therapies can ameliorate splenomegaly in PMF mainly through nonspecific myelosuppression, thereby decreasing the immature circulating myeloid pool accumulating in the spleen. Busulfan, chlorambucil, 6-thioguanine, radioactive phosphorus, melphalan, interferon-α, and hydroxyurea have each been used for this purpose.

Hydroxyurea. Hydroxyurea (hydroxycarbamide, HU) is a nonalchylating anti-neoplastic agent, which interrupts the normal mechanism of reduction of ribonucleotides and deoxyribonucleotides through the inactivation of ribonucleotide reductase, limiting DNA biosynthesis. It is usually well tolerated, and the dose is easy to be titrated to achieve the benefit for splenomegaly by lowering the leukocyte count as best tolerated. In old studies which used no comparable response criteria, up to 40% response on splenomegaly has been reported.

The response to HU has been analyzed recently according to the IWG-MRT criteria (Table 6.2) by Sirhan and colleagues in a cohort of 69 patients with PMF, 68% of whom were treated for symptomatic splenomegaly [25]. With a median HU starting daily dose of 1 g (range 250 mg to 3 g), the response was documented in 19 (28%) patients: 16 achieved clinical improvement and 3 partial response. The response rate was 48% in *JAK2*V617F positive patients as opposed to only 8% in mutation negative cases, and the presence of the V617F mutation retained significance on the multivariable analysis. The phenomenon of HU sensitivity in *JAK2*V617F mutation positive patients is supposed to simply be a reflection of quantitatively and qualitatively different myeloproliferation in mutation-positive, as opposed to mutation-negative, patients.

HU may carry more or less severe side effects: macrocytosis, neutropenia, leg and oral ulcers, cutaneous rash, skin dryness, nail pigmentation, cystitis, fever, and gastrointestinal symptoms. Moreover, a slight increase in skin cancer has been reported in patients on HU. Finally, the possible relationship between long-term therapy with HU and leukemic transformation is still a matter of debate.

Oral alkylators. The use of oral alkylators such as melphalan and busulphan as initial treatment to reduce splenomegaly in PMF has been limited by the increased risk of blast transformation and unfavorable toxicity profile. However, in 2002, Petti and coworkers [26] evaluated the use of low-dose melphalan in 99 patients with PMF, with a response rate of 66.7% and with 54% of patients achieving a response on splenomegaly. They used 2.5 mg three times a week, with progressive increase up to a maximum of 2.5 mg daily. However, it was concerning that blast transformation occurred in 26% of the study cohort. Based on these results, Chee and coworkers [27] in 2006 reported their experience with administering melphalan to a cohort of eight patients with PMF at a dose of 2 mg daily three times a week, and increasing the dosage to a maximum of 2 mg daily five times a week in nonresponders or patients who had relapsed. After a median follow-up duration of 21.5 months, the overall response ratio was 75%. In terms of effect on splenomegaly, among seven evaluable patients, a response was seen in four patients (57.1%). There was a trend towards more effective reduction in spleen size if initial splenomegaly was less marked.

The mode of action of melphalan in improving cytopenias and splenomegaly in PMF is likely multifactorial in nature; a combination of cytolytic effects on clonal cell proliferation and modulation of the immune response that affects hematopoiesis.

Oral busulphan has been used in PMF when classically used in the treatment of chronic myeloid leukemia in pre-imatinib era. Anecdotal reports signify its ability to reverse nonresponses with HU.

Interferons. Interferons (IFNs) have a wide range of biological activities, most of which provide a rationale for use in PMF. IFN-α (alpha) inhibits in vitro proliferation of hematopoietic progenitors, particularly the megakaryocytic lineage. Furthermore, IFN-α (alpha) is able to directly repress megakaryopoiesis by inhibiting thrombopoietin-induced MPL receptor signaling. Finally, IFN-α (alpha) antagonizes platelet-derived growth factor and inhibits the growth of marrow-derived fibroblasts.

Many clinical studies have been performed in PMF using various commercial forms of IFN-α (alpha) (Table 6.6) [28–32]. Most of the studies published to date used standard IFN-α (alpha)2a or 2b that were the first ones available for therapy. It can be noted that none of these forms is registered as yet by FDA, EMEA, or the health agencies of other countries for Ph-negative MPNs. Summarizing IFN studies that included more than 10 patients, the results have been disappointing. In 30% of the cases, spleen size decreased on treatment, whereas in almost the same proportion of patients, it did increase. Importantly, IFN toxicity in these studies was high, leading to rapid treatment discontinuation in more than 50% of the patients. IFN toxicity included common flu-like

Table 6.6 Published trials of standard IFN in PMF [27].

Author, year	Number of patients	Response rate (%)	Spleen size reduction (% of patients)	Discontinuation (%)	Type of IFN
Gilbert, 1998 [29]	22	NA	58	46	a2b
Tefferi et al., 2001 [30]	11	0	18	64	a2
Heis-Vahidi-Fard et al. 2001 [31]	9	0	20	67	γ
Radin et al. 2003 [32]	31	3	33	NA	a2

Abbreviations: *IFN* interferon, *NA* data not available

symptoms, worsening of cytopenias, fatigue, musculoskeletal pain, and development of auto-immune abnormalities.

More recently, pegylated forms of IFN have been developed. The addition of a polyethyleneglycol (peg) tail enhances plasma half-life with lower toxicity and increased drug stability and solubility, without affecting the therapeutic activity. These changes translate into improvement for patients, mainly because of longer intervals between administrations (weekly instead of every 24–48 h). The use of pegylated IFN (Peg-IFN) in PMF was reported in two different trials with quite divergent results [33–34]. In Jabbour and coworkers study (2000) with Peg-IFN-α (alpha) 2b, only 1 patient out of 11 achieved a complete response [33]. On the contrary, in a multicenter retrospective study with 18 patients treated with Peg-INF-α (alpha) 2a in seven French centers, the results favor a true efficacy [34]. All of the patients except two responded to achieve either complete remission or major response according to the EUMNET criteria, and only two patients stopped treatment because of the loss of efficacy. However, splenomegaly appeared sensitive to the drug only in two out of the 18 patients (11%).

The divergent results to IFN treatment are poorly understood. Acquisition of resistance to IFN-α (alpha) therapy had been dissected in molecular terms in a patient who received Peg-IFN-α (alpha) [35]. At the start of therapy, bone marrow DNA samples revealed the sole presence of *MPL*W515L mutation (60% mutant allelic ratio). The *MPL*W515L mutation burden decreased significantly during IFN-α (alpha) therapy. A del20 was acquired between months 6 and 123 of the therapy, at the time of IFN-α (alpha) clinical resistance. These findings are in line with the clinical observations that IFN-α (alpha) is more effective in the early stage of the disease.

Splenic Radiotherapy

Spleen radiotherapy has been used for treatment of the big spleen syndrome of PMF. Irradiation in fractions of 0.15–1 Gy administered daily or by an intermittent fractionation schedule (i.e., two or three times per week) to a total dose per treatment course of 2.5–6.5 Gy may be effective. In general, the experience from the literature is similar to what has been recently reported in a series of 23 patients by the Mayo Clinic [36]. These patients received a median of 277 cGy (range 30–1,365) over a median of 7.5 fractions (range 2–17). Initial response was 93.9% in terms of reduction in spleen size that lasted for a median of 6 months. However, treatment was associated with substantial myelosuppression in 43.5% of the patients that proved to be fatal in 13%. Nine patients (39.1%) were subsequently splenectomized and five suffered major perioperative complications including abdominal bleeding. Some patients were successfully treated with repeated treatment courses.

Splenectomy

In principle, all the patients with symptomatic splenomegaly who have been treated with cytoreductive therapy without sustained improvement are candidates to splenectomy. However, the decision for splenectomy is the result of a trade-off exercise between the expected benefits and the risk of mortality and morbidity.

A large number of series have reported the outcomes of splenectomy in PMF. The collection of 314 cases from the Mayo Clinic in three decades of experience provides the most representative figures of outcomes [37]. In that series, half of the patients were enrolled to splenectomy for symptomatic splenomegaly after a median time from the diagnosis of 26 months. Transfusion-dependent anemia, portal hypertension, and severe refractory thrombocytopenia were the other indications for splenectomy. Perioperative complications occurred in 27.7% of the patients and included bleeding (14%), thrombosis (9.9%), and infection (9.9%). The majority of post-operative bleeding occurred from the abdominal wound, while the great majority of post-operative thrombotic events occurred in the portal vein (67.8%).

High incidence of acute post-splenectomy portal vein thrombosis is probably due to local surgical factors, like the fact that the splenic vein remnant is attached to the portal vein. However, systemic factors can cooperate in PMF, like hypercoagulability, platelet activation, disturbance, and activation of the endothelium. In a series of 71 patients from different centers in Italy reported in 1993 [38], in which the cumulative incidence of thrombotic or hemorrhagic complications was 16.9%, new hemorrhagic or thrombotic events were predicted by age less than 50 years, a normal to high platelet count (>200 × 10^9/L) and huge splenomegaly (larger than 16 cm from the costal margin).

It is important to point out that neither in the series from Mayo Clinic nor in the Italian experience, an active diagnostic procedure (ecodoppler sonography) was mentioned as a tool for revealing post-splenectomy splanchnic vein thrombosis. By using an active screening, in a survey of the splenectomies in PMF performed in the last decade (64 patients), we discovered a 57% incidence of splanchnic vein thromboses (splenic vein, portal vein, and superior mesenteric vein). Most of the events were asymptomatic, thus not discoverable through clinical monitoring only (nonpublished observation).

In the Mayo Clinic series, surgical mortality was 6.7%. Surgical deaths consisted of infections (2.6%), hemorrhagic (2.2%), thrombotic (0.6%), or other complications (1.6%). Surgical mortality decreased between the three decades, so that in the last decade it was 5.5%. Among the survivors, 81% experienced a palliative benefit for their primary surgical indication, i.e., symptomatic splenomegaly, 50% for the indication of anemia, and 40.4% for the indication of portal hypertension. Among the patients who underwent splenectomy for refractory thrombocytopenia, 77% experienced a durable benefit.

Post-splenectomy rates of thrombocytosis (21%), accelerated hepatomegaly (8%), and leukemic transformation (11%) did not vary across the three decades during which the procedure was performed. Extensive and symptomatic hepatomegaly after splenectomy need high doses of cytoreductive agents. Benefit from the purine nucleoside analog, 2-chlorodeoxyadenosine (2-CdA), has been reported by the Mayo Clinic [39]. The drug has been successfully used with either of the two schedules commonly employed for this agent (4–6 monthly cycles of treatment with either 0.1 mg/kg/day intravenously by continuous infusion for 7 days or 5 mg/m^2 intravenously over 2 h for 5 consecutive days). In a recent update of the Mayo experience, responses were observed in 55% of patients for hepatomegaly. Responses were frequently durable and lasted for a median of 6 months after discontinuation of treatment.

Post-splenectomy refractory hepatomegaly can be exceptionally treated with fractionated radiotherapy (RT) to the liver in order to obtain symptom control and to prevent severe symptom recurrence. After 2 Gy fractionated RT to a treatment field encompassing nearly the whole liver, symptoms may improve and liver size decrease without severe side effects [40].

An unexpectedly high rate of blast transformation has been reported after splenectomy, with a relative risk in splenectomized patients increasing from 2.2 at 48 months to 14.3 at 12 years from diagnosis [41]. It appeared to be independent of factors related to spleen removal assignment. However, it is now known that patients with *JAK2*V617F mutation have a higher propensity to develop large splenomegaly, to be submitted to splenectomy, and to evolve towards blast transformation, as a result of accumulation of mutated alleles [42]. This recent evidence could allow us to interpret the high incidence of blast transformation after splenectomy as the result of the natural history of disease in patients with high V617F allele burden.

Current evidence would suggest that splenectomy should be considered primarily in patients with significant symptoms from the mass of the spleen, high RBC transfusion requirements, and symptomatic portal hypertension. However, the association of splenomegaly with cytopenias that worsen the disease burden and prevent adequate cytoreductive therapies reinforces the indication to splenectomy (Table 6.7).

Splenectomy preceding allogeneic stem cell transplantation has been documented to speed engraftment but without a significant improvement in outcomes. Given the risks of splenectomy, routine pretransplantation splenectomy is not recommended.

Given the potential dangers of splenectomy, the procedure should be considered only for patients who meet the criteria of adequate surgical candidates. The risk of incurring in post-operative thrombosis or hemorrhage should be deeply evaluated. A manifest or occult coagulopathy and a history of the previous portal thrombosis are the major risks for new thrombotic episodes or recurrence of thrombosis after splenectomy, respectively.

Treatment Strategy for Splenomegaly

Splenic enlargement must be treated when pressure symptoms ensue, or when it is progressive in order to prevent the development of massive, unmanageable splenomegaly. Medical therapy is the cornerstone therapeutic option for symptomatic splenomegaly in patients with PMF. HU has an efficacy and toxicity profile that renders the drug as the most common initial medical therapy used to decrease splenomegaly. Since treatment failures occur

Table 6.7 Indications to splenectomy in PMF.

Major
- Symptomatic and refractory splenomegaly with severe, transfusion-dependent anemia
- Symptomatic and refractory splenomegaly without cytopenias when substantial, i.e., significantly interfering with quality of life
- Symptomatic splenomegaly with thrombocytopenia or neutropenia when cytopenia is a major obstacle to splenomegaly treatment

Minor
- Severe, transfusion-dependent, and refractory anemia without significant splenomegaly
- Severe, life threatening, and refractory thrombocytopenia
- Portal hypertension

Uncertain
- Large splenomegaly before allogeneic stem cell transplantation

in approximately 60% of the cases, more aggressive approaches should be considered as a second line therapy. A role of alkylating agents, like melphalan and busulphan, as a second therapy after failure of HU has been claimed. However, evidence accumulated on the use of alkylating agents in ET discourages using HU and alkylators sequentially due to high risk of leukemia. A range of different myelosuppressive therapies most typically used for acute leukemia or higher risk MDS had been used anecdotally to treat PMF patients with refractory splenomegaly. Low-dose subcutaneous cytarabine and danorubicin administered as a single agent are included in this group. These strategies, however, have not vetted through structured clinical trials. Experimental therapies or allogeneic stem cell transplantation should better be considered in these cases. Splenectomy remains the choice in cases where no such options are feasible or the patient results refractory to experimental therapies and is not a candidate to transplantation. Spleen radiation therapy should be considered as a temporary measure to be employed in patients who are too ill to tolerate splenectomy.

Treatment of Extramedullary Nonhepato-splenic Hematopoiesis

The cornerstone therapy for extramedullary nonhepato-splenic hematopoiesis is radiotherapy. Myeloid progenitor cells that comprise EMH are radiosensitive, thus suitable for external beam radiotherapy. The diffuse infiltrative nature of EMH limits surgical resection, and medical therapy can be of palliative benefit but is neither always effective nor associated with a prompt response.

Abdominal irradiation has been utilized for control of ascites created by peritoneal seeding from EMH. In a recent series of 14 patients with advanced disease, a median of 150 cGy/course (range 50–1,000) was given in approximately six fractions [43]. Symptomatic relief (e.g., reduction in ascites or mass effect) was subjectively reported in 86% of the patients. Objective reduction in the ascites was achieved in 80% of the cases. Paraspinal EMH, as a potential cause of spinal cord compression, should be considered in all patients with PMF, and early recognition is critical to minimize neurologic dysfunction. MRI is currently the diagnostic modality of choice, and confirmation by biopsy is useful for excluding other possible causes (i.e., metastatic cancer). However, biopsy is not always necessary and decompressive therapy should not wait for histologic confirmation in the patient with cord compression. Decompression can be successfully accomplished through external beam radiotherapy, along with high-dose corticosteroid therapy to decrease associated edema.

Symptomatic EMH can arise in any number of other locations including the pleural space causing pleural effusions, the pericardium causing pericardial effusions, or the pelvis causing ureteral obstruction. Management of these complex situations requires early recognition, histologic diagnosis, and prompt therapy, which is usually radiotherapy.

Treatment of Pulmonary Hypertension

PMF patients with symptoms consistent with pulmonary hypertension should be evaluated for occult pulmonary EMH after excluding post-thrombotic or other causes of pulmonary hypertension. The current management of PH includes vasodilator including phosphodiesterase-type five inhibitors (which increase nitric oxide levels, e.g., sildenafil) and prostacyclin analogues. The Mayo Clinic has recently reported the experience with single fraction, low-dose (100 cGy), external beam radiation to the lungs for palliating PMF-associated pulmonary hypertension [44]. Currently a total of seven patients have received such treatment, and the majority have achieved improvement in performance status, decreased pulmonary artery pressures on echocardiography, and decreased pulmonary EMH on lung technitium^{99m}-sulfur colloid scans.

Management of Leukemic Transformation

Mesa et al. reported the most extensive experience with the management of PMF in leukemic transformation [2]. Supportive care alone or noninduction chemotherapy had similar outcomes to that of aggressive induction chemotherapy. However, a subset of patients (41% of those receiving induction chemotherapy) reverted their marrow to a chronic phase of MMM.

Experimental Therapies

In the last years, significant efforts have been undertaken to develop new agents that will positively affect survival in PMF. The most significant new therapeutic target was JAK-STAT pathway, based on the demonstrated role of the *JAK2*V617F mutation on the pathogenesis of PMF and MPNs as a whole. This subject matter is expanded in an accompanying chapter of this book. However, research goals were also to target other candidate pathogenetic pathways of PMF, most of them known to be involved in other MPNs or MDS.

Interferon in the Early Phase of the Disease

An experimental objective of PMF treatment, as for all MPNs, should be eradication of the malignant clone and cure of the disease. This goal has been recently envisaged in polycythemia vera (PV) placing high expectation on the therapeutic efficacy of IFN [45]. The reasons of such an expectation is that in vitro studies suggested that clonal MPN progenitors may be more sensitive to IFN-α (alpha) than their normal counterparts and that in vivo studies showed reversion from monoclonal to polyclonal patterns of hematopoiesis, or disappearance of a chromosomal abnormality in IFN-α (alpha)-treated patients. Recently, Kiladjian and colleagues could also show that IFN-α (alpha) was able to markedly decrease the proportion of circulating V617F-mutated cells in PV patients [45]. An additional argument is that IFNα may have immunological properties by inducing immune responses to candidate tumor antigens, among which the recently identified PV-associated tumor antigens may represent targets for immune effectors [46].

The experimental idea in PMF is that an early treatment with IFN could reverse the evolution of the disease by directly repressing the malignant clone. This principle was exploited by Silver and Vandris [47] who reported the use of IFN in 13 PMF patients with an early phase of the disease, i.e., with hematopoietic foci occupying at least 30% of the marrow biopsy, and no more than grade 2 reticulin or collagen fibrosis. Before the treatment, nine patients had a Lille risk score of 0, three had a score of 1, and one patient had a score of 2. None of the patients required transfusions. rIFN-α (alpha)2b at 500,000–1,000,000 units, subcutaneously, thrice weekly, was the starting dose. As a result of the treatment, the median spleen size that was 7.0 cm below the costal margin (range 0–24 cm) before treatment, reversed to 0 cm (range 0–20 cm) at the last follow-up. Reduction of abnormal marrow morphology occurred in five of nine patients. Reticulin and collagen fibrosis diminished in three of five patients, and was virtually absent in two. A trend toward normalization of megakaryocytic atypia and increased normal hematopoiesis was observed. However, only one out of four patients had a sequential decrease in *JAK2*V617F allele burden from 45.6 to 11.2% over 3 years. IFN was well tolerated. Grade-1 toxicity occurred in six of the 13 patients, including mild depression, dry skin, cough, myalgia, and asthenia, which did not require dose reduction. Nine patients experienced mild cytopenias.

Testing More Potent Immunomodulators: Lenalidomide and Pomalidomide

Lenalidomide and pomalidomide are second generation more potent immunomodulators that are created by chemical modification of thalidomide with the intent to reduce toxicity and enhance anti-cancer and immunological activities. Lenalidomide is approved by the US FDA for use in MDS and in multiple myeloma.

Lenalidomide was evaluated as a single agent in a total of 68 patients with symptomatic MF [48]. Oral lenalidomide at 10 mg/d for 3–4 months gave an overall response rate of 22% for anemia and 50% for thrombocytopenia. Lenalidomide was effective in patients where prior treatment with thalidomide had failed. High-toxicity profile of lenalidomide as a single agent was, however, evidenced mostly consisting of myelosupression. This prompted to evaluate the safety and efficacy of the combination of lenalidomide and prednisone in patients with PMF. In a phase II study, the MD Anderson Cancer Center investigators treated 40 patients [49]. The therapy consisted of lenalidomide 10 mg/d (5 mg/d if baseline platelet count <100 × 10^9/L) on days 1–21 of a 28-day cycle for six cycles, in combination with prednisone 30 mg/d orally during cycle 1, 15 mg/d during cycle 2, and 15 mg/d every other day during cycle 3. According to the IWG-MRT criteria (Table 6.2), three patients (7.5%) had partial response and nine patients (22.5%) had clinical improvement. The overall response rates were 30% for anemia and 42% for splenomegaly. Moreover, 10 of the 11 assessable responders who started therapy with reticulin fibrosis grade 4 experienced reductions to at least a score of 2. All the eight *JAK2*V617F-positive responders experienced a reduction of the baseline mutant allele burden, which was greater than 50% in four, including one of whom the mutation became undetectable. Grade 3–4 hematologic adverse events included neutropenia (58%), anemia (42%), and thrombocytopenia (13%).

Pomalidomide was evaluated in a phase II randomized, multicenter, double-blind, adaptive design study, with 84 patients with PMF-associated anemia [45]. Four treatment arms were evaluated: pomalidomide (2 mg/d) plus placebo, pomalidomide (2 mg/d) plus prednisone, pomalidomide (0.5 mg/d) plus prednisone, and prednisone plus placebo. Response in anemia according to the IWG criteria was documented in 20 patients (20/84), including 15 who became transfusion-independent. Response rates in the four treatment arms for patients receiving ≥3 cycles of treatment ($n = 62$) were 38%, 23%, 40%, and 25%, respectively. Response to pomalidomide with or without prednisone was durable and significantly better in the absence of leukocytosis. *JAK2*V617F or cytogenetic status did not affect the response. Grade ≥3 toxicities were infrequent and included neutropenia, thrombocytopenia, and thrombosis.

Addressing Nonspecific Molecular Targets: Antifarnesyl Transferase and Antiproteasome Agents

Tipifarnib (R115777 or Zarnestra™) is an orally bioavailable nonpeptidomimetic inhibitor of farnesyltransferase (FT), the enzyme that transfers the 15-carbon farnesyl group to the carboxyl terminal end of the selected polypeptides. FT inhibitors were originally synthesized and tested based on the premise that they would inhibit the membrane targeting and function of oncogenic *ras* mutants. Subsequent studies, however, have demonstrated that FT inhibitors inhibit proliferation of transformed cells in vitro and in vivo even if ras mutations were absent. FT inhibitors proved to have efficacy in acute leukemias. A phase II trial with tipifarnib was undertaken in symptomatic PMF patients by Mesa and colleagues [46]. Patients were treated with 300 mg of tipifarnib orally twice daily for the first 21 days of a 28-day cycle. Among the 34 patients enrolled in the trial, tipifarnib resulted in little improvement in anemia. In contrast, R115777 did result in clinically relevant decreases in organomegaly in 11 patients (33%), many of whom had previously failed HU. Responses observed did not significantly correlate with the reductions in bone marrow fibrosis, osteosclerosis, neoangiogenesis, or resolution of baseline karyotypic abnormalities.

The proteasome inhibitor bortezomib (Velcade™) is a modified dipeptidyl boronic acid indicated as a powerful candidate for antitumor activity. It directly induces tumor cell death by inhibiting the degradation of several critical intracellular proteins involved in cell cycle regulation. It also inhibits degradation of IkB and hence blocks multifunctional transcription factor nuclear factor-kappa B (NFkB) leading to reduced levels of growth factors such as interleukin-6, vascular endothelial growth factor (VEGF), cell adhesion molecules, and particularly transforming growth factor beta-1 (TGF-β (beta)1). In addition, bortezomib indirectly inhibits angiogenesis and prevents tumor adaptation to hypoxia by functional inhibition of hypoxia-inducible factor 1-alpha (HIF-1α (alpha)). With these targets, bortezomib has been approved by FDA for the therapy of multiple myeloma and mantle cell lymphoma and has shown a clinical activity in the treatment of a number of hematological malignancies. NF-kB signaling pathway and angiogenesis are candidate targets for bortezomib in PMF. In the TPO^HIGH mouse model of myelofibrosis, bortezomib proved able to reduce fibrosis both in bone marrow and in spleen, and to impair osteosclerosis development reducing TGF-β (beta) levels [52]. With these premises, Mesa and coworkers reported the results of a pilot phase II study with bortezomib in nine patients with PMF and two with systemic mastocytosis or chronic myelomonocytic leukemia, showing lack of any clinical efficacy of the drug [53]. The MPD Research Consortium reported the results of a phase I–II study performed in 12 adults with PMF, refractory, or not suitable to first-line chemotherapy

[54]. Bortezomib was given at day 1, 4, 8, and 11 from 0.8 to 1.3 mg/m^2, every 21 days × 6 cycles. Dose-limiting toxicity occurred in one patient treated with bortezomib in the 1.3 mg/m^2 cohort, consisting of respiratory distress syndrome. The maximum-tolerated dose was 1.3 mg/m^2 for 4 days every 3 weeks. No complete, major, or moderate responses according to the EUMNET response criteria were documented. One minor response was documented due to complete response in the platelet count.

Targeting Neoangiogenesis

Although increased angiogenesis is almost universally present in hematologic malignancies, the degree of increase is most pronounced in PMF. On this basis, a compound built on the rationale of angiogenesis inhibition is the small molecule tyrosine kinase inhibitor of the receptor for the VEGF PTK787/ZK 222584 (PTK/ZK). PTK/ZK also inhibits a broad array of additional tyrosine kinases including platelet-derived growth factor receptor (PDGFR), c-kit, and c-fms. Although in theory this agent should have been quite active, Giles and coworkers from MD Anderson Cancer Center, in a study with 29 patients, observed responses that were quite modest with mainly the clinical improvement [55]. Additionally, decreases in intramedullary angiogenesis were really not observed with only modest reductions in marrow hypercellularity described.

Targeting Epigenetics

Epigenetic changes are cell-heritable, potentially modifiable abnormalities that affect gene expression through the two classic mechanisms of DNA methylation and acetylation of histone proteins. Studies on epigenetic gene regulation in PMF are still scanty and have been focused on single genes credited as being potentially involved in the pathogenesis of the disorder. Thus, hypermethylation of p15^{INK4B}, p16^{INK4A}, retinoic acid receptor β, calcitonin, SOCS3, and CXCR4 has been observed in PMF. A short-term treatment with 5-Aza reduced promoter methylation, increased membrane expression of CXCR4, and resulted in improved migration of CD34+ cells in response to SDF-1 in vitro. Similar findings have been reported after long-term incubation of PMF CD34+ cells exposed to 5-Aza followed by trichostatin A, and this treatment corrected bone marrow seeding of treated cells once infused in NOD/SCID mice.

The hypomethylating agents, azacitidine and decitabine, have been tested in PMF patients with a goal of improving cytopenias and splenomegaly or delaying blast transformation. Azacitidine was first approved by FDA in 2004, while decitabine was approved by FDA in the 2006 for the treatment of MDS. The experience with azacitidine was derived from two phase II trials in patients with refractory/relapsed PMF and post-PV/post-essential thrombocythemia MF [56]. The trials differed in the drug scheduling. In the first, 34 patients were given azacitidine at 75 mg/m^2 daily for 7 days every 4 weeks subcutaneously (total cycle dose, 525 mg/m^2). In the second trial a 5-day weekly schedule (total dose 375 mg/m^2) was employed in 10 patients. No patient among those receiving the reduced dosage schedule achieved even a clinical improvement, the lowest response according to the IWG-RT criteria. In the higher-dose trial, responses were observed in ten patients (29%), including complete response in one, partial response in seven, and hematological improvement in two.

Neutropenia was the main adverse effect with grade 3–4 severity in 29% of the patients, and in thrombocytopenia all the grades occurred in 9%. Grade 3–4 non-neutropenic infections were reported in 26% of the patients.

In a phase II multicenter study with decitabine in 21 patients with PMF, 7 patients (37%) responded, including 2 with blast phase MF [57]. There was one complete response, two partial responses, and four hematological improvements. There was a 61% reduction in the count of circulating CD34+ cells that distinguished responders from nonresponders.

Many histone deacethylase (HDAC) inhibitors are currently available, e.g., depsipeptide, SAHA (Vorinostat), trichostatin A, valproic acid, ITF 2357 (Givinostat), and LBH589. ITF2357 was shown to selectively inhibit the *JAK*2V617F-carrying HEL cell growth at an IC50 of 1 nM. The safety and efficacy of ITF2357 in the treatment of patients with PMF and other MPN have been evaluated in a phase II study with patients refractory to HU or young patients who are in need of cytotoxic therapy [58]. The drug was given orally at a starting daily dose of 50 mg b.i.d. that could be escalated to 50 mg t.i.d. in the absence of toxicity. In MF patients (*n* = 13), the hematological response, as evaluated by EUMNET criteria, was 33%, and a partial response for splenomegaly was seen in 23%.

In a patient with a *JAK*2V617F-positive post-essential thrombocythemia MF vorinostat produced improvement in transfusion-dependent anemia and thrombocytopenia [59]. Modest improvement of anemia and reduction of transfusions was also serendipitously observed in a patient with PMF who had received valproic acid for epilepsy prophylaxis.

Concluding Remarks

Experimental treatment modalities with drugs which have a non-PMF-specific molecular target, such as anti-pharnesyltransferase, anti-proteasome, and anti-VEGF receptor agents, have documented the futility of such an approach. Treating patients with small doses of rIFN-α (alpha)2b in the early stage of PMF resulted in a regression of clinical and histological disease manifestations in a significant proportion of patients. However, appropriate patient selection for early phase clinical trials requires a more than superficial definition of early phase PMF and understanding of the natural history of this disorder. Results of the first trials with epigenetic agents have been dismal. It is conceivable that combining epigenetic therapy with other drugs might be worthwhile and more efficacious. One could imagine the opportunity to associate epigenetic therapy either with cytotoxic drugs or with the novel specific JAK2 inhibitors. Pomalidomide as a single agent and the combination of lenalidomide and prednisone resulted in active and well-tolerated novel immunomodulators. They should enter phase III clinical trials for the prospect of becoming first-line therapy for anemia in a disease orphan of very active or safe drug therapies for this indication.

References

1. Di Tucci AA, Matta G, Deplano S, et al. Myocardial iron overload assessment by T2* magnetic resonance imaging in adult transfusion dependent patients with acquired anemias. Haematologica. 2008;93:1385–1388.

2. Mesa RA, Li CY, Ketterling RP, et al. Leukemic transformation in myelofibrosis with myeloid metaplasia: a single-institution experience with 91 cases. Blood. 2005;105:973–977.

3. Tefferi A, Barosi G, Mesa RA, et al. IWG for Myelofibrosis Research and Treatment (IWG-MRT). International Working Group (IWG) consensus criteria for treatment response in myelofibrosis with myeloid metaplasia, for the IWG for Myelofibrosis Research and Treatment (IWG-MRT). Blood. 2006;108:1497–1503.

4. Barosi G, Bordessoule D, Briere J, et al. Response criteria for myelofibrosis with myeloid metaplasia: results of an initiative of the European Myelofibrosis Network (EUMNET). Blood. 2005;106:2849–2853.

5. Besa EC, Nowell PC, Geller NL, Gardner FH. Analysis of the androgen response of 23 patients with agnogenic myeloid metaplasia: the value of chromosomal studies in predicting response and survival. Cancer. 1982;49:308–313.

6. Shimoda K, Shide K, Kamezaki K, et al. The effect of anabolic steroids on anemia in myelofibrosis with myeloid metaplasia: retrospective analysis of 39 patients in Japan. Int J Hematol. 2007;85:338–343.

7. Cervantes F, Alvarez-Larran A, Domingo A, et al. Efficacy and tolerability of danazol as a treatment for the anaemia of myelofibrosis with myeloid metaplasia: long-term results in 30 patients. Br J Haematol. 2005;129:771–775.

8. Cervantes F, Alvarez-Larran A, Hernandez-Boluda JC, et al. Erythropoietin treatment of the anaemia of myelofibrosis with myeloid metaplasia: results in 20 patients and review of the literature. Br J Haematol. 2004;127:399–403.

9. Tefferi A, Strand JJ, Lasho TL, et al. Respective clustering of unfavorable and favorable cytogenetic clones in myelofibrosis with myeloid metaplasia with homozygosity for JAK2(V617F) and response to erythropoietin therapy. Cancer. 2006;106:1739–1743.

10. Tsiara SN, Chaidos A, Bourantas LK, et al. Recombinant Human Erythropoietin for the treatment of anaemia in patients with chronic idiopathic myelofibrosis. Acta Haematol. 2006;117:156–161.

11. Huang J, Tefferi A. Erythropoiesis stimulating agents have limited therapeutic activity in transfusion-dependent patients with primary myelofibrosis regardless of serum erythropoietin level. Eur J Haematol. 2009;83:154–155.

12. Cervantes F, Alvarez-Larran A, Hernandez-Boluda JC, et al. Darbepoetin-alpha for the anaemia of myelofibrosis with myeloid metaplasia. Br J Haematol. 2006;134:184–186.

13. Merup M, Kutti J, Birgerard G, et al. Negligible clinical effects of thalidomide in patients with myelofibrosis with myeloid metaplasia. Med Oncol. 2002;19:79–86.

14. Barosi G, Elliott M, Canepa L, et al. Thalidomide in myelofibrosis with myeloid metaplasia: a pooled-analysis of individual patient data from 5 studies. Leuk Lymph. 2002;43:2301–2307.

15. Mesa RA, Steensma DP, Pardanani A, et al. A phase II trial of combination of low-dose thalidomide and prednisone for the treatment of myelofibrosis with myeloid metaplasia. Blood. 2003;101:2534–2541.

16. Strupp C, Germing U, Scherer A, et al. Thalidomide for the treatment of idiopathic myelofibrosis. Eur J Haematol. 2004;72:52–57.

17. Marchetti M, Barosi G, Balestri F, et al. Low-dose thalidomide ameliorates cytopenias and splenomegaly in myelofibrosis with myeloid metaplasia: a phase II trial. J Clin Oncol. 2004;22:424–431.

18. Abgrall JF, Guibaud I, Bastie JN, et al. Thalidomide versus placebo in myeloid metaplasia with myelofibrosis: a prospective, randomized, double-blind, multi-center study. Haematologica. 2006;91:1027–1032.

19. Thomas DA, Giles FJ, Albitar M, et al. Thalidomide therapy for myelofibrosis with myeloid metaplasia. Cancer. 2006;106:1974–1984.

20. Weinkove R, Reilly JT, McMullin MF, et al. Low-dose thalidomide in myelofibrosis. Haematologica. 2008;93:1100–1101.
21. Leitch HA, Chase JM, Goodman TA, et al. Improved survival in red blood cell transfusion dependent patients with primary myelofibrosis (PMF) receiving iron chelation therapy. Hematol Oncol. 2010;28:40–48
22. Tefferi A, Mesa RA, Pardanani A, et al. Red blood cell transfusion need at diagnosis adversely affects survival in primary myelofibrosis-increased serum ferritin or transfusion load does not. Am J Hematol. 2009;84:265–267.
23. Di Tucci AA, Murru R, Alberti D, et al. Correction of anemia in a transfusion-dependent patient with primary myelofibrosis receiving iron chelation therapy with deferasirox (Exjade, ICL670). Eur J Haematol. 2007;78:540–542.
24. Messa E, Cilloni D, Messa F, et al. Deferasirox treatment improved the hemoglobin level and decreased transfusion requirements in four patients with the myelodysplastic syndrome and primary myelofibrosis. Acta Haematol. 2008;120:70–74.
25. Sirhan S, Lasho TL, Hanson CA, et al. The presence of JAK2V617F in primary myelofibrosis or its allele burden in polycythemia vera predicts chemosensitivity to hydroxyurea. Am J Hematol. 2008;83:363–365.
26. Petti MC, Latagliata R, Spadea T, et al. Melphalan treatment in patients with myelofibrosis with myeloid metaplasia. Br J Haematol. 2002;116:576–581.
27. Chee L, Kalnins R, Turner P. Low dose melphalan in the treatment of myelofibrosis: a single centre experience. Leuk Lymphoma. 2006;47:1409–1412.
28. Kiladjian JJ, Chomienne C, Fenaux P. Interferon-alpha therapy in bcr-abl-negative myeloproliferative neoplasms. Leukemia. 2008;22:1990–1998.
29. Gilbert HS. Long term treatment of myeloproliferative disease with interferon-alpha-2b:feasibility and efficacy. Cancer. 1998;83:1205–1213.
30. Tefferi A, Elliot MA, Yoon SY, et al. Clinical and bone marrow effects of interferon alfa therapy in myelofibrosis with myeloid metaplasia. Blood. 2001;97:1896.
31. Heis-Vahidi-Fard N, Forberg E, Eichinger S, et al. Ineffectiveness of interferon-gamma in the treatment of idiopathic myelofibrosis: a pilot study. Ann Hematol. 2001;80:79–82.
32. Radin AI, Kim HT, Grant BW, et al. Phase II study of alpha2 interferon in the treatment of the chronic myeloproliferative disorders (E5487): a trial of the Eastern Cooperative Oncology Group. Cancer. 2003;98:100–109.
33. Jabbour E, Kantarjian H, Cortes J, et al. PEG-IFN-alpha-2b therapy in BCR-ABL-negative myeloproliferative disorders: final result of a phase 2 study. Cancer. 2007;110:2012–2018.
34. Ianotto JC, Kiladjian JJ, Demory JL, et al. PEG-IFN-alpha-2a therapy in patients with myelofibrosis: a study of the French Groupe d'Etudes des Myelofibroses (GEM) and France intergroupe des syndromes Myéloprolifératifs (FIM). Br J Haematol. 2009;146:223–225.
35. Buxhofer-Ausch V, Gisslinger H, Berg T, et al. Acquired resistance to interferon alpha therapy associated with homozygous MPL-W515L mutation and chromosome 20q deletion in primary myelofibrosis. Eur J Haematol. 2009;82:161–163.
36. Elliott MA, Chen MG, Silverstein MN, Tefferi A. Splenic irradiation for symptomatic splenomegaly associated with myelofibrosis with myeloid metaplasia. Br J Haematol. 1998;103:505–511.
37. Mesa RA, Nagorney DS, Schwager S, Allred J, Tefferi A. Palliative goals, patient selection, and perioperative platelet management: outcomes and lessons from 3 decades of splenectomy for myelofibrosis with myeloid metaplasia at the Mayo Clinic. Cancer. 2006;107:361–370.
38. Barosi G, Ambrosetti A, Buratti A, et al. Splenectomy for patients with myelofibrosis and myeloid metaplasia: Pretreatment variables and outcome prediction. Leukemia. 1993;7:200–206.

39. Faoro LN, Tefferi A, Mesa RA. Long-term analysis of the palliative benefit of 2-chlorodeoxyadenosine for myelofibrosis with myeloid metaplasia. Eur J Haematol. 2005;74:117–120.

40. Riesterer O, Gmür J, Lütolf U. Repeated and preemptive palliative radiotherapy of symptomatic hepatomegaly in a patient with advanced myelofibrosis. Onkologie. 2008;31:325–327.

41. Barosi G, Ambrosetti A, Centra A, et al. Splenectomy and risk of blast transformation in myelofibrosis with myeloid metaplasia. Italian Cooperative Study Group on Myeloid with Myeloid Metaplasia. Blood. 1998;91:3630–3636.

42. Barosi G, Bergamaschi G, Marchetti M, et al. JAK2 V617F mutational status predicts progression to large splenomegaly and leukemic transformation in primary myelofibrosis. Blood. 2007; 110:4030–4036.

43. Tefferi A, Jiménez T, Gray LA, et al. Radiation therapy for symptomatic hepatomegaly in myelofibrosis with myeloid metaplasia. Eur J Haematol. 2001;66:37–42.

44. Steensma DP, Hook CC, Stafford SL, Tefferi A. Low-dose, single-fraction, whole-lung radiotherapy for pulmonary hypertension associated with myelofibrosis with myeloid metaplasia. Br J Haematol. 2002;118:813–816.

45. Kiladjian JJ, Cassinat B, Chevret S, et al. Pegylated interferon-alfa-2a induces complete hematologic and molecular responses with low toxicity in polycythemia vera. Blood. 2008;112:3065–3072.

46. Xiong Z, Yan Y, Liu E, et al. Novel tumor antigens elicit anti-tumor humoral immune reactions in a subset of patients with polycythemia vera. Clin Immunol. 2007;122:279–287.

47. Silver RT, Vandris K. Recombinant interferon alpha (rIFN alpha-2b) may retard progression of early primary myelofibrosis. Leukemia. 2009;23:1366–1369.

48. Tefferi A, Cortes J, Verstovsek S, et al. Lenalidomide therapy in myelofibrosis with myeloid metaplasia. Blood. 2006;108:1158–1164.

49. Quintás-Cardama A, Kantarjian H, Manshouri T, et al. Lenalidomide plus prednisone results in durable clinical, histopathologic, and molecular responses in patients with myelofibrosis. J Clin Oncol. 2009;27:4760–4766.

50. Tefferi A, Verstovsek S, Barosi G, et al. Pomalidomide is active in the treatment of anemia associated with myelofibrosis. J Clin Oncol. 2009; 27:4563–4569.

51. Mesa RA, Camoriano JK, Geyer SM, et al. A phase II trial of tipifarnib in myelofibrosis: primary, post-polycythemia vera and post-essential thrombocythemia. Leukemia. 2007;21:1964–1970.

52. Wagner-Ballon O, Pisani DF, Gastinne T, et al. Proteasome inhibitor bortezomib impairs both myelofibrosis and osteosclerosis induced by high thrombopoietin levels in mice. Blood. 2007;110:345–353.

53. Mesa RA, Verstovsek S, Rivera C, et al. Bortezomib therapy in myelofibrosis: a phase II clinical trial. Leukemia. 2008;22:1636–1638.

54. Barosi G, Gattoni E, Barbui T et al., A Phase I study of the proteasome inhibitor bortzomib in patients with myelofibrosis. Blood. 2007;110:1036a.

55. Giles FJ, List AF, Carroll M, et al. PTK787/ZK 222584, a small molecule tyrosine kinase receptor inhibitor of vascular endothelial growth factor (VEGF), has modest activity in myelofibrosis with myeloid metaplasia. Leuk Res. 2007;7:891–897.

56. Mesa RA, Verstovsek S, Rivera C, et al. 5-Azacitidine has limited therapeutic activity in myelofibrosis. Leukemia. 2009;23:180–182.

57. Danilov AV, Relias V, Feeney DM, et al. Decitabine is an effective treatment of idiopathic myelofibrosis. Br J Haematol. 2009;145:131–132.

58. Rambaldi A, Della Casa CM, Salmoiraghi S, et al. A phase 2A study of the histone deacetylase inhibitor ITF2357 in patients with Jak2 V617F positive chronic myeloproliferative neoplasms. Blood. 2008;112:100a.

59. Lee J. Clinical efficacy of vorinostat in a patient with essential thrombocytosis and subsequent myelofibrosis. Ann Hematol. 2009;88:699–700.

Chapter 7

Hematopoietic Cell Transplantation for Myelofibrosis

Daniella M.B. Kerbauy and H. Joachim Deeg

Keywords: Chronic idiopathic myelofibrosis • Agnogenic myeloid metaplasia • Primary myelofibrosis (PMF) • Hematopoietic cell transplantation

Introduction

Chronic idiopathic myelofibrosis, also known as agnogenic myeloid metaplasia, and now referred to as primary myelofibrosis (PMF), is a clonal chronic myeloproliferative disease of the bone marrow. PMF is characterized by progressive marrow fibrosis, apparently due to signals derived from clonal hematopoietic cells, extramedullary hematopoiesis with splenomegaly, anemia or pancytopenia, and a leukoerythroblastic peripheral blood picture. The median survival of patients after diagnosis of PMF is 3.5–5 years. PMF is a heterogenous disease with regard to presenting symptoms and disease evolution.

The median age at diagnosis is in the seventh decade of life, and patients may either be diagnosed incidentally or present with severe constitutional symptoms. However, PMF can also occur in younger patients. Leukemic transformation occurs in about 20% of the patients. Dependent upon presentation and patient age, treatment strategies range from palliation of symptoms to an aggressive, potentially curative approach using allogeneic hematopoietic cell transplantation (HCT). As discussed elsewhere in this volume, drugs such as androgens, hydroxyurea, busulfan, corticosteroids, interferon, erythropoietin, thalidomide, lenalidomide, anagrelide, and others have been used for the treatment of PMF. Splenectomy and splenic irradiation have been carried out to relieve symptoms related to splenomegaly. Patients subjected to splenectomy who eventually undergo HCT show faster hematopoietic recovery after transplantation (see below), but splenectomy is not generally recommended and may be indicated only in patients who are severely symptomatic and do not respond to other interventions.

More recently, a V617F mutation in the Janus Kinase 2 (JAK2) tyrosine kinase has been observed in about 50% of PMF patients. This finding offers the opportunity to test the potential efficacy of anti-JAK2-targeted therapy in these patients. Those studies and the use of other drugs of potential interest are discussed elsewhere.

S. Verstovsek and A. Tefferi (eds.), *Myeloproliferative Neoplasms: Biology and Therapy*,
Contemporary Hematology, DOI 10.1007/ 978-1-60761-266-7_7,
© Springer Science+Business Media, LLC 2011

The only currently available treatment with proven curative potential is allogeneic HCT. However, this approach is also associated with potentially fatal complications, and treatment decisions must take into consideration life expectancy and quality of life without transplantation. Thus, a careful disease risk assessment and evaluation for the presence of co-morbidities are essential when deciding about optimal clinical management.

Several risk scores have been developed for the classification of PMF (discussed in detail elsewhere). These scoring systems include several prognostic factors such as anemia, leukocyte count, constitutional symptoms, circulating myeloblasts, platelet and monocyte count, age, and gender. Although these models typically provide assessment at a given time point and do not consider disease evolution, they are very helpful in identifying patients who would benefit from HCT.

In this chapter we will address several aspects of transplantation, including patient selection, donor selection, transplant strategies, and outcome. We will also include in this review patients who developed marrow fibrosis following antecedent polycythemia vera (PV) or essential thrombocythemia (ET), as most of the reports in the literature also include cohorts of patients in these two categories. Specific issues with regard to transplant outcome such as pre-transplant splenectomy and evaluation of residual disease after HCT will be discussed briefly.

Autologous HCT

Although autologous HCT is not expected to cure patients with PMF, it can relieve symptoms and may offer prolonged life expectancy for patients who are not eligible for allogeneic HCT. Only a few studies describing small numbers of patients are available. In one series, 21 received high-dose chemotherapy (busulfan) followed by peripheral blood progenitor cell (PBPC) infusion [1]. Fifteen of the 21 patients experienced clinical improvement. Seven of ten with anemia, seven of ten with symptomatic splenomegaly, and six of eight with thrombocytopenia improved symptoms and cell counts; marrow fibrosis regressed in six patients. Actuarial survival was 61% at 2 years. PBSC mobilization was possible in all but one patient. In fact, the concentration of CD34+ cells spontaneously circulating in peripheral blood in these patients is rather high. In this particular study a minimum of 4.8×10^6 CD34+ cells/kg was collected. More recently, Cervantes et al. [2] showed that patients treated with high-dose treosulfan achieved successful hematopoietic reconstitution following autologous PBSC infusion.

Allogeneic HCT

High-Dose (Conventional) Conditioning HCT for Patients with Myelofibrosis

Despite initial concerns that extensive marrow fibrosis would interfere with engraftment, first successful reports were presented in the 1990s. In a small series, engraftment of allogeneic cells was documented, and fibrosis was shown to resolve after HCT [3, 4]. A large retrospective study showed no significant impact of marrow fibrosis on engraftment and hematopoietic reconstitution [5].

Additional larger series confirmed the curative potential of allogeneic HCT for myelofibrosis. Two studies, each including more than 50 patients, showed 5-year overall survival rates of 47% and 3-year overall survival of 58%, respectively; non-relapse mortality (NRM) was 27% and 20%, respectively [6, 7]. In Guardiola's cohort most patients received marrow grafts from HLA-identical related donors. Patients were conditioned with high-dose TBI-containing regimens. The absence of splenectomy and the presence of osteomyelosclerosis were associated with a longer time to neutrophil and platelet recovery. Hemoglobin levels ≤100 g/dl and the presence of osteomyelosclerosis before transplant negatively affected outcome. In the Seattle cohort, the source of stem cells was marrow in 33 and PBPC in 23 patients. In contrast to the Guardiola study a large proportion of patients (20 of 56) were transplanted from unrelated donors. Conditioning regimens consisted of targeted busulfan and cyclophosphamide (tBUCY) ($n = 44$) or high-dose TBI plus chemotherapy ($n = 12$). In this series, patients conditioned with tBUCY were more likely to survive (76%; Fig. 7.1). There was no significant difference in transplant outcomes between patients transplanted from HLA-identical siblings and HLA-matched unrelated donors. As observed before, the presence of splenectomy resulted in a shorter time to granulocyte and platelet engraftment. In agreement with an earlier report [6], clinical stage by Dupriez score, cytogenetic abnormalities, and degree of marrow fibrosis significantly influenced transplant outcome. Moreover, the inclusion of pre-transplant platelet count and degree of marrow fibrosis along with the Dupriez score significantly improved prognostic accuracy.

The report of the largest cohort to date, from a single center, confirmed the curative potential of allogeneic HCT, with some patients now followed in complete remission for 15 years or longer [8]. In that series of 104 patients, median age at HCT was 49 years, and the estimated 7-year survival was 61%. The tBUCY conditioning regimen was superior to other regimens with regard to long-term outcome. Dupriez score, low platelet count, older patient age, and higher co-morbidity score [9] were significantly associated with increased mortality. However, in a multivariate regression model, the Dupriez score lost its impact, while conditioning regimen (tBUCY), high platelet count at transplantation, younger age, and decreased co-morbidity score were significant for improved survival. Marrow fibrosis in this series had a less pronounced effect on transplant outcome than reported previously. This may have been due to the sampling variation and the interpretation based on single marrow biopsies. However, it is also possible that patients were referred for HCT at different stages of their disease course.

Assessment of marrow fibrosis resolution after HCT should be done with caution when based on single needle biopsies. Nevertheless, results with magnetic resonance imaging (MRI) showed a good correlation between biopsy and MRI findings at specific sites, although MRI of the skeleton provides a better overall evaluation of fibrosis status of the marrow [10] (Fig. 7.2).

The above study in 104 patients was the first to address the impact of co-morbidity on transplant outcome in patients with myelofibrosis. As most patients are diagnosed in the sixth or seventh decade of life, application of co-morbidity scores (HCT-CI) may be useful in selecting patients for one or

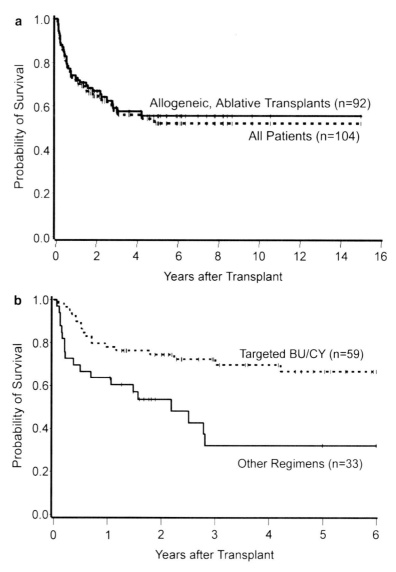

Fig. 7.1 *Overall survival among 104 patients transplanted from related or unrelated donors.* (**a**) All patients (Ablative indicates high dose conditioning); (**b**) By conditioning regimen (targeted BUCY [(t)BUCY] compared with other regimens, including high-dose total body irradiation). Surviving patients are indicated by tick marks [34]

another HCT approach, with the intent of minimizing the risk of toxicity and NRM. The NRM rates have varied from 30 to 40% in published studies. In the latest report by the Seattle team the projected NRM at 5 years was 34%. The non-relapse causes of death were: pneumonia/pulmonary failure; multiorgan failure; hemolytic uremic syndrome; thrombotic thrombocytopenic purpura; invasive aspergillosis; GVHD; sepsis; and encephalitis.

The Gruppo Italiano Trapianto di Midollo Osseo – GITMO – recently evaluated their HCT results in patients with myelofibrosis over a 20-year period [11]. The overall outcome in that cohort was inferior to that in the previous reports, with an NRM of 43%, and a 3-year overall survival of 42%. However, the

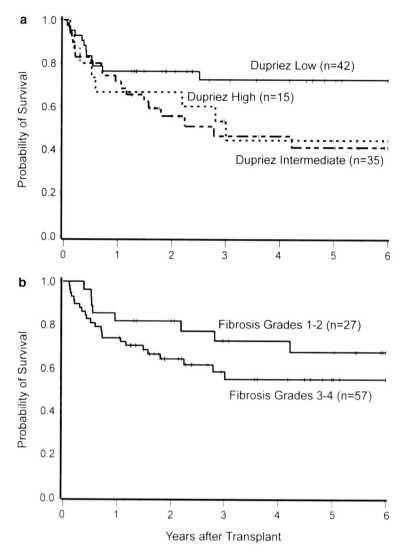

Fig. 7.2 *Impact of disease parameters on survival.* (**a**) Effect of Dupriez (Lille) score. (**b**) Effect of the degree of marrow fibrosis [8]

heterogeneous study population and accrual over two decades during which considerable progress has been made explain these results. In fact, this analysis showed progressive improvement in HCT outcome over the time interval studied. There was a significant reduction in NRM rates after 1996, which had a positive impact on overall survival and relapse-free survival, although the differences did not reach statistical significance.

Another important variable to consider is time from diagnosis to HCT. In this retrospective Italian study, time between diagnosis and transplant was the only clinical factor significantly associated with outcome in univariate analysis and for NRM in a multivariate regression model. As this analysis included intermediate and high-risk patients as determined by the Dupriez score, those findings could suggest that HCT should be offered earlier in the disease course. In the latest Seattle update, the median

Table 7.1 Selected series of allogeneic hematopoietic stem cell transplantation for myelofibrosis after high-dose (conventional) conditioning.

Reference	Number of patients	Age (years), median (range)	Related/ unrelated donor	Overall survival (%)/follow-up (years)	Non-relapse mortality (%) at years	Graft failure (%)
Guardiola et al. [6]	55	42 (4–53)	49/6	47/5	27 at 1	9
Deeg et al. [7]	56	43 (10–66)	36/26	58/3	32 at 3	5
Kerbauy et al.[a] [8]	104	49 (18–70)	59/45	61/7	34 at 5	10
Patriarca et al.[a] [11]	100	49 (21–68)	82/18	42/3	43 at 3	12

[a]Including reduced intensity conditioning regimens

disease duration before HCT was 15 months (compared to 33 months in earlier studies), and a larger proportion of patients had low Dupriez scores, which may well have contributed to improved outcome. Thus, the optimum timing of HCT must be determined in the context of several clinical features and the prognostic score to optimize HCT outcome. A summary of results from studies using high-dose conditioning for allogeneic HCT is provided in Table 7.1.

Reduced Intensity Conditioning HCT for Myelofibrosis

Reduced intensity conditioning (RIC) HCT is associated with reduced acute toxicity. However, the question has been raised whether such an approach provides effective treatment for myelofibrosis patients. "RIC" comprises a number of regimens with different intensities, and transplant outcome in this setting must be carefully evaluated under consideration of the regimen that was used to prepare the patient for HCT.

Rondelli et al. [12] reported results in 21 patients transplanted at several institutions over an extended time interval; the median age was 54 years, and patients had intermediate or high-risk Dupriez scores. RIC regimens varied, most included fludarabine. All but one patient achieved full donor cell engraftment. The overall survival was 86% at 2.7 years. Complete remission was achieved in 76% of patients, and most patients showed regression of splenomegaly and a decrease of marrow fibrosis. Moreover, the rate of acute GVHD was low, which contributed to decreased NRM. In a prospective study of RIC in 21 patients of similar ages (median 53 years), Kroger et al. observed an NRM of 16% and an overall survival of 84% [13].

A multicenter retrospective study comparing high-dose conditioning and RIC in myelofibrosis patients suggested that both strategies offer the potential of cure. Although patients receiving RIC were older, with lower performance status, NRM was lower than among patients conditioned with high-dose regimens ($P = 0.08$) [14]. There was no difference in relapse rates or disease progression between the two groups, and a trend toward better progression-free survival and overall survival for patients transplanted with RIC regimens was noted [14]. Another multicenter study showed higher NRM among patients conditioned with high-dose regimens (30%) than in the RIC group (10%); however, there was no difference in survival [15].

The degree of marrow fibrosis and splenomegaly are good parameters to evaluate clinical response to HCT. A report on 24 patients transplanted with an RIC regimen showed advanced marrow fibrosis before HCT, and rapid regression of fibrosis after HCT [16]. Regression of marrow fibrosis occurred in 59% at day +100, in 90% at day +180, and in 100% at day +360. The impact of splenomegaly was evaluated in 10 patients undergoing RIC HCT and classified as intermediate or high risk; spleen longitudinal diameters ranged from 12 to 34 cm at diagnosis. Neutrophil engraftment occurred later in patients with spleens larger than 30 cm. All patients showed at least a 50% reduction in spleen size following HCT in parallel with progressive resolution of marrow fibrosis. Reduction of splenomegaly after HCT may be due to the conditioning regimen and a result of the graft-versus-myelofibrosis effect [17]. Results from several studies are conflicting with regard to the adverse impact of splenomegaly on transplant outcome. There is agreement that patients who underwent splenectomy (for various reasons) engrafted earlier, regardless of the intensity of the conditioning regimen [8, 17, 18]. Splenectomy had no impact on overall survival in either report. The potential benefit of earlier engraftment, however, does not justify the potential morbidity and mortality associated with splenectomy.

Recently, salvage and preemptive immunotherapy with donor lymphocyte infusion (DLI) has been reported to hold promise for patients showing clinical or molecular relapse after HCT. The phenomenon of a graft-versus-myelofibrosis effect is well documented in reports on relapsed patients after allogeneic HCT, who showed a reduction of marrow fibrosis after DLI [19, 20]. Kroger et al. [21] presented data on 17 patients with myelofibrosis with clinical relapse (salvage DLI) or residual disease as evidenced by the presence of the JAK2 mutation in peripheral blood cells [22]. All patients given DLI for molecular relapse responded with complete molecular remissions, while remissions were seen in only four patients (44%), who were in clinical relapse. Thus, DLI for molecular relapse after HCT appears to offer excellent results.

In summary, RIC regimens offer good results in patients transplanted for myelofibrosis. This is of note, in particular, since most patients transplanted had intermediate or high-risk disease, and co-morbidities were frequent. The overall survival ranged from 56% at 1 year to 85% at 2.5 years, and NRM was less than 20% in most reports. A summary of results is shown in Table 7.2.

Table 7.2 Selected series of allogeneic hematopoietic stem cell transplants for myelofibrosis after reduced intensity conditioning.

Reference	Number of patients	Age (years), median (range)	Related/ unrelated donor	Overall survival (%)/follow-up (years)	Non-relapse mortality at 1 year (%)	Graft failure
Rondelli et al. [32]	21	54 (27–68)	19/2	85/2.5	10	1
Kroger et al. [13]	21	53 (32–63)	8/13	84/3	16	–
Merup et al. [15]	10	58	20[a]/7	61/7	10	–
Snyder et al.[a] [33]	9	54	2/7	56/1	40	1

[a]One related donor was a haplo-identical parent

What to Consider When Advising Patients with Myelofibrosis on Transplantation

Prognostic Score Models

Several prognostic scoring systems have been developed. They are discussed in detail elsewhere in this volume. The Lille (or Dupriez) score [23] is the most widely used score and distinguishes three risk categories: low, intermediate, and high (based on hemoglobin and leucocyte count) with median survivals of 93, 26, and 13 months, respectively. Other reports have introduced constitutional symptoms and circulating blasts [24, 25]. The Mayo Clinic group has added monocyte and platelet counts to the risk assessment [26]. The International Working Group for Myelofibrosis Research and Treatment proposed yet another scoring system based on their findings in 1,054 patients from seven centers [27]. In multivariate analysis, age greater than 65 years was a predictor of short survival. The other risk parameters for shorter survival were constitutional symptoms, hemoglobin level less than 10 g/dl, leukocyte count greater than $25 \times 10^9/l$, and circulating blasts 1% or greater. The presence of none (low), one (intermediate-1), two (intertmediate-2), or three or more factors (high risk) segregated the patients into groups with significantly different median survivals of 135, 95, 48, and 27 months, respectively. In this cohort, 409 patients had assessable metaphases, and the presence of clonal cytogenetic abnormalities was associated with hemoglobin less than 10 g/dl and shorter survival. Interestingly, the independent prognostic contribution was restricted to patients in the intermediate-risk group [27]. The negative prognostic impact of an abnormal karyotype has been reported by different groups [28]. In one analysis, unfavorable impact was restricted to trisomy 8 and deletion of 12p, while deletions of 13q and 20q had no influence in survival. Assessment of cytogenetic abnormalities can be difficult in myelofibrosis patients due to the inability to aspirate marrow. Thus, data are limited with regard to cytogenetic impact on transplant outcome.

The Role of JAK2 Mutations

The impact of a mutated JAK2 on prognosis has yet to be defined, particularly in HCT. However, monitoring for the JAK2 mutation after HCT may be of clinical value [22, 29, 30]. Minimal residual disease kinetics after transplantation can be determined using a highly sensitive real-time PCR to detect the JAK2-V617F mutation. As clinical remission criteria (e.g. disappearance of fibrosis) may not be reached, monitoring JAK-2 positivity by PCR can add important information with regard to depth of remission and can identify patients who may benefit from adoptive immunotherapy, such as DLI [31].

Conclusions

HCT using either high-dose or RIC regimens has curative potential for patients with myelofibrosis. The most appropriate treatment plan in a patient with myelofibrosis must be based on a comprehensive clinical evaluation. Patients should be evaluated according to prognostic scoring systems in order to determine optimum management. However, a clinical evaluation should go beyond that in specific cases where risk stratification could be difficult. Thus, assessment of marrow fibrosis by means of biopsy and MRI studies, karyotype evaluation, can add information on the likely clinical evolution.

a Transplant Evaluation (traditional)

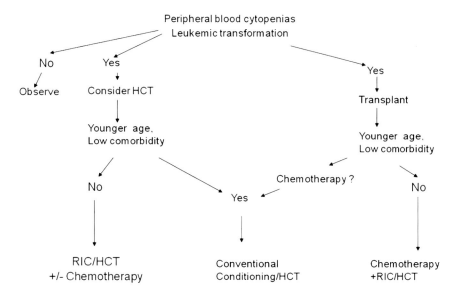

b Transplant Evaluation (based on score)

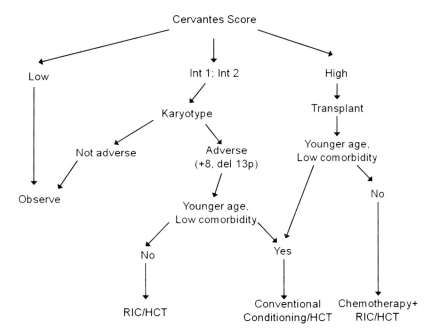

Fig. 7.3 *Decision tree for hematopoietic cell transplantation in patients with myelofibrosis.* (**a**) Traditional transplant evaluation. (**b**) Transplant evaluation based on Cervantes score (adapted from [27])

In view of a lack of randomized trials the decision regarding a conditioning regimen for HCT should be based on patient age, co-morbidities, prior treatment, and type of donor among others. Disease duration and potential prior treatment may be additional factors. Figure 7.3 provides flow diagrams to guide transplant decision making, based on traditional criteria (a) and the more recently developed scoring system by Cervantes et al. [27] (b).

Acknowledgment Supported in part by HL036444, CA15704, and CA18029; D.M.B.K. is also supported by FAPESP 2009/05449-0.

References

1. Anderson JE, Tefferi A, Craig F, et al. Myeloablation and autologous peripheral blood stem cell rescue results in hematologic and clinical responses in patients with myeloid metaplasia with myelofibrosis. Blood 2001;98(3):586–593.
2. Cervantes F. Modern management of myelofibrosis (Review). Br J Haematol 2005;128(5):583–592.
3. Dokal I, Jones L, Deenmamode M, Lewis SM, Goldman JM. Allogeneic bone marrow transplantation for primary myelofibrosis. Br J Haematol 1989;71:158–160.
4. Creemers GJ, Lowenberg B, Hagenbeek A. Allogeneic bone marrow transplantation for primary myelofibrosis. Br J Haematol 1992;82:772–773.
5. Soll E, Massumoto C, Clift RA, et al. Relevance of marrow fibrosis in bone marrow transplantation: a retrospective analysis of engraftment. Blood 1995;86(12): 4667–4673.
6. Guardiola P, Anderson JE, Bandini G, et al. Allogeneic stem cell transplantation for agnogenic myeloid metaplasia: a European Group for Blood and Marrow Transplantation, Société Française de Greffe de Moelle, Gruppo Italiano per il Trapianto del Midollo Osseo, and Fred Hutchinson Cancer Research Center collaborative study. Blood 1999;93(9):2831–2838.
7. Deeg HJ, Gooley TA, Flowers MED, et al. Allogeneic hematopoietic stem cell transplantation for myelofibrosis. Blood 2003;102(12):3912–3918.
8. Kerbauy DMB, Gooley TA, Sale GE, et al. Hematopoietic cell transplantation as curative therapy for idiopathic myelofibrosis, advanced polycythemia vera, and essential thrombocythemia. Biol Blood Marrow Transplant 2007;13(3):355–365.
9. Yeni PG, Hammer SM, Carpenter CC, et al. Antiretroviral treatment for adult HIV infection in 2002: updated recommendations of the International AIDS Society-USA Panel (Review) [erratum appears in JAMA. 2003 Jan-Feb;11(1):32]. JAMA 2002;288(2):222–235.
10. Sale GE, Deeg HJ, Porter BA. Regression of myelofibrosis and osteosclerosis following hematopoietic cell transplantation assessed by magnetic resonance imaging and histologic grading. Biol Blood Marrow Transplant 2006;12:1285–1294.
11. Patriarca F, Bacigalupo A, Sperotto A, et al. Allogeneic hematopoietic stem cell transplantation in myelofibrosis: the 20-year experience of the Gruppo Italiano Trapianto di Midollo Osseo (GITMO). Haematologica 2008;93(10):1514–1522.
12. Rondelli D, Barosi G, Bacigalupo A, et al. Allogeneic hematopoietic stem-cell transplantation with reduced-intensity conditioning in intermediate- or high-risk patients with myelofibrosis with myeloid metaplasia. Blood 2005;105(10):4115–4119.
13. Kroger N, Zabelina T, Schieder H, et al. Pilot study of reduced-intensity conditioning followed by allogeneic stem cell transplantation from related and unrelated donors in patients with myelofibrosis. Br J Haematol 2005;128(5):690–697.
14. Gupta V, Kroger N, Aschan J, et al. A retrospective comparison of conventional intensity conditioning and reduced-intensity conditioning for allogeneic hematopoietic cell transplantation in myelofibrosis (Letter to the Editor). Bone Marrow Transplant 2009;44(5):317–320.
15. Merup M, Lazarevic V, Nahi H, et al. Different outcome of allogeneic transplantation in myelofibrosis using conventional or reduced-intensity conditioning regimens. Br J Haematol 2006;135(3):367–373.

16. Kroger N, Thiele J, Zander A, et al. Rapid regression of bone marrow fibrosis after dose-reduced allogeneic stem cell transplantation in patients with primary myelofibrosis. Exp Hematol 2007;35(11):1719–1722.

17. Ciurea SO, Sadegi B, Wilbur A, et al. Effects of extensive splenomegaly in patients with myelofibrosis undergoing a reduced intensity allogeneic stem cell transplantation. Br J Haematol 2008;141(1):80–83.

18. Li Z, Gooley T, Appelbaum FR, Deeg HJ. Splenectomy and hemopoietic stem cell transplantation for myelofibrosis (Letter to the Editor). Blood 2001;97(7): 2180–2181.

19. Byrne JL, Beshti H, Clark D, et al. Induction of remission after donor leucocyte infusion for the treatment of relapsed chronic idiopathic myelofibrosis following allogeneic transplantation: evidence for a "graft vs. myelofibrosis" effect. Br J Haematol 2000;108(2):430–433.

20. Cervantes F, Rovira M, Urbano-Ispizua A, Rozman M, Carreras E, Montserrat E. Complete remission of idiopathic myelofibrosis following donor lymphocyte infusion after failure of allogeneic transplantation: demonstration of a graft-versus-myelofibrosis effect. Bone Marrow Transplant 2000;26(6):697–699.

21. Kroger N, Badbaran A, Lioznov M, et al. Post-transplant immunotherapy with donor-lymphocyte infusion and novel agents to upgrade partial into complete and molecular remission in allografted patients with multiple myeloma. Exp Hematol 2009;37(7):791–798.

22. Kroger N, Badbaran A, Holler E, et al. Monitoring of the JAK2-V617F mutation by highly sensitive quantitative real-time PCR after allogeneic stem cell transplantation in patients with myelofibrosis. Blood 2007;109(3):1316–1321.

23. Dupriez B, Morel P, Demory JL, et al. Prognostic factors in agnogenic myeloid metaplasia: a report on 195 cases with a new scoring system. Blood 1996;88(3): 1013–1018.

24. Cervantes F, Pereira A, Esteve J, et al. Identification of "short-lived" and "long-lived" patients at presentation of idiopathic myelofibrosis. Br J Haematol 1997;97(3):635–640.

25. Cervantes F, Barosi G, Demory JL, et al. Myelofibrosis with myeloid metaplasia in young individuals: disease characteristics, prognostic factors and identification of risk groups. Br J Haematol 1998;102(3):684–690.

26. Dingli D, Schwager SM, Mesa RA, Li CY, Tefferi A. Prognosis in transplant-eligible patients with agnogenic myeloid metaplasia: a simple CBC-based scoring system. Cancer 2006;106(3):623–630.

27. Cervantes F, Dupriez B, Pereira A, et al. New prognostic scoring system for primary myelofibrosis based on a study of the International Working Group for Myelofibrosis Research and Treatment. Blood 2009;113(13):2895–2901.

28. Tefferi A, Mesa RA, Schroeder G, Hanson CA, Li CY, Dewald GW. Cytogenetic findings and their clinical relevance in myelofibrosis with myeloid metaplasia. Br J Haematol 2001;113(3):763–771.

29. Steckel NK, Koldehoff M, Ditschkowski M, Beelen DW, Elmaagacli AH. Use of the activating gene mutation of the tyrosine kinase (VAL617Phe) JAK2 as a minimal residual disease marker in patients with myelofibrosis and myeloid metaplasia after allogeneic stem cell transplantation. Transplantation 2007;83(11):1518–1520.

30. Ditschkowski M, Elmaagacli AH, Trenschel R, Steckel NK, Koldehoff M, Beelen DW. No influence of V617F mutation in JAK2 on outcome after allogeneic hematopoietic stem cell transplantation (HSCT) for myelofibrosis. Biol Blood Marrow Transplant 2006;12(12):1350–1351.

31. Benjamini O, Koren-Michowitz M, Amariglio N, Kroger N, Nagler A, Shimoni A. Relapse of postpolycythemia myelofibrosis after allogeneic stem cell transplantation in a polycythemic phase: successful treatment with donor lymphocyte infusion directed by quantitative PCR test for V617F-JAK2 mutation. Leukemia 2008;22(10):1961–1963.

32. Rondelli D, Barosi G, Bacigalupo A, Prchal JT, Popat U, Alessandrino EP, et al. Non-myeloablative allogeneic HSCT in high risk patients with myelofibrosis [abstract]. Blood 2003;102(11):199a.
33. Snyder DS, Palmer J, Stein AS, et al. Allogeneic hematopoietic cell transplantation following reduced intensity conditioning for treatment of myelofibrosis. Biol Blood Marrow Transplant 2006;12(11):1161–1168.
34. Tidball JG, Wehling-Henricks M. Evolving therapeutic strategies for Duchenne muscular dystrophy: targeting downstream events (Review). Pediatr Res 2004;56(6):831–841.

Chapter 8

JAK2 Inhibitors for Therapy of Myeloproliferative Neoplasms

Fabio P.S. Santos and Srdan Verstovsek

Keywords: Polycythemia vera • Essential thrombocythemia • Myelofibrosis • JAK2 inhibitor • JAK2 V617F

Introduction

The classical Philadelphia chromosome-negative myeloproliferative neoplasms (Ph-negative MPNs) are hematopoietic stem cell disorders and include poly-cythemia vera (PV), essential thrombocythemia (ET), and primary myelofi-brosis (PMF) [1]. MF can also develop secondarily in patients with PV and ET (post-PV or -ET MF). Patients with PV and ET have close to normal life expectancy, but present with an increased risk for thrombosis [2]. They are usually treated with cytoreductive agents (e.g. hydroxyurea, anagrelide, ^{32}P, busulphan, and pipobroman) which can effectively control elevated blood cell counts and decrease the risk of thrombotic phenomena, but may also be associated with an increased risk of transformation to acute myeloid leukemia (AML) and/or post-PV/ET MF [2–4]. Therefore, apart from hydroxyurea, there are few drugs available for treating these patients without incurring significant side effects. There are also few treatment options available for patients with MF [5]. Patients with MF suffer from different signs and symp-toms, including massive splenomegaly, peripheral blood cytopenias, and con-stitutional symptoms such as fever, fatigue, and cachexia [5, 6]. Treatment is palliative and symptom-directed. Some of the available drugs that are used in practice include hydroxyurea, hematopoietic growth factors, immunomodula-tory drugs (e.g. thalidomide, lenalidomide), and conventional chemotherapeutic agents such as daunorubicin and melphalan [5]. However, no medication is approved as therapy for MF. Hematopoietic stem cell transplantation (HSCT) is a potential curative option for patients with MF [7]. However, it is only applicable in a minority of patients, mainly younger patients with available donors. It also carries a significant risk of morbidity and mortality (12–38% in recent series) [7], which precludes widespread application of this therapy. Thus, there is need for effective therapies for patients with MF, which poten-tially may change the natural history of this disease.

S. Verstovsek and A. Tefferi (eds.), *Myeloproliferative Neoplasms: Biology and Therapy*, Contemporary Hematology, DOI 10.1007/ 978-1-60761-266-7_8, © Springer Science+Business Media, LLC 2011

Recently, an activating mutation of the JAK2 tyrosine kinase (TK) (JAK2 V617F) was described in patients with Ph-negative MPNs [8–11]. The discovery of the JAK2 V617F mutation opened up the prospect for developing JAK2 inhibitors for use in patients with MPNs, akin to the development of imatinib that targets BCR-ABL1 in chronic myeloid leukemia (CML). Several JAK2 inhibitors are being tested in preclinical and clinical studies, and we summarize here the most recent clinical results seen with these compounds.

The JAK Family of Tyrosine Kinases

The JAK family of TK (named after the two-faced Roman god Janus) was first described in 1989 [12]. There are four members of the JAK family: JAK1, JAK2, JAK3, and TYK. JAKs are cytoplasmic kinases that associate with the intracellular portion of cytokine receptors that do not possess intrinsic kinase activity, such as receptors for hematopoietic growth factors (erythropoietin receptor [EPOR], G-CSF receptor [GCSFR], and thrombopoietin receptor [c-MPL]) [13]. Binding of the putative ligand leads to receptor dimerization and subsequent approximation of two JAK kinases, which trans-phosphorylate and activate each other, initiating intracellular signaling pathways (Fig. 8.1a).

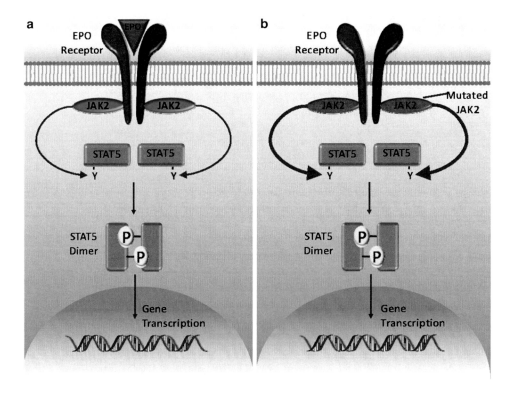

Fig. 8.1 *Activation of wild-type and mutated JAK2.* In *panel* (**a**), binding of the ligand (EPO) to the receptor leads to activation of JAK2 tyrosine kinases, which bind to the intracytoplasmic portion of the EPO receptor. Activation of JAK2 leads to phosphorylation of several intracellular signaling molecules, such as STAT5, depicted here. Phosphorylation of STAT5 leads to dimerization and translocation to the nucleus, where the STAT5 dimer acts as a transcription factor and induces gene expression. In *panel* (**b**), the mutated JAK2 (JAK2 V617F or exon 12 mutations) is constitutively active, even in the absence of the ligand, thus leading to continuous intracellular signaling

One of the most important intracellular signaling pathways activated by JAKs is the JAK-STAT (signal transducer and activator of transcription) pathway [13]. STATs are latent, cytoplasmic transcription factors [14]. JAKs phosphorylate STATs tyrosine residues, leading to STAT dimerization, translocation to the nucleus, and activation of transcription. Aberrant activation of STAT3 and STAT5 has been linked to neoplastic transformation [14]. Other signaling pathways which can be activated by JAKs include the Ras/Raf/MAPK pathway and the PI3K/Akt pathway. Activation of these pathways leads to increased cellular proliferation and resistance to apoptosis, and deregulation could cause the development of hematological malignancies.

Structurally, JAKs consists of seven different domains (Fig. 8.2) [15]. The tyrosine kinase domain (JAK homology domain 1, [JH1]) and the pseudokinase domain (JH2) are located in the C-terminal portion of the molecule. The kinase domain has all the features of an active TK domain, while the pseudokinase domain has no kinase activity [16]. It is believed that the JH2 domain interacts and inhibits the activity of the kinase domain, as deletion of the JH2 domain leads to increased kinase activity [17]. Residue V617 is located in a loop connecting two β-strands of the JH2 domain which interact with the activation loop of the JH1 domain [18]. The JAK2 V617F mutation possibly leads to increased kinase activity by disrupting this interaction and the inhibitory activity of the JH2 domain. Domains JH3–JH4 have a structure similar to SH2 (Src-homology 2) domains [19]. The JH5–JH7 domains are located in the N-terminus and contain a FERM (Band 4.1, ezrin, radixin, and moesin) motif. The FERM motif is essential for binding of the JAK kinase to the intracytoplasmic portion of the cytokine receptor [15].

Mouse knockout models and studies of patients with primary immunodeficiencies have provided important insights into the primary roles of JAKs. JAK1-deficient mice die at birth from neuronal defects and an inability from suckling [20]. Deficiency of JAK1 also leads to a severe impairment in lymphocyte development from defective interleukin (IL)-7 signaling. JAK1–/– cells revealed that JAK1 is essential for signaling by receptors containing the common γc chain (e.g. IL-2 and IL-7 receptors), class II cytokine receptors (including Interferons [IFN]-α, -β, and -γ), and cytokine receptors containing gp130 (e.g. IL-6 receptor) [20]. Deficiency of JAK2 is lethal to mice embryos due to the absence of definitive erythropoiesis [21, 22]. JAK2 is essential for signaling through the EPOR and c-MPL receptors, as well as cytokine receptors that utilize the common β-chain (IL-3 receptor and granulocyte–macrophage colony stimulating factor [GM-CSF] receptor) and IFN-γ receptors [21]. There is normal lymphoid development, however [22]. Thus, JAK2 is important for signaling pathways that control erythroid and myeloid, but not lymphoid,

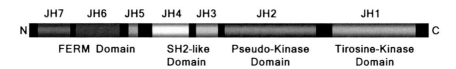

Fig. 8.2 *Structure of JAK tyrosine kinases.* JAK kinases are composed of seven different homology domains (JH1–JH7). Domain JH1 is the tyrosine kinase domain, while domain JH2 is the pseudokinase domain, responsible for regulating activity of the JH1 domain. Domains JH3–JH4 have a structure similar to SH2 (Src-Homology 2 domains), which bind to phosphorylated tyrosine residues. Domains JH5–JH7 have a FERM-like motif and are responsible for binding to the intracytoplasmic portion of cytokine receptors

development. JAK3 is only activated by cytokines of the γc family (IL-2, IL-4, IL-7, IL-9, IL-15, and IL-21), and deficiency of JAK3 leads to severe impairment in lymphoid development, with reductions in numbers of T and B lymphocytes and NK-cells [23, 24]. Mutations in JAK3 have been described in patients with severe combined immunodeficiency (SCID) [25, 26]. Mice that are deficient in TYK2 are phenotypically normal but exhibit an increased susceptibility to viral infections and a reduced response to IL-12 [27, 28].

The JAK2 V617F Mutation

Initial clues to the role of JAK2 pseudokinase domain mutations in myeloproliferative neoplasms came from studies with the fruit fly *Drosophila melanogaster*. A point mutation (E695K) located in the JH2 domain of the gene *Hopscotch*, the JAK equivalent of *Drosophila*, leads to increased kinase activity and development of a leukemia-like picture with increased numbers of hemocytes (fly blood cells) [29]. There was also increased activation of STAT92E (STAT equivalent of *Drosophila*). A homologous mutation in murine JAK2 also leads to increased kinase activity and STAT5 activation in mammalian cells [29].

The JAK2 V617F mutation was first described by several groups in 2005. It was identified primarily in patients with PV (90–97%), ET (60%), and PMF (50%) [8–11]. Subsequent studies revealed that the mutation is also found, albeit more rarely, in selected cases of chronic myelomonocytic leukemia, atypical CML and AML [30]. Recent studies have revealed that the presence of a germline JAK2 haplotype (46/1) predisposes to the development of the JAK2 V617F mutation [31–33]. The JAK2 V617F mutation leads to constitutive activation of the JAK2 TK (Fig. 8.1b), and expression of the mutated kinase in BaF/3 cells expressing EPOR conferred EPO hypersensitivity and EPO-independent growth and survival [11]. Animal models showed that expression of the JAK2 V617F TK in hematopoietic stem cells leads to a phenotype similar to PV with later progression to fibrotic changes in the bone marrow [34, 35].

Despite this important advance, several questions still remain regarding the role of JAK2 V617F in MPNs. The mechanism through which a single mutation can give rise to diseases with different phenotypes is still unknown. Patients with JAK2-mutated ET are usually heterozygous for the mutation [36], and the presence of JAK2 V617F is associated with a "PV-like phenotype" and a higher propensity to evolve into PV [37, 38]. Patients with PV are usually homozygous for JAK2 V617F [36]. Animal models have demonstrated that expression of the mutation at a lower level than the wild-type JAK2 leads to a phenotype more similar to ET [39]. Conversely, expression of the mutated TK at a high level generates a phenotype more akin to PV [39]. This suggests that JAK2 V617F-positive PV/ET form a biological continuum. The allelic burden of the JAK2 V617F mutation may also have prognostic significance. In PV, greater than 75% allelic burden is associated with higher hematocrit, white blood cell (WBC) count, and higher incidence of splenomegaly and thrombotic events. Patients with primary MF who are JAK2 V617F-positive may have higher hemoglobin and WBC count and a higher risk of leukemic transformation and of developing massive splenomegaly [40]. However, other studies suggested that survival is worse in patients with JAK2 V617F-positive primary MF who have low allelic ratio of the mutation [41, 42].

Another unanswered question pertains to those patients with JAK2 V617F-negative MPNs. Search for other mutations led to the discovery of JAK2 exon 12 mutations in 3% of PV patients [43] and mutations of c-MPL (MPL W515K/L) in 8.5% of ET and 10% of MF patients [44, 45]. These mutations also lead to increased cellular proliferation and hypersensitivity or independency to hematopoietic growth factors. While the JAK2 V617F and related mutations certainly contribute to the pathogenesis of MPNs, they are probably a secondary genetic event, and not the disease-initiating mutation [46]. Indeed, JAK2 V617F-negative erythroid colonies from patients with PV can grow in the absence of erythropoietin [46]. Recent studies have revealed other mutations in patients with MPNs, such as *TET2* mutations which are found in 12% of patients [47]. In some patients *TET2* mutations preceded the appearance of the JAK2 V617F mutation. Additionally, several reports described patients with JAK2 V617F-positive MPNs who developed JAK2 V617F-negative AML [48]. Thus, it appears that a single mutation (JAK2 V617F) cannot explain the complex heterogeneity of MPNs. Identification of other mutations and potential therapeutic targets in MPNs is the current subject of intense investigation.

Rationale for Targeting JAK2 in Myeloproliferative Neoplasms

The discovery of the BCR-ABL1 inhibitor imatinib and its unprecedented success in the therapy of CML ushered cancer medicine into the era of kinase inhibitors [49]. These drugs target kinases that are abnormally activated in cancer cells, with the objective of blocking cellular proliferation and inducing apoptosis [49]. The JAK2 V617F mutation generates a constitutively active TK, and so there was a rationale for developing JAK2 inhibitors for treating patients with MF and other MPNs. However, a few points should be mentioned. First, it must be remembered that ATP (adenosine tri-phosphate) is the source of phosphate groups utilized by TK for phosphorylating protein targets, and most TK inhibitors (TKI) in current development are small molecules that act by competing with ATP for the ATP-binding catalytic site in the TK domain [49]. Since the JAK2 V617F mutation occurs outside of the TK domain, it is likely that most JAK2 inhibitors will target both the mutated and wild-type kinase. Inhibition of wild-type JAK2 will lead to myelosuppression, as JAK2 is an important mediator of hematopoietic growth factor signaling. On the other hand, JAK2 inhibitors might function in patients with both mutated and unmutated MPNs. Suppression of erythropoiesis and thrombopoiesis might also be seen as a desired side effect if these drugs are used in patients with PV and ET. Second, based on the complex biology of MF, and on results already seen with these compounds, it is likely that therapy with JAK2 inhibitors will not lead to clonal eradication in this disorder, as is seen in patients with CML treated with imatinib. These drugs may also act by suppressing signaling by inflammatory cytokines [50]. MF is a disease characterized by excessive production of proinflammatory cytokines [51], and normalization of this inflammatory milieu improves patients' systemic symptoms, leading to weight gain, improvement in fatigue, and reduction of spleen size. Thus, there is great therapeutic benefit for employing these drugs to achieve symptom control and improve the quality of life of patients with MPNs. A better knowledge of how these drugs work in MF and other MPNs is needed to capitalize on their efficacy.

Clinical Trials with JAK2 Inhibitors

The results of clinical studies with five different JAK2 inhibitors in MF have already been presented (Tables 8.1 and 8.2; Fig. 8.3). While varying in their efficacy and toxicity profile, a few common features have been seen. Most responses consist in improvement in spleen size and constitutional symptoms. Some compounds have lead to a decrease in the burden of JAK2-mutated clones, but none have achieved major molecular eradication. Also, no improvement is usually seen in bone marrow fibrosis and cytopenias. The majority of studies have focused on patients with MF, due to their worse survival and lack of adequate therapy, but some recent studies are also being conducted in patients with PV and ET who are refractory or intolerant to conventional therapy with hydroxyurea.

CEP-701

CEP-701 (also known as a lestaurtinib) is a TKI which belongs to the chemical class of indocarbazole alkaloids. CEP-701 is a FLT3 inhibitor and is being evaluated in clinical trials of FLT3-positive AML [52]. Preclinical data showed CEP-701 to be a potent inhibitor of both wild-type and mutant JAK2, with an IC50 of 1 nM against wild-type JAK2 [53]. CEP-701 inhibited the proliferation of JAK2 V617F-positive cells xenografted in nude mice, demonstrating in vivo activity [53].

The first clinical trial reported with CEP-701 was a single-center phase II study that recruited 22 patients with JAK2 V617F-positive primary MF or post-PV/ET MF [54]. Patients recruited required therapy, including either previously treated patients that were relapsed, intolerant, or refractory to therapy or if newly diagnosed then with intermediate or high risk according to Lille scoring system [55]. Patients received CEP-701 as a liquid formulation at a dose of 80 mg twice daily. Responses were graded by the International Working Group (IWG) on Myelofibrosis Research and Treatment response criteria [56]. Median age was 61 years (range 38–83) and median number of prior therapies was 3 (range 0–6). Responses were seen in six patients (27%). All responses consisted of clinical improvements (CI): three patients had a reduction in spleen size, two patients achieved transfusion independency, and one patient had a reduction in spleen size associated with improvement in cytopenias. Median time to response was 3 months and median duration of response 14+ months. There was no change in bone marrow fibrosis, JAK2 V617F allelic burden, and cytokine levels. Responders had significant

Table 8.1 In vitro kinase inhibition profile of current JAK2 inhibitors.

Drug	Company	Current phase	Target(s)	IC50 Value (nM) JAK2	JAK1	JAK3
CEP-701	Cephalon	I/II	JAK2, FLT3	1	?	?
INCB018424	Incyte	III	JAK2, JAK1	2.8	3.3	322
SB1518	S*Bio	I	JAK2, FLT3	23	1280	520
TG101348	TargeGen	II	JAK2, FLT3	3	105	996
XL019	Exelixis	Discontinued	JAK2	2	132	250

Table 8.2 Preliminary clinical results of trials with JAK2 inhibitors in patients with MF.

Reference	Treatment	N	Major clinical responses and side effects
Santos et al. [54]	CEP-701 80 mg twice daily (Phase II)	22	Improvement in splenomegaly; GI toxicity and cytopenias
Hexner et al. [58]	CEP-701 80–160 mg twice daily (Phase I)	26	Reduction in splenomegaly; GI toxicity
Verstovsek et al. [61]	INCB018424 10–25 mg twice daily (Phase I/II)	153	Reduction in splenomegaly, fatigue, weight loss, and exercise capability; cytopenias
Verstovsek et al. [67]	SB1518 100–600 mg once daily (Phase I/II)	43	Improvement in splenomegaly and systemic symptoms; GI toxicity
Pardanani et al. [70]	TG101348 30–800 mg once daily (Phase I/II)	59	Reduction in splenomegaly, improvement in systemic symptoms, elevated WBC, and platelet counts; GI toxicity and cytopenias
Shah et al. [72]	XL019 25–300 mg once daily or 25 mg thrice a week (Phase I/II)	30	Improvement in splenomegaly, systemic symptoms; neurotoxicity

MF myelofibrosis, *CI* clinical improvement, *IWG* International Working Group, *GI* gastrointestinal, *WBC* white blood cell count

downregulation of phosphorylated STAT3, a known downstream messenger of JAK2. Main toxicity was myelosuppression (grade 3–4 anemia 14%; grade 3–4 thrombocytopenia 23%) and gastrointestinal disturbances (diarrhea, any grade 72%, grade 3–4 9%; nausea, grade 1–2 only, 50%; and vomiting, grade 1–2 only, 27%).

The dose of 80 mg that was utilized in the trial above was based on the results from the studies conducted in patients with FLT3-positive AML [57]. A phase I/II trial led by the Myeloproliferative Diseases Research Consortium explored the possibility that higher doses might have a better efficacy in MF and also evaluated a capsule formulation of CEP-701. The phase I results of this study were recently reported [58]. Twenty-six patients with JAK2 V617F-positive MF (primary or post-PV/ET) were recruited in a classic 3 + 3 dose escalation design trial. CEP-701 was administered at doses ranging from 80 to 100 mg twice daily in 7 patients (liquid formulation) and 100 to 160 mg twice daily in 19 patients (capsule formulation). The maximum tolerated dose (MTD) was not reached, and currently there are six patients enrolled at the highest dose level (160 mg twice daily). Dose-limiting toxicity (DLT) was grade 3 diarrhea observed in one patient in the liquid cohort and in the capsule cohort each. Diarrhea (grade 1–2 only) was seen in 71% of patients in the liquid cohort and 37% of patients in the capsule cohort. Other significant side effects include nausea (grade 1–2 29% liquid cohort, 37% capsule cohort). Spleen size was reduced in six patients (median 5.8 cm). In four patients with

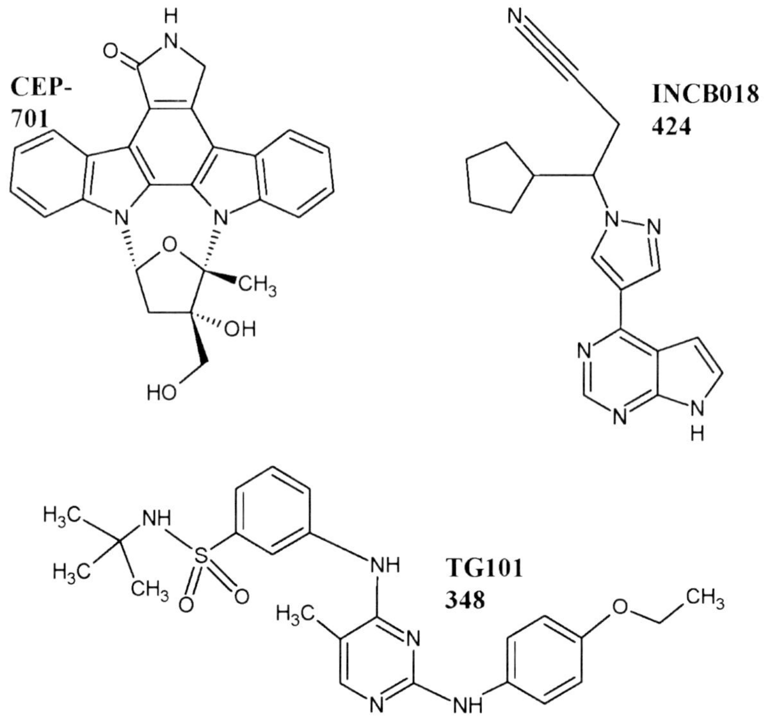

Fig. 8.3 Chemical structure of selected JAK2 tyrosine kinase inhibitors

paired baseline and week 24 samples, reduction of JAK2 V617F allelic burden was seen in three patients (range 6–41.5%).

CEP-701 is also being studied in a phase II trial of high-risk patients with JAK2 V617F-positive PV or ET [59]. Inclusion criteria for PV included neutrophil count above 7 × 10⁹/L and/or prior use of hydroxyurea; inclusion criteria for ET included prior use of hydroxyurea. Patients received a starting dose of 80 mg twice daily of CEP-701 with possible escalation to 120 mg twice daily. Overall, 39 patients were recruited (PV = 27; ET = 12). Fifteen patients have completed 18 weeks of treatment. A reduction in spleen size to nonpalpable was seen in 83% of patients. Improvement in pruritus was seen in 5/5 patients. Three patients (out of five) with phlebotomy dependence had a reduction in phlebotomy requirements. However, there was no concomitant reduction in WBC count or platelet count. JAK2 V617F allelic burden had a greater than 15% decrease in three of 15 evaluable patients. Severe adverse events reported included deep venous thrombosis (four patients) and arterial thrombosis (two patients).

INCB018424

INCB018424 is a potent, selective, and orally available JAK2 inhibitor currently being evaluated in clinical trials in patients with MF and PV/ET. Preclinical studies demonstrated that INCB018424 inhibits JAK2 at 2.8 nM in kinase assays and it inhibited proliferation of BaF/3 cells expressing JAK2 V617F with an IC50 value of 127 nM [60]. It also inhibits JAK1 (IC50 3.3 nM). Inhibition of proliferation correlated with reduced levels of phosphorylated

JAK2 and STAT5. In contrast, no inhibition of cells expressing BCR-ABL1 or mutated c-KIT was seen. INCB018424 also inhibited the cytokine-independent growth of erythroid-colony-forming units from patients with PV (IC50 67 nM), while colony formation from normal donors was inhibited with an IC50 value > 400 nM [60]. This suggests that INCB018424 has greater potency against the mutated form of JAK2. Oral administration of INCB018424 significantly decreased spleen and liver size and improved survival in a murine model of MPN [60]. This was accompanied by a decrease in circulating levels of inflammatory cytokines.

A phase I/II clinical trial was conducted in patients with primary or post-PV/ET MF [61]. The phase I portion of the trial determined that the MTD was 25 mg twice daily or 100 mg once daily, and the DLT was thrombocytopenia. The study was expanded into phase II with different doses and schedules and has accrued 153 patients. Median age of patients was 65 years, and 93% had intermediate-2/high-risk by IWG criteria [62]. Forty-five percent had karyotypic abnormalities and 34% were transfusion-dependent. Median time on therapy is 15 months, and 75% of patients (115/153) remain on therapy. Most frequent nonhematological toxicities were diarrhea (grade 1–2: 5.9%), fatigue (grade 1–2: 3.3%; grade 3: 1.6%), and headache (grade 1–2: 3.3%). No grade 4 nonhematological toxicity was recorded. Since not all patients could tolerate a starting dose of 25 mg twice daily due to hematological toxicity (mainly thrombocytopenia), an optimized dose regimen was tested in 35 patients. Patients received a starting dose of 15 mg twice daily (10 mg twice daily if platelets <200 × 10^9/L) followed by slow titration over the first months to 20 and 25 mg twice daily if no response was seen and there was no major toxicity. Use of this optimized dose regimen significantly decreased the rate of hematological toxicity (grade 3–4 anemia 8.3%; grade 3–4 thrombocytopenia 2.9%) compared with the conventional dose of 25 mg twice daily (grade 3–4 anemia 26.3%; grade 3–4 thrombocytopenia 29.4%). Importantly, there was no decrease in efficacy. Significant reductions in spleen size (>50%) were observed in the majority of patients as early as 1 month after therapy start. A ≥35% reduction in spleen volume by magnetic resonance imaging (MRI), which corresponds to a greater than 50% reduction in spleen length by physical exam, was seen in 48% of patients at 6 months of therapy who were on the optimized dose schedule cohort. Spleen size reduction occurred independently of disease subtype (primary or post-PV/ET MF) and of JAK2 V617F mutational status. There was also significant improvement in systemic symptoms. After 6 months of therapy 58% of patients had ≥50% reduction in a symptom score based on MF symptoms (fatigue, abdominal discomfort/pain, bone/muscle pain, night sweats, and pruritus) [63]. Importantly, improvement in systemic symptoms and spleen size was accompanied by a significant reduction in plasma level of proinflammatory cytokines (e.g. IL-1, macrophage inflammatory protein-1β (beta) [MIP-1β (beta)], tumor necrosis factor-α (alpha) [TNF-α], IL-6, and vascular endothelial growth factor [VEGF]). There was also improvement in exercise capacity, with an improvement from baseline in the 6-min walking test of 34, 57, and 71 m after 1, 3, and 6 months of therapy. One hundred and ten patients had available data on JAK2 V617F burden after 3 months of treatment. Median allelic burden at baseline was 70%. There was an average decrease in the allele burden of 11% at 1 year and 18% at 2 years. A greater than 25% reduction was seen in 19 patients and a greater than 50%

reduction was seen in 8 patients only. Only three patients transformed to AML (rate of 0.016 patients/year), which is less than expected based on historical cohorts [40]. INCB018424 is a potent JAK2 inhibitor which leads to significant improvements in spleen size, exercise capacity, and systemic symptoms in patients with MF. These effects are accompanied by a reduction in proinflammatory cytokine levels, which suggests that INCB018424 mechanism of action is related in part to the inhibition of cytokine signaling mediated by JAK1. Randomized controlled phase III trials of INCB018424 in patients with MF are currently in progress.

Another trial evaluated INCB018424 in patients with PV/ET [64]. Inclusion criteria included refractoriness or intolerance to hydroxyurea; additional inclusion criteria included hematocrit >45% or dependence on phlebotomies (for patients with PV) and platelet count >650 × 10^9/L (for patients with ET). Responses were assessed by the European LeukemiaNet criteria [65]. In the first part of the trial, patients were randomized between three doses (10 mg twice daily, 25 mg twice daily, and 50 mg once daily). In the second part of the study the best dose cohort (PV: 10 mg twice daily; ET 25 mg twice daily) was expanded. Seventy-three patients have been recruited (PV – 34; ET – 39). In the PV cohort, median age of patients was 58 years, median hematocrit was 46.4%, and median WBC count was 13.2 × 10^9/L. Splenomegaly was seen in 74% of patients and median spleen size by palpation was 9 cm below left costal margin. All patients were positive for the JAK2 V617F mutation. Therapy with INCB018424 resulted in rapid and durable normalization of the hematocrit. At 6 months, median hematocrit was 39%. Only two patients required phlebotomies in the first 2 weeks after starting the drug, and none ever since. There was also rapid and sustained normalization of WBC and platelet counts. Patients experienced significant reductions in spleen size; at 6 months 80% of patients with palpable splenomegaly had a greater than 50% reduction in spleen size, and in 52% it was no longer palpable. This was accompanied by improvements in systemic symptoms (pruritus, bone pain, and night sweats). The response rate was 97%, including 45% complete remission and 52% partial response. In patients with ET, the median age was 51 years. Median platelet count was 884 × 10^9/L and 67% were positive for the JAK2 V617F mutation. Therapy with INCB018424 significantly reduced platelet counts, with a median platelet count of 553 × 10^9/L at 6 months. There were also significant reductions in WBC, splenomegaly, and systemic symptoms. The overall response rate was 90%, including 13% complete remission and 77% partial response. INCB018424 was very well tolerated in patients with PV/ET, and only three patients have discontinued therapy due to adverse events. Ninety-two percent of patients remain on study. The most common toxicity was anemia (PV – grade 2: 12%; ET – grade 2: 18%). Most common grade 3 toxicity was thrombocytopenia (PV: 3%) and leukopenia (ET: 5%). No grade 4 toxicities were recorded. Overall, therapy with INCB018424 was highly effective in patients with PV/ET who were refractory or intolerant to hydroxyurea, with minimal side effects.

SB1518

SB1518 is a newly developed TKI that has activity as a JAK2 inhibitor [66]. SB1518 inhibits both wild-type (IC50 = 22 nM) and mutated JAK2 (IC50 = 19 nM). SB1518 also has activity as an FLT3 inhibitor. Preclinical data demonstrated that SB1518 inhibited proliferation of BaF/3 cells transfected with the EPOR and the JAK2 V617F mutation and decreased phosphorylation of JAK2 and STAT5. In a murine model of MPN, administration of SB1518 to nude mice xenografted with JAK2 V617F-positive cells led to normalization of elevated WBC count, reduction of GFP-labeled BaF/3 cells in the peripheral blood, improvement in cytopenias and hepatosplenomegaly, reduction of phosphorylated-STAT5 in involved organs, and increased survival. Data on the phase I clinical trial conducted in patients with MF and AML were recently presented [67]. Overall, 43 patients were recruited, including 36 with MF and 7 with AML. SB1518 was administered at doses ranging from 100 to 600 mg orally once daily continuously in 28-days cycles. Median age was 70 years, and 78% were positive for the JAK2 V617F mutation. Twenty-eight patients had a greater than 5 cm splenomegaly, and median spleen size in these patients was 13 cm. Median time on study drug was 111 days, and the MTD was 500 mg. DLT were observed in three of six patients receiving 600 mg and mostly included gastrointestinal symptoms (abdominal pain, diarrhea). Symptoms subsided after drug interruption and all the three patients restarted SB1518 at a lower dose. Most common toxicities were diarrhea (all grades: 33%; grade 3: 4%), nausea (grade 1–2 only: 13%), and thrombocytopenia (grades 3–4: 4%). There were 25 patients with MF who had baseline splenomegaly greater than 5 cm and had a follow-up assessment by physical examination. Of these, seven patients (28%) had a marked (>50%) and durable reduction in spleen size. Seven additional patients had a 35–50% reduction in spleen size. Marked spleen reduction was observed both in JAK2 V617F-positive (6/23) and -negative (1/2) patients. Among the seven patients with AML, three had evidence of clinical benefit, including one patient with >50% spleen reduction after 28 days and two patients with stable disease. Correlative studies demonstrated that as early as 2 h after oral dosing there was a decrease in levels of phosphorylated JAK2 and STAT5, consistent with target inhibition. Development of SB1518 will continue with the dose of 400 mg once daily recommended for the phase 2 trial.

TG101348

TG101348 is a selective JAK2 inhibitor with IC50 values of 3 nM, having less potency against JAK3 (335× less potent) and JAK1 (35× less potent) (Table 8.1). TG101348 also inhibits FLT3 at 15 nM. In preclinical evaluation TG101348 inhibited proliferation of JAK2 V617F-positive HEL cells and BaF/3 cells transduced with JAK2 V617F [68]. TG101348 also inhibited erythroid colony formation by JAK2 V617F-positive human progenitor cells and engraftment in xenotransplant studies [69]. Activity of TG101348 was accompanied by a reduction in phosphorylated STAT5, indicating inhibition of the JAK-STAT signaling pathway [69]. In a murine model of PV, administration of TG101348 led to improvement in hematocrit, reduction in spleen and liver size, normalization of spleen architecture with elimination of extramedullary hematopoiesis, and improved survival and reversal of bone marrow fibrosis in some instances [68].

A phase 1 clinical trial was conducted in patients with MF who were intermediate/high-risk and had symptomatic splenomegaly [70]. The trial was designed as a phase I, open label study with dose escalation, followed by expansion of the cohort once MTD was determined. Fifty-nine patients with MF (primary MF or post-PV/ET MF) were enrolled, including 40 in the expanded cohort. Median age of patients was 64 years. JAK2 V617F mutation was positive in 86% of patients, and 98% had splenomegaly. Patients received TG101348 at doses ranging from 30 to 800 mg once daily in 28-day cycles. Intrapatient dose escalation was allowed after three courses. The MTD was determined to be 680 mg daily. DLT observed at 800 mg included grade 3–4 hyperamylasemia (6%) and hyperlipasemia (13%). Other grade 3–4 laboratory abnormalities observed included hypocalcemia (8%), elevated liver enzymes (8%), and hyperkalemia (8%). Laboratory abnormalities were usually transient and reversible upon drug discontinuation. Most common nonhematological toxicities observed were mainly gastrointestinal in nature, including diarrhea (all grades: 76%; grade 3: 13%), nausea (all grades: 70%; grade 3: 5%), vomiting (all grades: 69%; grade 3: 3%), and anorexia (all grades: 21%; grade 3: 3%). Grade 3–4 hematological toxicities at MTD included neutropenia (grade 3: 15%), thrombocytopenia (grade 3–4: 33%), and new-onset transfusion-dependent anemia (67%). So far, 75% of patients remain on trial receiving the drug, and median treatment duration is 6 months. Efficacy of TG101348 was confirmed by marked reductions in splenomegaly. Clinical improvement based on reduction of spleen size was observed in 49% of total patients, 56% of patients by 3 months, and 100% of patients by 5 months. Among patients who presented with elevated ($>11 \times 10^9$/L) WBC count, 73% had a normal WBC count at last follow-up (median time 6 months). A similar decrease was observed in patients who presented with thrombocytosis ($>450 \times 10^9$/L). TG101348 also led to improvement in systemic symptoms, including pruritus, night sweats, fatigue, and early satiety. However, different from other JAK2 inhibitors, this was not accompanied by a reduction in proinflammatory cytokine levels. A reduction in JAK2 V617F allelic burden was observed in 59% of patients who carried the mutation. Preliminary observations in selected patients also showed improvement in bone marrow cellularity and fibrosis. The results observed with TG101348 in the phase I trial suggest that its mechanism of action is a direct consequence of JAK2 V617F inhibition [70]. Longer follow-up and larger studies are needed to confirm these observations.

XL019

XL019 is a potent and reversible inhibitor of JAK2 TK (IC50 = 2 nM) [71]. XL019 also demonstrated excellent selectivity against JAK2 (minimum >50-fold selectivity against >120 different kinases including other members of the JAK2 family) (Table 8.1). XL019 inhibited STAT5 in both primary human erythroid progenitor cells stimulated with EPO (IC50 = 64 nM) and cell lines carrying mutated JAK2 (IC50 = 623 nM in HEL 92.1.7 cells) [71]. In a xenograft tumor model of HEL 92.1.7 cells, XL019 suppressed STAT5 phosphorylation (IC50 = 42 mg/kg) and led to tumor growth inhibition, tumor cell apoptosis, and reduction in tumor vasculature [71]. A phase I study evaluated XL019 in patients with primary or post-PV/ET MF [72]. Initial dose escalation started at 100 mg once daily for 21 days of 28-days cycles. However, reversible peripheral neuropathy developed in all patients receiving ≥100 mg daily doses of XL019. This led to dose modification to 25–50 mg once daily and 25 mg three times a week. Thirty patients have been recruited, and 21 have received doses ≤50 mg. A greater than 50% reduction in spleen size was observed in five of 12 evaluable patients. Improvements in anemia, WBC counts, pruritus, and fatigue were also observed in some patients. Four patients had a preleukemic stage of MF, with elevated (10–19%) blast counts in the peripheral blood and/or bone marrow. Therapy with XL019 led to blast count reduction in three of these patients. Interestingly, no hematological side effects were observed. Most common side effects were neurological in nature, including peripheral neuropathy, formication, paresthesia, and balance disorder. Due to the presence of neurotoxicity even at low doses of the compound, the study was discontinued and no further evaluation of XL019 is planned.

Future Perspectives

JAK2 inhibitors have initiated the development of targeted therapies for patients with MF and other MPNs. Clinical results seen with these compounds demonstrate improvement in splenomegaly and systemic symptoms in the majority of patients being treated, and these compounds could become an important part of the armamentarium to treat patients with these disorders. However, several challenges still lay ahead.

The true mechanism of action of these drugs in MF is still not fully elucidated. Their beneficial effect could be due to a nonspecific inhibition of cytokine signaling, to inhibition of aberrant TK in the neoplastic clone, and maybe both. Host genetic variants could influence response to treatment. Also, even though all compounds target JAK2, they vary in their potency and specificity. It will be important to compare results of drugs with less specificity for JAK2 (e.g. INCB018424 which is a JAK1 and JAK2 inhibitor) with compounds more specific for targeting JAK2 to better ascertain the value of selectivity for JAK2.

In most clinical trials so far, no consistent reduction in JAK2 allelic burden has been observed. The reason for this is unknown, and it could be that just targeting one mutated kinase is not sufficient to lead to clonal eradication. However, longer follow-up is still needed, as most drugs have been in clinical trials for only 1–2 years so far. It must be remembered that both patients with mutated- and unmutated-JAK2 derive benefit from these compounds. Determining biomarkers for response could be useful for selecting patients for treatment with these drugs.

In conclusion, JAK2 inhibitors are a novel class of agents with promising results for treating patients with MF. Further studies are needed to better understand their role in the treatment of MPNs.

References

1. Tefferi A, Gilliland G. Classification of chronic myeloid disorders: from Dameshek towards a semi-molecular system. *Best Pract Res Clin Haematol.* 2006;19(3):365–385.
2. Finazzi G, Barbui T. Evidence and expertise in the management of polycythemia vera and essential thrombocythemia. *Leukemia.* 2008;22(8):1494–1502.
3. Finazzi G, Caruso V, Marchioli R, et al. Acute leukemia in polycythemia vera: an analysis of 1638 patients enrolled in a prospective observational study. *Blood.* 2005;105(7):2664–2670.
4. Harrison CN, Campbell PJ, Buck G, et al. Hydroxyurea compared with anagrelide in high-risk essential thrombocythemia. *N Engl J Med.* 2005;353(1):33–45.

5. Mesa RA, Barosi G, Cervantes F, Reilly JT, Tefferi A. Myelofibrosis with myeloid metaplasia: disease overview and non-transplant treatment options. *Best Pract Res Clin Haematol.* 2006;19(3):495–517.

6. Mesa RA, Niblack J, Wadleigh M, et al. The burden of fatigue and quality of life in myeloproliferative disorders (MPDs): an international Internet-based survey of 1179 MPD patients. *Cancer.* 2007;109(1):68–76.

7. Kroger N, Holler E, Kobbe G, et al. Allogeneic stem cell transplantation after reduced-intensity conditioning in patients with myelofibrosis: a prospective, multicenter study of the Chronic Leukemia Working Party of the European Group for Blood and Marrow Transplantation (EBMT). *Blood.* 2009;114(26): 5264–5270.

8. Baxter EJ, Scott LM, Campbell PJ, et al. Acquired mutation of the tyrosine kinase JAK2 in human myeloproliferative disorders. *Lancet.* 2005;365(9464):1054–1061.

9. James C, Ugo V, Le Couedic JP, et al. A unique clonal JAK2 mutation leading to constitutive signalling causes polycythaemia vera. *Nature.* 2005;434(7037):1144–1148.

10. Kralovics R, Passamonti F, Buser AS, et al. A gain-of-function mutation of JAK2 in myeloproliferative disorders. *N Engl J Med.* 2005;352(17):1779–1790.

11. Levine RL, Wadleigh M, Cools J, et al. Activating mutation in the tyrosine kinase JAK2 in polycythemia vera, essential thrombocythemia, and myeloid metaplasia with myelofibrosis. *Cancer Cell.* 2005;7(4):387–397.

12. Wilks AF. Two putative protein-tyrosine kinases identified by application of the polymerase chain reaction. *Proc Natl Acad Sci U S A.* 1989;86(5):1603–1607.

13. Leonard WJ, O'Shea JJ. Jaks and STATs: biological implications. *Annu Rev Immunol.* 1998;16:293–322.

14. Yu H, Jove R. The STATs of cancer – new molecular targets come of age. *Nat Rev Cancer.* 2004;4(2):97–105.

15. Giordanetto F, Kroemer RT. Prediction of the structure of human Janus kinase 2 (JAK2) comprising JAK homology domains 1 through 7. *Protein Eng.* 2002;15(9):727–737.

16. Wilks AF, Harpur AG, Kurban RR, Ralph SJ, Zurcher G, Ziemiecki A. Two novel protein-tyrosine kinases, each with a second phosphotransferase-related catalytic domain, define a new class of protein kinase. *Mol Cell Biol.* 1991;11(4):2057–2065.

17. Saharinen P, Silvennoinen O. The pseudokinase domain is required for suppression of basal activity of Jak2 and Jak3 tyrosine kinases and for cytokine-inducible activation of signal transduction. *J Biol Chem.* 2002;277(49):47954–47963.

18. Lindauer K, Loerting T, Liedl KR, Kroemer RT. Prediction of the structure of human Janus kinase 2 (JAK2) comprising the two carboxy-terminal domains reveals a mechanism for autoregulation. *Protein Eng.* 2001;14(1):27–37.

19. Radtke S, Haan S, Jorissen A, et al. The Jak1 SH2 domain does not fulfill a classical SH2 function in Jak/STAT signaling but plays a structural role for receptor interaction and up-regulation of receptor surface expression. *J Biol Chem.* 2005;280(27):25760–25768.

20. Rodig SJ, Meraz MA, White JM, et al. Disruption of the Jak1 gene demonstrates obligatory and nonredundant roles of the Jaks in cytokine-induced biologic responses. *Cell.* 1998;93(3):373–383.

21. Parganas E, Wang D, Stravopodis D, et al. Jak2 is essential for signaling through a variety of cytokine receptors. *Cell.* 1998;93(3):385–395.

22. Neubauer H, Cumano A, Muller M, Wu H, Huffstadt U, Pfeffer K. Jak2 deficiency defines an essential developmental checkpoint in definitive hematopoiesis. *Cell.* 1998;93(3):397–409.

23. Nosaka T, van Deursen JM, Tripp RA, et al. Defective lymphoid development in mice lacking Jak3. *Science.* 1995;270(5237):800–802.

24. Thomis DC, Gurniak CB, Tivol E, Sharpe AH, Berg LJ. Defects in B lymphocyte maturation and T lymphocyte activation in mice lacking Jak3. *Science.* 1995;270(5237):794–797.

25. Macchi P, Villa A, Giliani S, et al. Mutations of Jak-3 gene in patients with autosomal severe combined immune deficiency (SCID). *Nature*. 1995;377(6544):65–68.

26. Russell SM, Tayebi N, Nakajima H, et al. Mutation of Jak3 in a patient with SCID: essential role of Jak3 in lymphoid development. *Science*. 1995;270(5237):797–800.

27. Karaghiosoff M, Neubauer H, Lassnig C, et al. Partial impairment of cytokine responses in Tyk2-deficient mice. *Immunity*. 2000;13(4):549–560.

28. Shimoda K, Kato K, Aoki K, et al. Tyk2 plays a restricted role in IFN alpha signaling, although it is required for IL-12-mediated T cell function. *Immunity*. 2000;13(4):561–571.

29. Luo H, Rose P, Barber D, et al. Mutation in the Jak kinase JH2 domain hyperactivates Drosophila and mammalian Jak-Stat pathways. *Mol Cell Biol*. 1997;17(3):1562–1571.

30. Jelinek J, Oki Y, Gharibyan V, et al. JAK2 mutation 1849G>T is rare in acute leukemias but can be found in CMML, Philadelphia chromosome-negative CML, and megakaryocytic leukemia. *Blood*. 2005;106(10):3370–3373.

31. Olcaydu D, Harutyunyan A, Jager R, et al. A common JAK2 haplotype confers susceptibility to myeloproliferative neoplasms. *Nat Genet*. 2009;41(4):450–454.

32. Kilpivaara O, Mukherjee S, Schram AM, et al. A germline JAK2 SNP is associated with predisposition to the development of JAK2(V617F)-positive myeloproliferative neoplasms. *Nat Genet*. 2009;41(4):455–459.

33. Jones AV, Chase A, Silver RT, et al. JAK2 haplotype is a major risk factor for the development of myeloproliferative neoplasms. *Nat Genet*. 2009;41(4):446–449.

34. Lacout C, Pisani DF, Tulliez M, Gachelin FM, Vainchenker W, Villeval JL. JAK2V617F expression in murine hematopoietic cells leads to MPD mimicking human PV with secondary myelofibrosis. *Blood*. 2006;108(5):1652–1660.

35. Wernig G, Mercher T, Okabe R, Levine RL, Lee BH, Gilliland DG. Expression of Jak2V617F causes a polycythemia vera-like disease with associated myelofibrosis in a murine bone marrow transplant model. *Blood*. 2006;107(11):4274–4281.

36. Scott LM, Scott MA, Campbell PJ, Green AR. Progenitors homozygous for the V617F mutation occur in most patients with polycythemia vera, but not essential thrombocythemia. *Blood*. 2006;108(7):2435–2437.

37. Campbell PJ, Scott LM, Buck G, et al. Definition of subtypes of essential thrombocythaemia and relation to polycythaemia vera based on JAK2 V617F mutation status: a prospective study. *Lancet*. 2005;366(9501):1945–1953.

38. Wolanskyj AP, Lasho TL, Schwager SM, et al. JAK2 mutation in essential thrombocythaemia: clinical associations and long-term prognostic relevance. *Br J Haematol*. 2005;131(2):208–213.

39. Tiedt R, Hao-Shen H, Sobas MA, et al. Ratio of mutant JAK2-V617F to wild-type Jak2 determines the MPD phenotypes in transgenic mice. *Blood*. 2008;111(8):3931–3940.

40. Barosi G, Bergamaschi G, Marchetti M, et al. JAK2 V617F mutational status predicts progression to large splenomegaly and leukemic transformation in primary myelofibrosis. *Blood*. 2007;110(12):4030–4036.

41. Guglielmelli P, Barosi G, Specchia G, et al. Identification of patients with poorer survival in primary myelofibrosis based on the burden of JAK2V617F mutated allele. *Blood*. 2009;114(8):1477–1483.

42. Tefferi A, Lasho TL, Huang J, et al. Low JAK2V617F allele burden in primary myelofibrosis, compared to either a higher allele burden or unmutated status, is associated with inferior overall and leukemia-free survival. *Leukemia*. 2008;22(4):756–761.

43. Scott LM, Tong W, Levine RL, et al. JAK2 exon 12 mutations in polycythemia vera and idiopathic erythrocytosis. *N Engl J Med*. 2007;356(5):459–468.

44. Pikman Y, Lee BH, Mercher T, et al. MPLW515L is a novel somatic activating mutation in myelofibrosis with myeloid metaplasia. *PLoS Med*. 2006;3(7):e270.

45. Beer PA, Campbell PJ, Scott LM, et al. MPL mutations in myeloproliferative disorders: analysis of the PT-1 cohort. *Blood*. 2008;112(1):141–149.

46. Nussenzveig RH, Swierczek SI, Jelinek J, et al. Polycythemia vera is not initiated by JAK2V617F mutation. *Exp Hematol.* 2007;35(1):32–38.
47. Delhommeau F, Dupont S, Della Valle V, et al. Mutation in TET2 in myeloid cancers. *N Engl J Med.* 2009;360(22):2289–2301.
48. Tam CS, Nussenzveig RM, Popat U, et al. The natural history and treatment outcome of blast phase BCR-ABL-myeloproliferative neoplasms. *Blood.* 2008;112(5):1628–1637.
49. Krause DS, Van Etten RA. Tyrosine kinases as targets for cancer therapy. *N Engl J Med.* 2005;353(2):172–187.
50. Vannucchi AM. How do JAK2-inhibitors work in myelofibrosis: an alternative hypothesis. *Leuk Res.* 2009;33(12):1581–1583.
51. Vannucchi AM, Migliaccio AR, Paoletti F, Chagraoui H, Wendling F. Pathogenesis of myelofibrosis with myeloid metaplasia: lessons from mouse models of the disease. *Semin Oncol.* 2005;32(4):365–372.
52. Levis M, Allebach J, Tse KF, et al. A FLT3-targeted tyrosine kinase inhibitor is cytotoxic to leukemia cells in vitro and in vivo. *Blood.* 2002;99(11):3885–3891.
53. Hexner EO, Serdikoff C, Jan M, et al. Lestaurtinib (CEP701) is a JAK2 inhibitor that suppresses JAK2/STAT5 signaling and the proliferation of primary erythroid cells from patients with myeloproliferative disorders. *Blood.* 2008;111(12):5663–5671.
54. Santos FP, Kantarjian HM, Jain N, et al. Phase 2 study of CEP-701, an orally available JAK2 inhibitor, in patients with primary or post-polycythemia vera/essential thrombocythemia myelofibrosis. *Blood.* 2010;115(6):1131–1136.
55. Dupriez B, Morel P, Demory JL, et al. Prognostic factors in agnogenic myeloid metaplasia: a report on 195 cases with a new scoring system. *Blood.* 1996;88(3):1013–1018.
56. Tefferi A, Barosi G, Mesa RA, et al. International Working Group (IWG) consensus criteria for treatment response in myelofibrosis with myeloid metaplasia, for the IWG for Myelofibrosis Research and Treatment (IWG-MRT). *Blood.* 2006;108(5):1497–1503.
57. Smith BD, Levis M, Beran M, et al. Single-agent CEP-701, a novel FLT3 inhibitor, shows biologic and clinical activity in patients with relapsed or refractory acute myeloid leukemia. *Blood.* 2004;103(10):3669–3676.
58. Hexner E, Goldberg JD, Prchal JT, et al. A multicenter, open label phase I/II study of CEP701 (Lestaurtinib) in adults with myelofibrosis; a report on phase I: a study of the Myeloproliferative Disorders Research Consortium (MPD-RC) [abstract]. *Blood.* 2009;114(22):754.
59. Moliterno AR, Hexner E, Roboz GJ, et al. An open-label study of CEP-701 in patients with JAK2 V617F-positive PV and ET: update of 39 enrolled patients [abstract]. *Blood.* 2009;114(22):753.
60. Quintas-Cardama A, Vaddi K, Liu P, et al. Preclinical characterization of the selective JAK1/2 inhibitor INCB018424: implications for the treatment of myeloproliferative neoplasms. *Blood* 2010;115(15):3109–3117.
61. Verstovsek S, Kantarjian H, Mesa RA, et al. Long-term follow up and optimized dosing regimen of INCB018424 in patients with myelofibrosis: durable clinical, functional and symptomatic responses with improved hematological safety [abstract]. *Blood.* 2009;114(22):756.
62. Cervantes F, Dupriez B, Pereira A, et al. New prognostic scoring system for primary myelofibrosis based on a study of the International Working Group for Myelofibrosis Research and Treatment. *Blood.* 2009;113(13):2895–2901.
63. Mesa RA, Schwager S, Radia D, et al. The Myelofibrosis Symptom Assessment Form (MFSAF): an evidence-based brief inventory to measure quality of life and symptomatic response to treatment in myelofibrosis. *Leuk Res.* 2009;33(9):1199–1203.
64. Verstovsek S, Passamonti F, Rambaldi A, et al. A phase 2 study of INCB018424, an oral, selective JAK1/JAK2 inhibitor, in patients with advanced Polycythemia

Vera (PV) and Essential Thrombocythemia (ET) refractory to hydroxyurea [abstract]. *Blood.* 2009;114(22):311.

65. Barosi G, Birgegard G, Finazzi G, et al. Response criteria for essential thrombocythemia and polycythemia vera: result of a European LeukemiaNet consensus conference. *Blood.* 2009;113(20):4829–4833.

66. Goh KC, Ong WC, Hu C, et al. SB1518: a potent and orally active JAK2 inhibitor for the treatment of myeloproliferative disorders [abstract]. *Blood.* 2007;110(11):538.

67. Verstovsek S, Odenike O, Scott B, et al. Phase I dose-escalation trial of SB1518, a novel JAK2/FLT3 inhibitor, in acute and chronic myeloid diseases, including primary or post-essential thrombocythemia/polycythemia vera myelofibrosis [abstract]. *Blood.* 2009;114(22):3905.

68. Wernig G, Kharas MG, Okabe R, et al. Efficacy of TG101348, a selective JAK2 inhibitor, in treatment of a murine model of JAK2V617F-induced polycythemia vera. *Cancer Cell.* 2008;13(4):311–320.

69. Geron I, Abrahamsson AE, Barroga CF, et al. Selective inhibition of JAK2-driven erythroid differentiation of polycythemia vera progenitors. *Cancer Cell.* 2008;13(4):321–330.

70. Pardanani AD, Gotlib JR, Jamieson C, et al. A phase I evaluation of TG101348, a selective JAK2 inhibitor, in myelofibrosis: clinical response is accompanied by significant reduction in JAK2V617F allele burden [abstract]. *Blood.* 2009;114(22):755.

71. Verstovsek S, Pardanani AD, Shah NP, et al. A phase I study of XL019, a selective JAK2 inhibitor, in patients with primary myelofibrosis and post-polycythemia vera/essential thrombocythemia myelofibrosis [abstract]. *Blood.* 2007;110(11):553.

72. Shah NP, Olszynski P, Sokol L, et al. A phase I study of XL019, a selective JAK2 inhibitor, in patients with primary myelofibrosis, post-polycythemia vera, or post-essential thrombocythemia myelofibrosis [abstract]. *Blood.* 2008;112(11):98.

Chapter 9

Blastic Transformation of Classic Myeloproliferative Neoplasms

Ruben A. Mesa

Keywords: Myeloproliferative disorder • Blast phase • Acute myeloid leukemia • Leukemic transformation

The BCR-ABL Negative MPNs

The BCR/ABL negative chronic myeloproliferative neoplasms (MPNs) (polycythemia vera (PV), essential thrombocythemia (ET), and primary myelofibrosis (PMF)), first described by William Dameshek in 1951 [1], are currently in a period of rapid discovery regarding their pathogenetic mechanisms. The watershed moment for MPNs occurred in 2005 with the heavily publicized discovery of the $JAK2^{V617F}$ mutation [2–5]. This latter point mutation, in the pseudo-kinase domain of JAK2 (a key component of the cell growth and differentiation JAK-STAT pathway), leads to constitutive activation of the pathway. Additional genetic mutations with potential pathogenetic implications have also been described including the $c\text{-}MPL^{W515L/K}$ (in 5% of PMF and 1% of ET) [6] and alternative mutations in the exon 12 of JAK2 in some of those PV patients previously identified as wild type for JAK2 [7].

The MPNs have a variable period of risk of vascular events, and a long-term risk of transformation to an overt myelofibrotic phase, acute leukemia, or death (Fig. 9.1). Current available therapies have rarely been able to impact this natural history beyond palliating symptoms or decreasing the risk of vascular events. In this chapter, we will focus on the most advanced clinical scenario for MPN patients, the biology, and consequence of blastic transformation.

Phenotype of Leukemic Transformation in the MPNs

Disease progression in MPNs is the development of overt acute leukemia with a variable risk (Table 9.1) amongst MPN patients (see Fig. 9.1) or most appropriately what is called a blast phase [8] (see Fig. 9.1). Clinically as patients progress, they tend to experience a decrease in the efficacy of intramedullary hematopoiesis as manifested by worsening thrombocytopenia, worsening constitutional

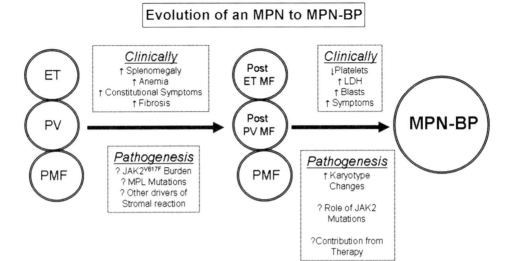

Fig. 9.1 Clinical and pathogenetic changes occurring during myeloproliferative disorder progression. *ET* essential thrombocythemia, *PV* polcythemia vera, *PMF* primary myelofibrosis, *Post-ET/PV MF* post-essential thrombocythemia/polycythemia vera myelofibrosis

Table 9.1 Risk factors at presentation of primary myelofibrosis which suggest high risk of eventual transformation (MPN-BP).

Risk factor	Association with developing MPN-BP	References
Demographics		
Age at diagnosis	None	[29]
Sex	None	[29]
Peripheral blood		
Hemoglobin	Yes – univariate only	[29, 30]
Leukocyte count	Yes (>15 × 10⁹/L) – univariate	[30]
Platelet count	<100 × 10⁹/L	[29]
Presence of blasts	Yes – univariate	[29]
Blast percentage	Yes (greatest when >3%)	[29]
Physical exam features		
Splenomegaly	None	[29]
Bone marrow		
Cellularity	None	[19]
Reticulin fibrosis	None	[19]
Blast percentage	Yes	[19]
Karyotypic abnormalities (complex >2 lesions)	Yes	[19]
Molecular lesions		
JAK2^V617F	Low allele burden	[13, 15]
MPL mutations	No data available	
Myelofibrosis prognostic scores		
Lille [55]	None	[29]
Cervantes [56]	Yes – univariate only	[29]
Mayo [57]	Yes – univariate only	[29]

symptoms, and the potential development of functional neutropenia [9]. Patients most commonly will reach a blast phase after first having gone through a myelofibrotic phase whether PMF or post-ET/PV MF [9]. However, patients with PV or ET have been known to develop a blast phase without a clearly distinct prodrome of myelofibrosis developing [10].

Pathogenesis of Blastic Transformation in MPNs

The pathogenetic mechanisms of transformation to MPN-BP remain unclear. Although a growing number of MPN-associated mutations lead to activation of the JAK-STAT pathway (i.e., JAK2^{V617F}, exon 12, and MPL mutations), it is unclear whether these are disease-initiating mutations [11]. The mechanisms by which these mutations can lead to a widely varying disease phenotypes, or what leads to disease progression (see Fig. 9.1) remain unclear [11]. Available evidence has shown in Table 9.1 that neither the presence of a JAK2-V617F mutant [12] nor an increased allele burden [13] is more common in those who undergo MPN-BP 2 and that the majority [14], but not all [15], isolated acute leukemia clones obtained from previous JAK2-V167F mutant patients will have reverted to a JAK wild type state. Clinical observations from series of MPN-BP patients further support that JAK2-V617F allele burden does not increase (or likely decreases) after transformation [16]. Recent observations further demonstrate that perhaps different pathways for leukemic transformation occur in MPNs (a MF phenotypic step in JAK2-V617F – mutated patients, a direct MPN-BP from ET/PV in JAK2 wild type patients) [17]. The pathways to MPN-BP remain complex with many key issues remaining to be determined.

The transformation of CML from CP to BP is typically associated with additional karyotypic abnormalities which are independent of the BCR-ABL translocation [18]. We have shown that patients with MPNs who eventually transform are more likely to have karyotypic abnormalities at diagnosis and develop new abnormalities prior to MPN-BP [9, 19]. The process of MPN-BP may mirror CML-BC in that chromosomal instability and additional mutations are crucial for blastic transformation.

Defining Blastic Transformation from the MPNs

WHO Definition of Acute Leukemia

The complex implications of BP in patients with a prior MPN, in part, arise from lack of clear diagnostic guidance as to what constitute acute leukemia in these patients. Patients with all chronic myeloid neoplasms exist in a spectrum of disease severity from the point of their diagnosis to acute leukemia. What constitutes this latter threshold in between is an arbitrary set point in a biological continuum. The World Health Organization (WHO)-updated classification in 2008 of myeloid neoplasms classified MPN-BP as acute myeloid leukemia with multilineage dysplasia [20]. This subgroup was further divided into those who had a prior case of MDS or an MPN/MDS overlap disorder [20]. This definition is most pertinent to those with an MPN/MDS overlap disorder (chronic myelomonocytic leukemia (CMML), atypical chronic myeloid leukemia (aCML), or MPN/MDS unclassifiable), yet does not really address those with prior PMF, post-ET/PV MF, or prior ET/PV.

The threshold for a diagnosis of achieving BP was either 20% blood or marrow blasts or the presence of a acute leukemia defining karyotypic lesions despite blast percentage (t(8;21)(q22:q22), inv(16)(p13q22), t(16;16)(p13;q22), or t(15;17)(q22;q12)) [20]. Problems with these criteria for MPN-BP are two-fold. The first is that although karyotypic abnormalities are quite common amongst patients with MPN-BP [9], it is less clear that these defining mutations play any role in a transformed MPN [9] as opposed to de novo AML.

Assessing the Importance of Peripheral Blast Percentage

Patients with MPNs, particularly PMF and post-ET/PV MF, are predisposed to circulating myeloblasts in the peripheral blood [21, 22]. This latter phenomenon is true even when there is not a clear increase in bone marrow blast percentage. Reasons for this phenomenon relate to the abnormal trafficking of immature myeloid cells in these patients which may originate from abnormalities of the marrow stroma and is likely responsible for the increased circulating CD34+ cells in these patients [23]. Clinically, patients have been shown to have increased peripheral blood blasts for long periods of time without evidence of BP occurring [24]. Based upon this phenomenon, the International Working Group for Myelofibrosis Research and Treatment (IWG-MRT) has included amongst their clinical trial criteria that a patient on a trial must have a sustained peripheral blood blast percentage >20% for 4 weeks sustained before acute leukemia can be declared [25]. Until more is known regarding the biological underpinnings of a change from an MPN to MPN-BP arbitrary, clinical cutoffs will remain somewhat cumbersome. Indeed, some patients can have a clinical phenotype of MPN-BP with 15% blasts and succumb to their disease while others with a higher blast "burden" may have a more indolent course.

Risk Factors for Blastic Transformation

Risk Factors at Presentation

Risk factors for development of MPN-BP have been of great interest for two main reasons. First, to identify patients at high risk of death from their disease in order to employ more aggressive therapy such as allogeneic stem cell transplantation earlier in the course of their disease [26]. Second, to avoid unnecessary introduction of therapy for these patients earlier in the course of their disease which could exacerbate this underlying predisposition to acute leukemia [10, 27]. Analyses of risk factors for MPN-BP are features present (i.e., intrinsic to their MPN) at diagnosis or during the course of disease (including therapy).

Prognostication for patients with MPNs, done at the time of diagnosis, can look at risk of vascular events (mainly for ET and PV), death, and development of blast phase (which unfortunately usually leads to rapid death). Of these latter endpoints, we will focus on mortality and transformation. The International Working Group for Myelofibrosis Research and Treatment (IWG-MRT) recently published an International Prognostic Scoring System (IPSS-MF) to aid in assessing MF prognosis. Five features are independently associated with decreased survival age (>65), anemia (hemoglobin <10 g/dL), leukocytes >25 × 10^9, constitutional symptoms (night sweats, fever, significant

Table 9.2 MPN therapies and their association with MPN-BP.

Therapy	Association	References
Medical		
Hydroxyurea	Only as combination therapy	[10]
Erythropoiesis stimulating agents	Higher rate of blastic transformation in PMF patients treated with ESAs	[29]
Androgens	Higher rates of transformation in PMF, especially with danazol	[29]
Melphalan	Higher rates of transformation in trial of patients with PMF	[33]
Pipobroman	Higher leukemia rates in treated PV patients	[34, 35]
Phosphorus-32	Clear and undisputed increased risk of transformation with use	[31, 32]
Thalidomide	No increase rate seen	[29]
Surgical		
Splenectomy	Conflicting reports, but no clear link established	[37, 38]

weight loss), and the presence of circulating blasts in the peripheral blood. The IPSS-MF defines four risk groups (zero, one, two, or more than two of the five adverse features) with projected survival medians for each group ranging from a median of 27 months for high risk to 135 months for low-risk disease [28].

Although limited data exist on predicting eventual leukemic transformation, our group has shown that (1) low JAK2^{V617F} allele burden [13], (2) peripheral blast percentage >3%[29], and (3) thrombocytopenia present at diagnosis [29] as associated with higher risk of MPN-BP in these patients. Analysis of our institutional experience of eventual MPN-BP in PV and ET patients demonstrated that PV patients with baseline leukocytosis and ET patients with baseline anemia as most predisposed to development of either post-ET/PV MF or MPN-BP [30]. Additionally, our IWG-MRT analysis would suggest that patients who eventually transform are more likely to have higher LDH levels and more karyotypic abnormalities [19]. No uniform prognostic score for MPN-BP exists yet (Table 9.1).

Influence of Therapy upon Development of MPN-BP

The potential of therapy to accelerate the development of MPN-BP has long been a concern in MPN patients. Therapy-related acute leukemia has long been a concern with chemotherapy of malignant neoplasms and is of greater concern in patients with underlying myeloid neoplasms (see Table 9.2). Specific to MPNs, the use of myelosuppressive therapy with radioactive phosphorus (P-32) [31, 32] is most clearly associated with increased risk of MPN-BP along with alkylator therapy such as melphalan [33] and pipobroman [34, 35]. Much controversy exists regarding the agent hydroxyurea, a valid and efficacious myelosuppressive agent demonstrated to decrease risk of vascular events in patients with ET and PV. Despite much discussion, evidence now suggests that single-agent hydoxyurea is not a significant contributor to leukemic transformation. Indeed, hydroxyurea has not been shown to be leukemogenic in the unrelated disorder of sickle cell anemia [36]. However, there may be a synergistic leukemogenic potential role of hydroxyurea in patients who then go on to receive other treatments [10]. In the end, there is

Table 9.3 Medical options for myeloproliferative neoplasms – blast phase (MPN-BP) [9].

Therapy	Composition	Median survival (months)* [9]
Supportive care	Transfusions ± Hydroxyurea ± Antibiotic Support	2.1 (1.1–3.4)
Noninduction chemo-therapy	Weekly vincristine Oral alkylators Low-dose cytarabine Oral etoposide	2.9 (0.8–5.3)
Induction chemo-therapy	Cytarabine + Anthracycline (7 day) High-dose cytarabine (>1,000 mg/m²/dose) Mitoxantrone/VP-16/high-dose cytarabine	3.9 (1.6–8.9)
Antibody therapy	Gemtuzumab	2.5 (0.7–3.5)

*Median survivals according to Mayo Clinic Series

no way to definitively negate a slight role of hydrea on the risk of leukemic transformation, and therefore patients should be counseled accordingly. There are other agents with no suggestion of leukemogenicity (aspirin, anagrelide, and interferon) [29]. Our recent analysis suggested an independently increased risk of MPN-BP amongst patients exposed to erythroid-stimulating agents (ESAs) and androgen (particularly danazol) [29]. This risk was independent of anemia and was significant in multifactorial analysis. Whether there is a causal role remains unclear, and these single-institution observations do require further validation. Finally, patients who have been splenectomized for PMF have been reported in some series to have higher rates of transformation [37], but it remains unclear whether this may be merely an association in patients with a more aggressive disease course [38].

Clinical Course and Therapy of MPN-BP

Once a patient progresses to MPN-BP, significant morbidity and mortality usually follow [9]. Clinically, patients will have all the challenging peripheral blood cytopenias typical in de novo acute leukemia. Additionally, they face the significant debilitation, cachexia, poor performance status already present from their MPN. Additionally, they will frequently have significant splenomegaly contributing symptomatically but also to transfusion resistance.

Patients with MPN-BP will frequently have multiple features which are considered characteristic of high-risk acute leukemia – specifically, advanced age, antecedent myeloid disorder, and complex and poor-risk karyotypic abnormalities [9]. Therefore, it is not surprising that therapy for these patients has been quite disappointing. We have previously demonstrated that aggressive therapy (with myelosuppressive induction intent) did not seem to offer any survival benefit over purely supportive care (transfusions ± hydroxyurea) (details of therapies and outcomes in Table 9.3). Patients who underwent induction therapy had a 40% chance of returning to a more chronic appearing phase of PMF, but without any clear impact on survival. Therefore, induction

Table 9.4 Novel therapies under investigation for MPNs which may have a role for MPN-BP.

Compound	Company	Indication	Stage of development	Mechanism of action
INCB018424	Incyte	MF, PV	III	Selective JAK2 inhibitor
TG101348	Targen	MF	I	Selective JAK2 inhibitor
SBio 1518	SBio	MF	I/II	Selective JAK2 inhibitor
CYT387	Cytopia	MF	I	Selective JAK2 inhibitor
CEP-701	Cephalon	MF, ET, PV	II	FLT3 and JAK2 inhibitor
ITF2357	Italfarmaco	MF, ET, PV	II	HDAC and JAK2 inhibitor
LBH539	Novartis	MF	II	HDAC and JAK2 inhibitor
Pomalidomide	Celgene	MF	III	IMID
Azacitidine	Celgene	MF	II	Hypomethylation
Decitabine	Eisai	MF	II	Hypomethylation

therapy may well only provide a cosmetic cytoreduction in blasts without meaningful impact [9]. Interestingly, an IWG-MRT analysis showed that patients who died from either MPN-BP or PMF complications had a similar survival from their PMF diagnosis [19].

The clinical experience with MPN-BP at MD Anderson Cancer Center showed a similar adverse prognosis with a median survival of 5 months after a diagnosis of MPN-BP [16]. Resolution of blasts through induction chemotherapy (given in 40%) was achieved in 46% of those in whom that therapy was delivered, with 8/40 patients undergoing stem cell transplant. Amongst these latter patients who were successfully transplanted, 73% were alive 31 months after transplant. These findings raise the approach of induction followed by transplant as a potential salvage option in MPN-BP, but one likely to be employable in a small number of these patients.

The reasons for the lack of success of therapy in MPN-BP are many and include intrinsic drug resistance, lack of tolerability, and death from exacerbation of comorbidities. Given the dire consequence of transformation, if aggressive disease altering therapy is to be employed (i.e., allogeneic stem cell transplant [39]), it should be used prior to developing MPN-BP. Indeed, even in transplant candidates, pretransplant induction might be needed for cytoreduction. It is an arduous and frequently unsuccessful path for a patient to have induction therapy followed by allogeneic stem cell transplant in MPN-BP.

Given the dire outcomes with MPN-BP therapy, the interest in novel therapeutic options is great. Many separate approaches are being investigated. The first is the use of JAK2 inhibitors, although all the testing to date has been done in the chronic phase of MF. The most mature clinical experience for a JAK2 inhibitor is for INCB018424 (Incyte Co, Wilmington, DE) (selective against JAK1 and JAK2) where the agent leads to significant reduction in splenomegaly and dramatic improvement in constitutional symptoms [40]. Additional drugs being tested are early in their results (TG101348 – selective

JAK2 inhibitor (TarGen, San Francisco, CA) [41], XL019 – selective JAK2 inhibitor (Exelexis, San Francisco, CA) [42], CEP-701 (Cephalon, Frazer, PA, USA) [43], ITF2357 (Italfarmaco, Italy) [44]), but preliminary results also report improvements in splenomegaly and symptoms in MF patients. No JAK2 inhibitor has yet reported a significant ability to improve cytopenias, fibrosis, or histologic changes associated with MF (see Table 9.4). Although it is unclear (as discussed) whether MPN-associated mutations may play a role in developing MPN-BP, perhaps inhibition here may still have some efficacy (i.e., analogous to imatinib mesylate from CML-BP [45]). More likely, however, these agents may play a role in preventing eventual transformation.

Utilization of agents tested for myelodysplastic syndrome or acute myeloid leukemia offers additional exploration for MPN-BP. Targeting epigenetics through hypomethylation agents (such as azacitidine [46, 47] and decitabine [48]) has been used with improvements in splenomegaly and cytopenias. Whether these latter agents can delay MPN-BP or impact survival as has been shown in MDS has not yet been tested in MPNs [49]. Additional testing of novel dosing strategies with these agents (such as 10 days of decitabine monthly at 20 mg/m^2/day as shown to be active in AML [50]) is potentially worth pursuing.

Additional lines of investigation have included agents tested in AML trials such as the farnesyltrasferase inhibitors (such as tipifarnib [51]) which have been active in elderly AML [52]. Clofarabine, active in high-risk AML and MDS, is also of interest and deserves investigation [53]. We have previously demonstrated that the heat shock protein 90 inhibitor (17-allylamino-17-demethoxygeldanamycin (17-AAG)) can help abrogate cytarabine resistance in primary cells of MPN-BP patients [54]. A multicenter phase I clinical trial is ongoing utilizing combination treatment with 17-AAG+cytarabine for patients with high-risk acute leukemia and MPN-BP. Patients with MPN-BP should be considered for appropriate high-risk acute leukemia trials, or if not a candidate offered supportive care given the lack of benefit with currently available agents.

Conclusions

The progression of patients to MPN-BP is an extremely serious development for patients both symptomatically and prognostically. Salvage of patients through induction chemotherapy followed by allogeneic stem cell transplant is possible, but likely an option only in a small number of MPN-BP patients. Although we have a partial understanding of risk factors for eventual transformation, we have an incomplete understanding as to the pathogenetic mechanisms of disease progression. Given the rapid mortality, and resistance to current therapies, seen in patients with MPN-BP, the need for novel and targeted therapy for these patients is great. A better understanding of mechanisms of clonal progression is required to identify valid therapeutic targets. Hopefully, blockade of JAK2 earlier in the course of an MPN will delay or inhibit disease progression, yet whether this will occur depends upon long-term follow-up on current JAK2 inhibitor trials. Given the uncertain role that the JAK-STAT pathway maintains in the process of leukemic transformation, the need for further study into mechanisms of disease progression is crucial.

References

1. Damashek W. Some speculations on the myeloproliferative syndrome. Blood. 1951;6:372–5.
2. Baxter EJ, Scott LM, Campbell PJ, et al. Acquired mutation of the tyrosine kinase JAK2 in human myeloproliferative disorders. Lancet. 2005;365:1054–61.
3. Kralovics R, Passamonti F, Buser AS, Teo SS, Tiedt R, Passweg JR, et al. A gain-of-function mutation of JAK2 in myeloproliferative disorders. N Engl J Med. 2005;352(17):1779–90.
4. James C, Ugo V, Le Couedic JP, Staerk J, Delhommeau F, Lacout C, et al. A unique clonal JAK2 mutation leading to constitutive signalling causes polycythaemia vera. Nature. 2005;434(7037):1144–8.
5. Levine RL, Wadleigh M, Cools J. Activating mutation in the tyrosine kinase JAK2 in polycythemia vera, essential thrombocythemia, and myelofibrosis with myeloid metaplasia. Cancer Cell. 2005;7:387–97.
6. Pardanani AD, Levine RL, Lasho T, Pikman Y, Mesa RA, Wadleigh M, et al. MPL515 mutations in myeloproliferative and other myeloid disorders: a study of 1182 patients. Blood. 2006;108(10):3472–6.
7. Scott LM, Tong W, Levine RL, Scott MA, Beer PA, Stratton MR, et al. JAK2 exon 12 mutations in polycythemia vera and idiopathic erythrocytosis. N Engl J Med. 2007;356(5):459–68.
8. Mesa RA, Verstovsek S, Cervantes F, Barosi G, Reilly JT, Dupriez B, et al. Primary myelofibrosis (PMF), post polycythemia vera myelofibrosis (post-PV MF), post essential thrombocythemia myelofibrosis (post-ET MF), blast phase PMF (PMF-BP): consensus on terminology by the international working group for myelofibrosis research and treatment (IWG-MRT). Leuk Res. 2007;31(6):737–40.
9. Mesa RA, Li CY, Ketterling RP, Schroeder GS, Knudson RA, Tefferi A. Leukemic transformation in myelofibrosis with myeloid metaplasia: a single-institution experience with 91 cases. Blood. 2005;105(3):973–7.
10. Finazzi G, Caruso V, Marchioli R, Capnist G, Chisesi T, Finelli C, et al. Acute leukemia in polycythemia vera: an analysis of 1638 patients enrolled in a prospective observational study. Blood. 2005;105(7):2664–70.
11. Levine RL, Pardanani A, Tefferi A, Gilliland DG. Role of JAK2 in the pathogenesis and therapy of myeloproliferative disorders. Nat Rev Cancer. 2007;7(9):673–83.
12. Mesa RA, Powell H, Lasho T, Dewald G, McClure R, Tefferi A. JAK2(V617F) and leukemic transformation in myelofibrosis with myeloid metaplasia. Leuk Res. 2006;30:1457–60.
13. Tefferi A, Lasho TL, Huang J, Finke C, Mesa RA, Li CY, et al. Low JAK2V617F allele burden in primary myelofibrosis, compared to either a higher allele burden or unmutated status, is associated with inferior overall and leukemia-free survival. Leukemia. 2008;22(4):756–61.
14. Theocharides A, Boissinot M, Girodon F, Garand R, Teo SS, Lippert E, et al. Leukemic blasts in transformed JAK2-V617F-positive myeloproliferative disorders are frequently negative for the JAK2-V617F mutation. Blood. 2007;110(1):375–9.
15. Swierczek SI, Yoon D, Prchal JT. Blast transformation in a patient with primary myelofibrosis initiated from JAK2 V617F progenitor. ASH Annual Meeting Abstracts. 2007;110(11):a4665.
16. Tam CS, Nussenzveig RM, Popat U, Bueso-Ramos CE, Thomas DA, Cortes JA, et al. The natural history and treatment outcome of blast phase BCR-ABL-myeloproliferative neoplasms. Blood. 2008;112(5):1628–37.
17. Beer P, Delhommeau F, LeCouédic J, Bareford D, Kušec R, McMullin M, et al. Two routes to leukemic transformation following a jak2 mutation positive myeloproliferative neoplasm. 14th European Hematology Association Meeting. 2009.
18. Vardiman JW, Brunning RD, Harris NL. WHO histological classification of chronic myeloproliferative diseases. In: Jaffe ES, Harris NL, Stein H, Vardiman

JW, editors. World Health Organization classification of tumors: Tumours of the haematopoietic and lymphoid tissues. Lyon, France: International Agency for Research on Cancer (IARC) Press; 2001; p. 17–44.

19. Mesa RA, Cervantes F, Verstovsek S, Tam C, Dupriez B, Reilly J, et al. Clinical evolution to primary myelofibrosis – blast phase: an International Working Group for Myelofibrosis Research and Treatment (IWG-MRT) collaborative retrospective analysis. ASH Annual Meeting Abstracts. 2007;110(11):682.

20. Vardiman JW, Thiele J, Arber DA, Brunning RD, Borowitz MJ, Porwit A, et al. The 2008 revision of the World Health Organization (WHO) classification of myeloid neoplasms and acute leukemia: rationale and important changes. Blood. 2009;114(5):937–51.

21. Cervantes F. Myelofibrosis: biology and treatment options. Eur J Haematol Suppl. 2007 (68):13–7.

22. Cervantes F, Mesa R, Barosi G. New and old treatment modalities in primary myelofibrosis. Cancer J. 2007;13(6):377–83.

23. Barosi G, Viarengo G, Pecci A, Rosti V, Piaggio G, Marchetti M, et al. Diagnostic and clinical relevance of the number of circulating CD34(+) cells in myelofibrosis with myeloid metaplasia. Blood. 2001;98(12):3249–55.

24. Cervantes F, Pereira A, Esteve J, Rafel M, Cobo F, Rozman C, et al. Identification of "short-lived" and "long-lived" patients at presentation of idiopathic myelofibrosis. Br J Haematol. 1997;97(3):635–40.

25. Tefferi A, Barosi G, Mesa RA, Cervantes F, Deeg HJ, Reilly JT, et al. International Working Group (IWG) consensus criteria for treatment response in myelofibrosis with myeloid metaplasia, for the IWG for Myelofibrosis Research and Treatment (IWG-MRT). Blood. 2006;108(5):1497–503.

26. Kroger N, Zabelina T, Schieder H, Panse J, Ayuk F, Stute N, et al. Pilot study of reduced-intensity conditioning followed by allogeneic stem cell transplantation from related and unrelated donors in patients with myelofibrosis. Br J Haematol. 2005;128(5):690–7.

27. Wolanskyj AP, Schwager SM, McClure RF, Larson DR, Tefferi A. Essential thrombocythemia beyond the first decade: life expectancy, long-term complication rates, and prognostic factors. Mayo Clin Proc. 2006;81(2):159–66.

28. Cervantes F, Dupriez B, Pereira A, Passamonti F, Reilly JT, Morra E, et al. A new prognostic scoring system for primary myelofibrosis based on a Study of the International Working Group for Myelofibrosis Research and Treatment. Blood. 2008;112(11):657.

29. Huang J, Li CY, Mesa RA, Wu W, Hanson CA, Pardanani A, et al. Risk factors for leukemic transformation in patients with primary myelofibrosis. Cancer. 2008;112(12):2726–32.

30. Tefferi A, Gangat N, Wolanskyj AP, Schwager S, Pardanani A, Lasho TL, et al. 20+ yr without leukemic or fibrotic transformation in essential thrombocythemia or polycythemia vera: predictors at diagnosis. Eur J Haematol. 2008;80(5):386–90.

31. Osgood EE. Contrasting incidence of acute monocytic and granulocytic leukemias in P32-treated patients with polycythemia vera and chronic lymphocytic leukemia. J Lab Clin Med. 1964;64:560–73.

32. Parmentier C. Use and risks of phosphorus-32 in the treatment of polycythaemia vera. Eur J Nucl Med Mol Imaging. 2003;30(10):1413–7.

33. Petti MC, Latagliata R, Spadea T, Spadea A, Montefusco E, Aloe Spiriti MA, et al. Melphalan treatment in patients with myelofibrosis with myeloid metaplasia. Br J Haematol. 2002;116(3):576–81.

34. Najean Y, Rain JD. Treatment of polycythemia vera: the use of hydroxyurea and pipobroman in 292 patients under the age of 65 years. Blood. 1997;90(9):3370–7.

35. Kiladjian JJ, Rain JD, Bernard JF, Briere J, Chomienne C, Fenaux P. Long-term incidence of hematological evolution in three French prospective studies of hydroxyurea and pipobroman in polycythemia vera and essential thrombocythemia. Semin Thromb Hemost. 2006;32(4 Pt 2):417–21.

36. Steinberg MH, Barton F, Castro O, Pegelow CH, Ballas SK, Kutlar A, et al. Effect of hydroxyurea on mortality and morbidity in adult sickle cell anemia: risks and benefits up to 9 years of treatment. JAMA. 2003;289(13):1645–51.

37. Barosi G, Ambrosetti A, Centra A, Falcone A, Finelli C, Foa P, et al. Splenectomy and risk of blast transformation in myelofibrosis with myeloid metaplasia. Italian Cooperative Study Group on Myeloid with Myeloid Metaplasia. Blood. 1998;91(10):3630–6.

38. Mesa RA, Nagorney DS, Schwager S, Allred J, Tefferi A. Palliative goals, patient selection, and perioperative platelet management: outcomes and lessons from 3 decades of splenectomy for myelofibrosis with myeloid metaplasia at the Mayo Clinic. Cancer. 2006;107(2):361–70.

39. van Besien K, Deeg HJ. Hematopoietic stem cell transplantation for myelofibrosis. Semin Oncol. 2005;32(4):414–21.

40. Verstovsek S, Kantarjian HM, Pardanani AD, Thomas D, Cortes J, Mesa RA, et al. The JAK inhibitor, INCB018424, demonstrates durable and marked clinical responses in primary myelofibrosis (PMF) and post-polycythemia/essential thrombocythemia myelofibrosis (Post PV/ETMF). Blood. 2008;112(11):abstract 1762.

41. Pardanani AD, Gotlib J, Jamieson C, Cortes J, Talpaz M, Stone RM, et al. A phase I study of TG101348, an orally bioavailable JAK2-selective inhibitor, in patients with myelofibrosis. Blood. 2008;112(11):97.

42. Shah NP, Olszynski P, Sokol L, Verstovsek S, Hoffman R, List AF, et al. A phase I study of XL019, a selective JAK2 inhibitor, in patients with primary myelofibrosis, post-polycythemia vera, or post-essential thrombocythemia myelofibrosis. ASH Annual Meeting Abstracts. 2008;112(11):98.

43. Verstovsek S, Tefferi A, Kornblau S, Thomas D, Cortes J, Ravandi-Kashani F, et al. Phase II study of CEP701, an orally available JAK2 inhibitor, in patients with primary myelofibrosis and post polycythemia vera/essential thrombocythemia myelofibrosis. ASH Annual Meeting Abstracts. 2007;110(11):3543.

44. Rambaldi A, Dellacasa CM, Salmoiraghi S, Spinelli O, Ferrari ML, Gattoni E, et al. A phase 2A study of the histone-deacetylase inhibitor ITF2357 in patients with Jak2V617F positive chronic myeloproliferative neoplasms. Blood. 2008;112(11):100.

45. Druker BJ, Sawyers CL, Kantarjian H, Resta DJ, Reese SF, Ford JM, et al. Activity of a specific inhibitor of the BCR-ABL tyrosine kinase in the blast crisis of chronic myeloid leukemia and acute lymphoblastic leukemia with the Philadelphia chromosome. N Engl J Med. 2001;344(14):1038–42.

46. Mesa RA, Verstovsek S, Rivera C, Pardanani A, Hussein K, Lasho T, et al. 5-Azacitidine has limited therapeutic activity in myelofibrosis. Leukemia. 2009;23(1):180–2.

47. Quintas-Cardama A, Tong W, Kantarjian H, Thomas D, Ravandi F, Kornblau S, et al. A phase II study of 5-azacitidine for patients with primary and post-essential thrombocythemia/polycythemia vera myelofibrosis. Leukemia. 2008;22(5):965–70.

48. Odenike OM, Godwin JE, van Besien K, Huo D, Stiff PJ, Sher D, et al. Phase II study of decitabine in myelofibrosis with myeloid metaplasia. ASH Annual Meeting Abstracts. 2006;108(11):a4923.

49. Fenaux P, Mufti GJ, Hellstrom-Lindberg E, Santini V, Finelli C, Giagounidis A, et al. Efficacy of azacitidine compared with that of conventional care regimens in the treatment of higher-risk myelodysplastic syndromes: a randomised, open-label, phase III study. Lancet oncol. 2009;10(3):223–32.

50. Blum WG, Klisovic R, Liu S, Kefauver C, Grever MR, Schaaf L, et al. Efficacy of a novel schedule of decitabine in previously untreated AML, age 60 or older. J Clin Oncol (Meeting Abstracts). 2009;27(15S):7010.

51. Mesa RA, Camoriano JK, Geyer SM, Wu W, Kaufmann SH, Rivera CE, et al. A phase II trial of tipifarnib in myelofibrosis: primary, post-polycythemia vera and post-essential thrombocythemia. Leukemia. 2007;21(9):1964–70.

52. Lancet JE, Gojo I, Gotlib J, Feldman EJ, Greer J, Liesveld JL, et al. A phase 2 study of the farnesyltransferase inhibitor tipifarnib in poor-risk and elderly patients with previously untreated acute myelogenous leukemia. Blood. 2007;109(4):1387–94.

53. Faderl S, Verstovsek S, Cortes J, Ravandi F, Beran M, Garcia-Manero G, et al. Clofarabine and cytarabine combination as induction therapy for acute myeloid leukemia (AML) in patients 50 years of age or older. Blood. 2006;108(1):45–51.

54. Mesa RA, Loegering D, Powell HL, Flatten K, Arlander SJ, Dai NT, et al. Heat shock protein 90 inhibition sensitizes acute myelogenous leukemia cells to cytarabine. Blood. 2005;106(1):318–27.

55. Dupriez B, Morel P, Demory JL, Lai JL, Simon M, Plantier I, et al. Prognostic factors in agnogenic myeloid metaplasia: a report on 195 cases with a new scoring system. Blood. 1996;88(3):1013–8.

56. Cervantes F. Prognostic factors and current practice in treatment of myelofibrosis with myeloid metaplasia: an update anno 2000. Pathol Biol (Paris). 2001;49(2):148–52.

57. Dingli D, Schwager SM, Mesa RA, Li CY, Tefferi A. Prognosis in transplant-eligible patients with agnogenic myeloid metaplasia: a simple CBC-based scoring system. Cancer. 2006;106(3):623–30.

Chapter 10

Eosinophilic Disorders: Differential Diagnosis and Management

Jason Gotlib

Keywords: Eosinophils • Differential diagnosis • Management of eosinophilic disorders • Reactive eosinophilias • Primary/clonal eosinophilia • Lymphocyte-variant hypereosinophilia • Idiopathic hypereosinophilic syndrome (HES)

Introduction

Eosinophils serve a central function in the host defense against helminth infections and undergo recruitment and activation in allergic and inflammatory responses. However, as part of the immune system's effort to maintain normal homeostasis, the potential for collateral tissue damage by eosinophils exists. This chapter focuses on the differential diagnosis and management of eosinophilic disorders, including reactive eosinophilias, primary/clonal eosinophilia, lymphocyte-variant hypereosinophilia, and idiopathic hypereosinophilic syndrome (HES). These entities share a common theme of abnormal persistent elevation of the eosinophil count, and although patients may remain asymptomatic from eosinophilia, the potential for substantial morbidity and mortality from organ complications exists. The study of pathologic hypereosinophilia originated in descriptive and morphologic investigations; however, with an increasingly sophisticated understanding of the cellular and molecular bases of these diseases, new biologically oriented classification schemes have now emerged which carry therapeutic implications.

Classification

The classification of acquired eosinophilia can be simplified into three broad categories: primary, secondary (reactive), and idiopathic. In 2001, the World Health Organization (WHO) adopted a step-wise approach for partitioning eosinophilic disorders into these subcategories (Table 10.1) [1]. The revised 2008 WHO classification (Table 10.2) has recognized the growing list of molecularly defined primary eosinophilias by creating the major category

S. Verstovsek and A. Tefferi (eds.), *Myeloproliferative Neoplasms: Biology and Therapy*,
Contemporary Hematology, DOI 10.1007/ 978-1-60761-266-7_10,
© Springer Science+Business Media, LLC 2011

Table 10.1 2001 World Health Organization classification of eosinophilic disorders.

Exclude all causes of reactive eosinophilia secondary to
  Allergy
  Parasitic disease
  Infectious disease
  Pulmonary diseases (hypersensitivity pneumonitis, Loeffler's, etc.)

Exclude all neoplastic disorders with secondary, reactive eosinophilia
  T-cell lymphomas, including mycosis fungoides, Sezary syndrome
  Hodgkin lymphoma
  Acute lymphoblastic leukemia/lymphoma
  Mastocytosis

Exclude other neoplastic disorders in which eosinophils are part of the neoplastic clone
  CML (Ph chromosome or BCR-ABL-positive)
  AML including those with inv(16), t(16;16) (p13;q22)
  Other myeloproliferative diseases (PV, ET, PMF)
  Myelodysplastic syndromes

Exclude T-cell population with aberrant phenotype and abnormal cytokine population

If there is no demonstrable disease that could cause eosinophilia, no abnormal T-cell population, and no evidence of a clonal myeloid disorder, diagnose HES.

If requirements 1–4 have been met, and if the myeloid cells demonstrate a clonal cytogenetic abnormality or clonality is shown by other means, or if blasts are present in the peripheral blood (>2%) or marrow (>5% but less than 19%), diagnose CEL

Table 10.2 2008 World Health Organization classification of eosinophilic disorders.

Diagnostic criteria of an MPN[a] with eosinophilia associated with FIP1L1-PDGFRA
A myeloproliferative neoplasm with prominent eosinophilia
And
Presence of a *FIP1L1-PDGFRA* fusion gene[b]

Diagnostic criteria of MPN associated with ETV6-PDGFRB fusion gene or other rearrangement of PDGFRB
A myeloproliferative neoplasm, often with prominent eosinophilia and sometimes with neutrophilia or monocytosis
And
Presence of t(5;12)(q31 ~q33;p12) or a variant translocation[c] or, demonstration of an *ETV6-PDGFRB* fusion gene or rearrangement of PDGFRB

Diagnostic criteria of MPN or acute leukemia associated with FGFR1 rearrangement
A myeloproliferative neoplasm with prominent eosinophilia and sometimes with neutrophilia or monocytosis
Or
Acute myeloid leukemia or precursor T-cell or precursor B-cell lymphoblastic leukemia/lymphoma (usually associated with peripheral blood or bone marrow eosinophilia)
And
Presence of t(8;13)(p11;q12) or a variant translocation leading to FGFR1 rearrangement demonstrated in myeloid cells, lymphoblasts, or both

Table 10.2 Continued

Diagnostic criteria of chronic eosinophilic leukemia, not otherwise specified[d]

There is eosinophilia (eosinophil count >1.5 × 10^9/L)

There is no Ph chromosome or BCR-ABL fusion gene or other myeloproliferative neoplasms (PV, ET, PMF) or MDS/MPN (CMML or atypical CML)

There is no t(5;12)(q31 ~q35;p13) or other rearrangement of PDGFRB

There is no FIP1L1-PDGFRA fusion gene or other rearrangement of PDGFRA

There is no rearrangement of FGFR1

The blast cell count in the peripheral blood and bone marrow is less than 20% and there is no inv(16)(p13q22) or t(16;16)(p13;q22) or other feature diagnostic of AML

There is a clonal cytogenetic or molecular genetic abnormality, or blast cells are more than 2% in the peripheral blood or more than 5% in the bone marrow

---

[a]Patients presenting with acute myeloid leukemia or lymphoblastic leukemia/lymphoma with eosinophilia and a FIP1L1-PDGFRA fusion gene are also assigned to this category

[b]If appropriate molecular analysis is not available, this diagnosis should be suspected if there is a Ph-negative MPN with the hematological features of chronic eosinophilic leukemia associated with splenomegaly, a marked elevation of serum vitamin B12, elevation of serum tryptase and increased bone marrow mast cells

[c]Because t(5;12)(q31 ~q33;p12) does not always lead to an ETV6-PDGFRB fusion gene, molecular confirmation is highly desirable. If molecular analysis is not available, this diagnosis should be suspected if there is a Ph-negative MPN associated with eosinophilia and with a translocation with a 5q31–33 breakpoint

[d]Idiopathic hypereosinophilic syndrome is diagnosed when the following entities are excluded: reactive eosinophilia, lymphocyte-variant hypereosinophilia, chronic eosinophilic leukemia, NOS, clonal myeloid neoplasms associated eosinophilia, and eosinophilia-associated MPNs with rearrangements of PDGFRA, PDGFRB, and FGR1. In addition, an eosinophil count of >1.5 × 10^9/L must persist for at least 6 months and tissue damage must be present. If there is no tissue damage, idiopathic hyerpeosinophilia is the preferred diagnosis

"myeloid and lymphoid neoplasms with eosinophilia and abnormalities of *PDGFRA, PDGFRB,* or *FGFR1*" [2]. In the 2008 WHO scheme, "chronic eosinophilic leukemia, not otherwise specified" (CEL, NOS) is a primary eosinophilia subcategory included under the umbrella of "myeloproliferative neoplasms" [3]. CEL, NOS is characterized by absence of the Philadelphia chromosome or a rearrangement involving *PDGFRA/B* and *FGFR1.* It is additionally defined by an increase in blasts in the bone marrow or blood (but fewer than 20% to exclude acute leukemia as a diagnosis), and/or there is evidence for clonality in the eosinophil lineage [3]. A diagnosis of idiopathic HES is based on the following criteria: primary and secondary causes of eosinophilia are excluded, there is no evidence for lymphocyte-variant hypereosinophilia (discussed below), the absolute eosinophil count is >1.5 × 10^9/L for greater than 6 months, and tissue damage is present [4]. Idiopathic hypereosinophilia is the preferred term when end-organ damage is absent

[2, 3]. The historical definition of HES that the eosinophilia persists for more than 6 months is not consistently embraced since some patients may require more urgent treatment and the modern evaluation of eosinophilia may proceed in a more timely fashion.

Secondary Eosinophilia

Secondary or reactive eosinophilia has numerous causes (Table 10.3) which require vetting to the best of one's diagnostic capability before consideration of primary eosinophilia, lymphocyte-driven hypereosinophilia, or the default designation "idiopathic." In developing countries, eosinophilia most commonly derives from infections, particularly tissue-invasive parasites [5]. Allergy/atopy and hypersensitivity conditions, drug reaction/DRESS, collagen-vascular disease, pulmonary eosinophilic diseases (e.g., idiopathic acute or chronic eosinophilia pneumonia, tropical pulmonary eosinophilia, allergic bronchopulmonary aspergillosis), allergic gastroenteritis (with associated peripheral eosinophilia), and adrenal insufficiency are diagnostic considerations in the appropriate clinical context [6–8]. Non-myeloid malignancies may be associated with secondary eosinophilia which results from the production of cytokines such as IL-3, IL-5, and GM-CSF which promote eosinophil differentiation and survival. These cytokines are elaborated from malignant cells in T-cell lymphomas [9], Hodgkin's disease [10], and acute lymphoblastic leukemias [11]. In conjunction with a dedicated review of the patient's travel history and physical examination, repeated ova and parasite testing, stool culture, and serologic testing for specific parasites are paramount for identifying infectious etiologies. Additional laboratory and imaging tests will be guided by the differential diagnosis entertained by the evaluating physician.

"Primary" or "Clonal" Eosinophilia

Eosinophilia in conjunction with a myeloid malignancy with or without a clonal cytogenetic or molecular abnormality establishes the presence of a primary eosinophilia. Well-characterized examples of eosinophils being derived from the malignant clone include systemic mastocytosis [12] BCR-ABL-positive chronic myelogenous leukemia, acute myelogenous leukemia French–American–British subtypes M4Eo (inv(16)(p13q22) or t(16;16) (p13;q22)) [13] and M2 (t(8;21)(q22;q22)) [14], and myelodysplastic syndrome (MDS), especially with t(1;7) or dic(1;7) karyotypes [15, 16]. If a clonal marker or increased blasts are not found, blood or bone marrow evaluation, or additional laboratory testing may provide clinicopathologic signs indicative of a myeloid malignancy: hepato/splenomegaly, bone marrow hypercellularity or fibrosis, dysplasia, monocytosis, myeloid immaturity, and elevated serum B12 or serum tryptase levels [17, 18]. Although not formally adopted in the nomenclature of the World Health Organization (WHO), the term "myeloproliferative variant of hypereosinophilia" has been used to refer to some of these marrow-derived eosinophilic myeloid malignancies because they may share one or more clinical or laboratory features characteristic of CML or the classic myeloproliferative neoplasms.

Table 10.3 Reactive causes of eosinophilia.

Allergic/hypersensitivity diseases

Asthma, rhinitis, drug reactions, allergic bronchopulmonary aspergillosis, allergic gastroenteritis

Infections

Parasitic

Strongyloidiasis, *Toxocara canis*, *Trichinella spiralis*, visceral larva migrans, filariasis, Schistosomiasis, *Ancylostoma duodenale*, *Fasciola hepatica*, *Echinococcus*, *Toxoplasma*, other parasitic diseases

Bacterial/mycobacterial

Fungal (coccidioidomycosis, cryptococcus)

Viral (HIV, HSV, HTLV-II)

Rickettsial

Connective tissue diseases

Churg–Strauss syndrome, Wegener's granulomatosis, rheumatoid arthritis, polyarteritis nodosa, systemic lupus erythematosus, scleroderma, eosinophilic fasciitis/myositis

Pulmonary diseases

Bronchiectasis, cystic fibrosis, Loeffler's syndrome, eosinophilic granuloma of the lung

Cardiac diseases

Tropical endocardial fibrosis, eosinophilic endomyocardial fibrosis or myocarditis

Skin diseases

Atopic dermatitis, urticaria, eczema, bullous pemphigoid, dermatitis herpetiformis, episodic angioedema with eosinophilia (Gleich syndrome)

Gastrointestinal diseases

Eosinophilic gastroenteritis, celiac disease

Malignancies

Hodgkin's and Non-Hodgkin's lymphoma, acute lymphoblastic leukemia, Langerhans cell histiocytosis, angiolymphoid hyperplasia with eosinophilia (Kimura's disease), angioimmunoblastic lymphadenopathy, solid tumors (e.g., renal, lung, breast, vascular neoplasms, female tract cancers)

Immune system diseases/abnormalities

Wiskott–Aldrich syndrome, hyper-IgE (Job's) syndrome, hyper-IgM syndrome, IgA deficiency

Metabolic abnormalities

Adrenal insufficiency

Other

Il-2 therapy, L-tryptophan ingestion, toxic oil syndrome, renal graft rejection

Originally published by Gotlib et al. [76]

Myeloid and Lymphoid Neoplasms with Eosinophilia and Abnormalities of PDGFRA, PDGFRB, or FGFR1

The incidence of these molecularly defined eosinophilias is not known, but they are considered rare disease entities with an incidence <1/100,000 persons. The median frequency of the *FIP1L1-PDGFRA* fusion in patients with hypereosinophilia across eight published series enrolling more than ten patients was 23% (range 3–56%) [19]. Larger studies conducted in developing countries support a *FIP1L1-PDGFRA*-positive disease incidence of up to 20% among patients presenting with idiopathic hypereosinophilia [20–22].

In most cases, patients expressing *PDGFRA*, *PDGFRB*, or *FGFR1* fusion genes will have an abnormal karyotype indicating a rearrangement of 4q12 (*PDGFRA*), 5q31–33 (*PDGFRB*) or 8p11–13 (*FGFR1*) [3]. It is important to perform karyotyping in cases with eosinophilia in order to identify patients with chromosomal rearrangements who may benefit from targeted therapy with specific kinase inhibitors such as imatinib. In addition to karyotyping, RT-PCR or FISH analysis with probes flanking the *PDGFRA*, *PDGFRB*, and *FGFR1* genes is relevant in cases with obvious chromosomal rearrangements to confirm that the breakpoints are within these genes, as well as in cases without these specific rearrangements to check for possible cryptic rearrangements of these kinases. The most important example is the cytogenetically occult 800-kilobase 4q12 deletion that causes the *FIP1L1-PDGFRA* fusion [23, 24]. FISH probes that hybridize to the region between the *FIP1L1* and *PDGFRA* genes are now commonly used to detect the presence of the deletion. Since the *CHIC2* gene is located in this region, this FISH test is often referred to as "FISH for the *CHIC2* deletion" [25].

In addition to the *FIP1L1-PDGFRA* fusion gene [23, 24], variant *PDGFRA* fusion genes [26–30], as well as different *PDGFRB* [31–44] genes have been described in MPNs with eosinophilia (Table 10.4) (reviewed in 19). In 1994, *ETV6-PDGFRB* was the first of these fusion genes described in patients with CMML with eosinophilia and t(5;12) [45]. Despite the rare frequency (<1%) of *PDGFRB* rearrangements in cytogenetically defined cases of CMML and other myeloid neoplasms (e.g., atypical CML, juvenile myelomonocytic leukemia, chronic basophilic leukemia, MDS/MPN overlap), their recognition is critical given their responsiveness to imatinib.

Eosinophilic disorders related to fusions involving the *FGFR1* gene are similarly rare. The association of t(8;13)(p11;q11) with lymphoblastic lymphoma with eosinophilia and myeloid hyperplasia (e.g., 8p11 myeloproliferative syndrome (EMS)) was initially described in 1995, followed by the discovery of the *ZNF198-FGFR1* fusion gene in 1998 by several groups [46–49]. Additional fusion partners for *FGFR1* have since been described (Table 10.4) [50–56]. The *FGFR1* rearrangement can be found in both myeloid and lymphoid cells, suggesting an origin in a multipotent hematopoietic progenitor, and thus the basis for the disease's historical label of "stem cell leukemia/lymphoma syndrome."

Clinical Presentations of FIP1L1-PDGFRA-Positive Disease

FIP1L1-PDGFRA is a clonal marker associated with myeloproliferative features of hypereosinophilia including organomegaly, hypercellular bone marrows with increased mast cells and/or myelofibrosis, and increased serum tryptase levels [18, 23]. These patients historically exhibited a poor prognosis before imatinib was used in this disease setting [18, 23, 57]. The Mayo group also linked *FIP1L1-PDGFRA* positivity to cases pathologically identified as systemic

Table 10.4 Molecularly-defined eosinophilias involving rearranged *PDGFRA*, *PDGFRB*, and *FGFR1*.

	Fusion partner	Chromosomal abnormality	Reference
PDGFRA	*FIP1L1*	del(4)(q12q12)	Cools et al. [23]; Griffin et al. [24]; and others
	BCR	t(4;22)	Trempat et al. [26]; Baxter et al. [27]; and others
	KIF5B	Complex karyotype involving chromosomes 3, 4 and 10	Score et al. [28]
	CDK5RAP2	ins(9;4)(q33;q12q25)	Walz et al. [29]
	ETV6	t(4;12)	Curtis et al. [30]
	STRN	t(2;4)(p24;q12)	Curtis et al. [30]
PDGFRB	*WDR48*	t(1;3;5)(p36;p21;q33)	Curtis et al. [31]
	GPIAP1	der(1)t(1;5)(p34;q33), der(5)t(1;5)(p34;q15), der(11)ins(11;5)(p12:q15q33)	Walz et al. [32]
	TPM3	t(1;5)(q21;q33)	Rosati et al. [33]
	PDE4DIP	t(1;5)(q23;q33)	Wilkinson et al. [34]
	PRKG2	t(4;5;5)(q23;q31;q33)	Walz et al. [32]
	GOLGA4	t(3;5)(p21–25;q31–35)	Curtis et al. [31]
	HIP1	t(5;7)(q33;q11.2)	Ross et al. [35]
	CCDC6	t(5;10)(q33;q21)	Schwaller et al. [36]; Kulkarni et al. [37]
	GIT2	t(5;12)(q31–33;q24)	Walz et al. [23]
	NIN	t(5;14)(q33;q24)	Vizmanos et al. [38]
	KIAA1509	t(5;14)(q33;q32)	Levine et al. [39]
	CEV14	t(5;14)(q33;q32)	Abe et al. [40]
	TP53BP1	t(5;15)(q33;q22)	Grand et al. [41]
	NDE1	t(5;16)(q33;p13)	La Starza et al. [42]
	RABEP1	t(5;17)(q33;p13)	Magnusson et al. [43]
	SPECC1	t(5;17)(q33;p11.2)	Morerio et al. [44]
FGFR1	*ZNF198*	t(8;13)(p11;q12)	Xiao et al. [46]; Reiter et al. [47]; Popovici et al. [48]; Smedley et al. [49]
	CEP110	t(8;9)(p11;q33)	Guasch et al. [50]
	FGFR1OP1	t(6;8)(q27;p11–12)	Popovici et al. [51]
	BCR	t(8;22)(p11;q11)	Demiroglu [52]
	TRIM24	t(7;8)(q34;p11)	Belloni et al. [53]
	MYO18A	t(8;17)(p11;q23)	Walz et al. [54]
	HERVK	t(8;19)(p12;q13.3)	Guasch et al. [55]
	FGFR1OP2	ins(12;8)(p11;p11p22)	Grand et al. [56]

mastocytosis with eosinophilia (SM-eo) [25]. The bone marrows of patients with *FIP1L1-PDGFRA*-positive SM-Eo exhibited less dense clusters of mast cells by tryptase immunostaining than are typically seen in SM, particularly cases with the common D816V *KIT* mutation which is identified in approximately 80% of cases [21]. The *FIP1L1-PDGFRA* fusion and D816V *KIT* mutation appear to be mutually exclusive oncogenic mutations, as they have not been simultaneously reported in the same patients with systemic mastocytosis [58]. The *FIP1L1-PDGFRA* fusion has also been identified in cases of AML and T-cell lymphoblastic non-Hodgkin lymphoma [59], which were characterized by eosinophilia either preceding or contemporaneous with these diagnoses, or because eosinophilia persisted despite hematologic remission after intensive chemotherapy.

Lymphocyte-Variant Hypereosinophilia

In the healthy state, the cytokines GM-CSF, IL-3, and IL-5 direct the proliferation, survival, and differentiation of eosinophils. IL-5 is a specific eosinophil differentiation factor which is overproduced (primarily from CD4+ T-cells) as part of the immune response leading to the hypereosinophilia observed in parasitic infection and atopy/allergic disorders [60].

Some patients may exhibit expansion of abnormal lymphocyte populations without any other recognized cause of their hypereosinophilia [60]. These patients typically have cutaneous signs and symptoms as the primary disease manifestation. The immunophenotype of these lymphocytes include double-negative, immature T-cells (e.g., CD3$^+$CD4$^-$CD8$^-$) or absence of CD3 (e.g., CD3$^-$CD4$^+$), a normal component of the T-cell receptor complex [61–63]. Additional immunophenotypic abnormalities include elevated CD5 expression on CD3$^-$CD4$^+$ cells, and loss of surface CD7 and/or expression of CD27 [60]. In patients with T-cell-mediated hypereosinophilia with elevated IgE levels, lymphocyte production of IL-5, and in some cases IL-4 and IL-13, suggests that these T-cells have a helper type 2 (Th2) cytokine profile [60, 61, 63–65]. In a study of 60 patients recruited primarily from dermatology clinics, 16 had a unique population of circulating T-cells with an abnormal immunophenotype [66]. Clonal rearrangement of T-cell receptor genes was demonstrated in half of these individuals (8/60 total patients). The abnormal T-cells secreted high levels of interleukin-5 in vitro and displayed an activated immunophenotype (e.g., CD25 and/or HLA-DR expression). Four of these patients were ultimately diagnosed with either T-cell lymphoma or Sézary syndrome, indicating that lymphocyte-variant hypereosinophilia can exhibit malignant potential. In some cases, accumulation of cytogenetic changes (e.g., partial 6q and 10p deletions, trisomy 7) in T-cells and proliferation of lymphocytes with the CD3$^-$CD4$^+$ phenotype have been observed with progression to lymphoma [65, 67–69].

Consensus criteria for the diagnosis of lymphocyte-variant hypereosinophilia have not been established. The finding of isolated T-cell clonality by PCR without T-cell immunophenotypic abnormalities or demonstration of Th2 cytokine production is not felt to be sufficient to make a diagnosis of this eosinophilia variant [70]. Despite a recent study demonstrating that a high proportion of idiopathic HES patients exhibit a clonal T-cell receptor gene rearrangement by PCR (18/42 patients, 43%), it is unclear whether such clonal T-cell populations are pathogenetically relevant to the disease process

[71]. Detection of elevated serum levels of TARC, a chemokine implicated in Th2-mediated diseases, in addition to the finding of increased in vitro production of cytokines from cultured peripheral blood mononuclear cells and/or T-cells (research-based assays), provides additional support for a diagnosis of lymphocyte-variant hypereosinophilia [70, 72].

Diagnostic Algorithm for Evaluation and Treatment of Hypereosinophilia

The discovery of targetable molecular lesions in patients facilitates the grouping of subsets of patients with hypereosinophilia (Fig. 10.1). In patients whose work-up is negative for secondary causes of eosinophilia, a reasonable next step in the diagnostic work-up is screening for the *FIP1L1-PDGFRA* gene fusion (by RT-PCR or interphase/metaphase FISH). In instances where *FIP1L1-PDGFRA* screening is not available, evaluation of the serum tryptase may be useful as a surrogate marker for *FIP1L1-PDGFRA*-positive disease since increased levels segregate with this molecular finding and the myeloproliferative variant of hypereosinophilia [18]. At this stage of the diagnostic work-up, it is important to rule out other molecularly defined eosinophilias, which can be inferred from overt karyotypic abnormalities, such as reciprocal translocations involving 5q31–33 (*PDGFRB*), 4q12 (*PDGFRA*), and 8p11–13 (*FGFR1*) [2]. A negative screen for both reactive and molecularly defined causes of eosinophilia should prompt consideration of two remaining diagnostic possibilities: (1) CEL, NOS if there is a non-specific clonal cytogenetic abnormality, demonstration of eosinophil clonality (research-based assay), or blast cells (>2% in the peripheral blood or >5% in the bone marrow, but <20% blasts in both compartments [3] and (2) lymphocyte-variant hypereosinophilia, consisting of patients with hypereosinophilia in whom an abnormal T-cell population is demonstrated with additional supporting evidence such as an aberrant T-cell immunophenotype and/or cytokine production in vitro. Such diagnostic groups may not be mutually exclusive; for example, some patients have been described with the *FIP1L1-PDGFRA* fusion and either concurrent non-specific cytogenetic abnormalities or a clonal T-cell population [23,71]. If none of the above disease entities are encountered, a diagnosis of idiopathic HES is made if organ damage is present. Figure 10.1 presents treatment options (both commercially available and investigational) based on these diagnostic groupings.

Therapy

Molecularly Defined Eosinophilias

The first report of successful imatinib treatment of HES was reported in an online medical journal in 2001 [72]. Several case reports and small case series followed in 2001–2002, highlighting the dramatic hematologic responses of patients with HES empirically treated with imatinib in the dose range of 100–400 mg daily [73–76]. Complete and rapid hematologic remissions, with normalization of eosinophilia, were observed in the overwhelming majority of patients. The presence of a normal karyotype in responding patients implicated

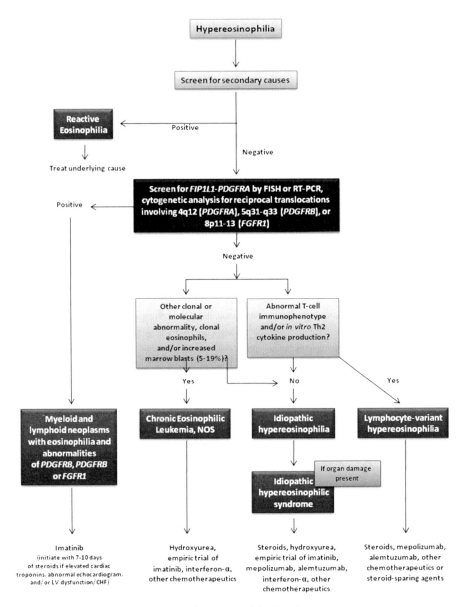

Fig. 10.1 Diagnostic and treatment algorithm for eosinophilic disorders

a cryptic mutation or rearrangement of a tyrosine kinase as the therapeutic target of imatinib, ultimately identified as FIP1L1-PDGFRα [23, 24]. The identification of this fusion in such cases, previously labeled as HES, would henceforth operationally define them as chronic eosinophilic leukemia.

Numerous studies have since confirmed the hematologic benefit of imatinib in *FIP1L1-PDGFRA*-positive CEL. Similar to CML, sensitive real-time quantitative PCR-based assays are used to follow in-depth molecular responses. Molecular remissions were first reported by the NIH group by PCR testing of the peripheral blood in five of six *FIP1L1-PDGFRA*-positive patients after 1–12 months of imatinib therapy [77]. Several additional reports have since described molecular remissions in imatinib-treated patients with *FIP1L1-PDGFRA* positive disease or after bone marrow transplantation.

The natural history of imatinib-treated *FIP1L1-PDGFRA*-positive chronic eosinophilic leukemia was reported by an Italian study which prospectively followed 27 patients for a median follow-up period of 25 months (range 15–60 months) [78]. Patients were dose escalated from an initial dose of 100 mg daily to a final dose of 400 mg daily after the first month. A complete hematologic remission was achieved in all patients within 1 month, and all patients became PCR negative for *FIP1L1-PDGFRA* after a median of 3 months of therapy (range 1–10 months). Patients who continued imatinib therapy remained PCR negative during a median follow-up period of 19 months (range 6–56+ months). A separate European study prospectively assessed the natural history of molecular responses to imatinib doses of 100–400 mg daily [79]. Among 11 patients with high pre-treatment transcript levels, all achieved a 3-log reduction in transcript levels by 1 year of therapy, and 9/11 patients achieved a molecular remission.

Although in-depth and durable molecular responses occur with imatinib, discontinuation of the drug can lead to relapse. In the Italian study, three patients who discontinued imatinib experienced rising *FIP1L1-PDGFRA* transcript levels; with re-initiation of treatment, fusion transcripts again became undetectable after 2–5 months of therapy [78]. In the European trial, withdrawal of imatinib in two patients was followed by a rapid rise in *FIP1L1-PDGFRA* fusion transcripts, with one of these patients achieving a second molecular remission after reinstitution of imatinib [79]. In a dose de-escalation trial of imatinib in five patients who had achieved a stable hematologic and molecular remission at 300–400 mg daily for at least 1 year, molecular relapse was observed in all patients after 2–5 months of either dose imatinib reduction or discontinuation [80]. Molecular remissions could be re-established with re-induction of imatinib in all cases at a dose range of 100–400 mg daily. Hematologic relapse was noted only several weeks after stoppage of imatinib in four patients in the Mayo series [81]. These data indicate that imatinib can suppress, but not eradicate, the *FIP1L1-PDGFRA* clone, and therefore ongoing imatinib treatment is recommended. Although 100 mg daily may be sufficient to achieve a molecular remission in some patients, others may require higher maintenance doses in the range of 300–400 mg daily. Maintenance dosing of 100–200 mg weekly may be sufficient to achieve a molecular remission in a proportion of patients [82]. For any patient, the ideal dose would be that which achieves and sustains a molecular remission.

FIP1L1-PDGFRA fusion-negative patients with hypereosinophilia may benefit from imatinib, usually administered at higher doses (>400 mg daily). However, hematologic responses in this group tend to be partial, short lived, and may reflect drug-related myelosuppression [23, 78]. Alternatively, some cases with complete responses may represent patients in which the *PDGFRA* or *PDGFRB* rearrangement (or other imatinib-sensitive tyrosine kinase target) remains undefined. Therefore, an empiric trial of imatinib in patients with hypereosinophilia but without detectable *PDGFR* rearrangements is considered a valid approach.

In patients with rearrangements of *PDGFRB* or *PDGFRA* variants other than F*IP1L1-PDGFRA*, case reports and series indicate that imatinib, usually at doses of 400 mg daily, can elicit durable hematologic and cytogenetic remissions [83]. The natural history of patients with 8p11 myeloproliferative disease related to *FGFR1* fusions follows an aggressive course usually terminating in AML in 1–2 years [3]. Therefore, intensive chemotherapy with regimens such as hyper-CVAD (directed to treatment of T- or B-cell lymphoma), followed by allogeneic transplantation, is recommended. Small molecule inhibition of the constitutively activated tyrosine kinase *ZNF198-FGFR1* fusion with PKC12 has been demonstrated in vitro, as well as in a patient who exhibited a hematologic and cytogenetic response [84]. These findings recapitulate the potential utility of small molecule inhibitors in historically poor-prognosis diseases.

Safety Profile of Imatinib in FIP1L1-PDGFRA Positive Disease

The safety profile of imatinib-treated patients with *FIP1L1-PDGFRA*-positive disease generally parallels the CML experience. However, several cases of cardiogenic shock have been reported in *FIP1L1-PDGFRA*-positive patients after initiation of imatinib [85, 86]. Early use of high-dose corticosteroids led to improvement of left ventricular dysfunction and clinical recovery. Currently, prophylactic use of steroids during the first 7–10 days of imatinib treatment is recommended for patients with known cardiac disease and/or elevated serum troponin levels [86].

Resistance to Imatinib in FIP1L1-PDGFRA Positive Disease

With over 7 years of experience with imatinib treatment of *FIP1L1-PDGFRA* positive disease, very few cases of acquired resistance have been reported [23, 87–89]. The first case of imatinib resistance was identified in a patient-advanced AML arising from CEL, who, after achieving a complete hematologic remission, relapsed after 5 months of therapy. Clinical relapse coincided with the identification of a T674I mutation within the ATP-binding domain of PDGFRα [23]. Ba/F3 cells transformed by the *FIP1L1-PDGFRα* T674I mutant were 1,000-fold more resistant to imatinib compared to cells transformed by the wild-type fusion [23]. Three additional cases of molecular resistance were similar due to the PDGFRα T674I mutation, all in the blast crisis phase of disease [87–89]. Lierman and colleagues reported a case of *FIP1L1-PDGFRα* T674I CEL in blast crisis that responded briefly to sorafenib, with subsequent rapid emergence of a *FIP1L1-PDGFRα* D842V mutant [89]. In vitro, the *FIP1L1-PDGFRα* D842V mutant was highly resistant to multiple tyrosine kinase inhibitors including sorafenib, imatinib, dasatinib, and PKC412 [89]. Recently, two novel tandem mutations, PDGFRα S601P and L629P, were identified in a *FIP1L1-PDGFRα*-positive patient, the first report of primary clinical resistance to imatinib in the chronic phase of the disease [90].

The *FIP1L1-PDGFRα* T674I mutation is analogous to the T315I BCR-ABL mutation in CML which confers broad-spectrum resistance to the tyrosine kinase inhibitors imatinib, dasatinib, and nilotinib [91]. PKC412, a potent FLT3 inhibitor that is in clinical development for the treatment of AML, was the first inhibitor with demonstrable activity against the *FIP1L1-PDGFRα* T674I mutant [92]. Using both in vitro and in vivo murine models, PKC412 could induce apoptosis in *FIP1L1-PDGFRα* T674I-transformed cells, and significantly reduced leukocytosis and splenomegaly in a *FIP1L1-PDGFRα* T674I mouse model [92]. Sorafenib, a BRAF and VEGFR inhibitor which is FDA approved for the treatment of renal cell and hepatocellular carcinoma, was also found to be a potent inhibitor of both the wild-type FIP1L1-PDGFRα and T674I mutant [93]. Nilotinib has also shown some activity against the wild-type and T674I mutant fusion [94, 95]. Imatinib-resistant disease related to specific *FIP1L1-PDGFR* mutants may therefore be amenable to alternative, structurally different small molecule kinase inhibitors.

Treatment of Idiopathic Hypereosinophilic Syndrome and Non-Molecularly Defined Eosinophilia

In patients with eosinophilia-related organ damage (e.g., heart, lungs, gastrointestinal, central nervous system, skin), therapy should be directed to the underlying reactive or clonal disorder. No clear data exist to support initiation of therapy based on a specific eosinophil count in the absence of organ disease, although an absolute eosinophil count of $1,500–2,000/mm^3$ has been recommended by some as a lower threshold for starting treatment [96]. Management algorithms have used serial monitoring of eosinophil counts, evaluation of clonality (e.g., T-cell receptor gene rearrangement, immunophenotyping), bone marrow aspiration and biopsy with cytogenetics, and directed organ assessment (eg., chest X-ray and/or CT thorax, echocardiography, cardiac troponin, pulmonary function testing, endoscopy, skin biopsy) in order to identify occult organ disease and alternative causes of eosinophilia which may slowly emerge after an initial diagnosis of idiopathic hypereosinophilia [97–99]. In patients with idiopathic HES, prednisone (1 mg/kg/day, tapered over 2–3 months) is indicated for organ involvement and is usually effective in producing rapid reductions in the eosinophil count [98, 100, 101]. Steroid refractoriness, which can be associated with lack of glucocorticoid receptor expression on eosinophils [102], warrants consideration of cytotoxic therapy. Hydroxyurea is an effective first-line chemotherapeutic for idiopathic HES which may be used in conjunction with corticosteroids or in steroid non-responders [98, 100, 101] Second-line agents, included vincristine [103–105], pulsed chlorambucil [98], cyclophosphamide [106], and etoposide [107–108]. Responses to cyclosporin-A [109, 110], and 2-chlorodeoxyadenosine have also been observed in HES [111].

Interferon-α (IFN-α) can elicit sustained hematologic and cytogenetic remissions in HES and CEL patients refractory to other therapies including prednisone and hydroxyurea [112–118]. Some have advocated its use as initial therapy for these eosinophilic disorders [117]. Remissions have been associated with improvement in clinical symptoms and organ disease, including hepatosplenomegaly [113, 117], cardiac and thromboembolic complications [112, 114], mucosal ulcers [116], and skin involvement [118]. The benefits of IFN-α derive from pleiotropic activities including inhibition of eosinophil proliferation and differentiation [119]. Inhibition of IL-5 synthesis from CD4+ helper T-cells may be relevant to its mechanism of action in lymphocyte-mediated hypereosinophilia [120]. IFN-α may also act more directly via IFN-α receptors on eosinophils, suppressing release of interleukin-5, and mediators of tissue injury such as cationic protein and neurotoxin [121].

Anti-IL-5 antibody approaches (e.g., mepolizumab, SCH55700) have been undertaken in HES based on the cytokine's role as a differentiation, activation, and survival factor for eosinophils. Mepolizumab is a fully humanized monoclonal IgG antibody that inhibits binding of IL-5 to the α chain of the IL-5 receptor expressed on eosinophils [122]. Treatment with mepolimuzab or SCH55700 could elicit rapid reductions in the periperhal blood eosinophil count within 48 h and/or decreases in serum levels of eosinophil mediators (e.g., cationic protein, eotaxin, TARC) [123–125]. Clinical benefit has included regression of constitutional symptoms, dermatologic lesions (including decreases in skin/tissue-infiltrating eosinophils), and improvements of FEV$_1$ measurements in patients with pulmonary disease [123–125].

Clinical and/or hematologic improvements have been observed for 30 days after a single dose of SCH55700 [125], and for 12 weeks after 3 monthly doses of mepolizumab [124]. Among the few patients studied, response has not been predicted by pre-treatment serum IL-5 levels or presence of the *FIP1L1-PDGFRA* fusion. Rebound eosinophilia, accompanied by increases in serum IL-5 levels, has been noted in some cases, and tachyphylaxis has been observed with repeated doses, not linked to the development of neutralizing antibodies to the recombinant antibody [125].

In phase I studies, anti-IL-5 therapy has been well tolerated except for mild infusional side effects [123–125]. In the largest study of HES patients to date, the safety and steroid-sparing effects of mepolizumab were evaluated in a multicenter, randomized, double-blind, placebo-controlled trial of 85 *FIP1L1-PDGFRAα*-negative patients [126]. Blood eosinophil levels were stabilized at <1,000 cells/mm^3 on 20–60 mg/day prednisone during a run-in period of up to 6 weeks. Patients were subsequently randomized to intravenous mepolizumab 750 mg or placebo every 4 weeks for 36 weeks. No adverse events were significantly more frequent with mepolizumab compared to placebo. A significantly higher proportion of mepolizumab-treated HES patients versus placebo were able to achieve the primary efficacy endpoint of a daily prednisone dose of ≤10 mg daily for at least eight consecutive weeks. The safety and efficacy of long-term administration of mepolizumab, as well as feasibility of maintenance infusions will need to be clarified with follow-up studies [127].

Alemtuzumab is an anti-CD52 monoclonal antibody, currently approved for treatment of B-cell chronic lymphocytic leukemia. It has been evaluated in refractory HES based on expression of the CD52 antigen on eosinophils [128, 129]. In one patient with an abnormal T-cell population and a markedly elevated serum IL-5 level, a dose of 30 mg sc weekly resulted in resolution of fever, improvement in painful skin lesions and left ventricular function, and normalization of the level of serum IL-5 [128]. In another HES patient who exhibited progressive disease despite a non-myeloablative peripheral blood stem cell transplant, alemtuzumab 20 mg weekly provided marked improvement in skin, joint, and cardiac complications, with striking transient eosinopenia after infusions of drug [129]. Durable control (6 months–2.5 years) was achieved in both cases with a maintenance regimen of 30 mg every 3 weeks.

In a study of 11 patients with refractory HES, intravenous alemtuzumab (5–30 mg) was administered intravenously once to thrice weekly [130]. Ten of eleven patients (91%) achieved normalization of the eosinophil count after a median of 2 weeks of therapy. The median duration of hematologic response was 3 months (1.5–17+ months), but seven of the ten patients relapsed, five while off treatment. In two patients, alemtuzumab re-challenge resulted in a second hematologic remission [130]. Adverse events included infusion-related symptoms, reactivation of cytomegalovirus infection, and one case of orbital lymphoma.

For patients with a FIP1L1-PDGFRA-negative WHO-defined myeloid malignancy with associated eosinophilia, therapy is directed according to the specific disease (e.g., myelodysplastic syndrome or systemic mastocytosis). For patients with CEL, NOS, hydroxyurea, interferon-alpha, an empiric trial of imatinib, or clinical trials with novel agents are all reasonable choices. For lymphocyte-variant hypereosinophilia, steroids are typically the first-line agent. As noted above, alemtuzumab has also demonstrated efficacy in this variant [128].

Bone marrow/peripheral blood stem cell allogeneic transplantation has been attempted in patients with aggressive/refractory HES. Disease-free survival ranging from 8 months to 5 years has been reported [131–135] with one patient relapsing at 40 months [136]. Allogeneic transplantation using non-myeloablative conditioning regimens have been reported in three patients, with remission duration of 3–12 months at the time of reported follow-up [137, 138]. In one patient who underwent an allogeneic stem cell transplantation from an HLA-matched sibling, the patient was disease free at 3 years, and there was no evidence of the FIP1L1-PDGFRA fusion which was present at diagnosis [139]. Despite success in selected cases, the role of transplantation in HES is not well established.

Advances in cardiac surgery have extended the life of patients with late-stage heart disease manifested by endomyocardial fibrosis, mural thrombosis, and valvular insufficiency [98, 100]. Mitral and/or tricuspid valve repair or replacement [140–144] and endomyocardectomy for late-stage fibrotic heart disease [141, 145] can improve cardiac function. Bioprosthetic devices are preferred over their mechanical counterparts because of the reduced frequency of valve thrombosis. Anticoagulants and anti-platelet agents have shown variable success in preventing recurrent thromboembolism [74, 146–148].

Conclusion

Recognition of reactive eosinophilia and directed treatment of culprit secondary causes remains of utmost importance for internists and subspecialists to whom such patients may be referred. The remaining pool of patients, most of whom have been historically categorized as idiopathic HES, has now contracted in size, partitioned into several pathophysiologically defined subtypes. These include the primary/clonal eosinophilias and lymphocyte-variant hypereosinophilia. Recognition of molecularly defined eosinophilias, whose pathobiology is linked to dysregulated tyrosine kinases, has bred substantial changes in the classification and treatment of these diseases. The exquisite sensitivity of PDGFRA/B-rearranged disorders to imatinib has translated into a fundamental reversal of the natural history of these once poor-prognosis diseases. The emergence of small molecule kinase inhibitors, as well as antibody therapy (e.g., mepolizumab, alemtuzumab) has ushered in new therapeutic horizons for eosinophilic disorders beyond traditional non-specific cytotoxics and corticosteroids.

References

1. Bain B, Pierre R, Imbert M, Vardiman JW, Brunning RD, Flandrin G. Chronic eosinophilic leukaemia and the hypereosinophilic syndrome. In: Jaffe ES, Harris NL, Stein H, Vardiman JW, eds. World Health Organization of Tumours: Tumours of Haematopoietic and Lymphoid Tissues. IARC Press: Lyon, France, 2001:29–31.
2. Bain BJ, Gilliland DG, Horny H-P, Vardiman JW. Myeloid and lymphoid neoplasms with eosinophilia and abnormalities of PDGFRA, PDGFRB, or FGFR1. In:

Swerdlow S, Harris NL, Stein H, Jaffe ES, Theile J, Vardiman JW (eds). World Health Organization Classification of Tumours. Pathology and Genetics of Tumours of Haematopoietic and Lymphoid Tissues. IARC Press: Lyon, France, 2008:68–73.

3. Bain BJ, Gilliland DG, Horny H-P, Vardiman JW. Chronic eosinophilic leukaemia, not otherwise specified. In: Swerdlow S, Harris NL, Stein H, Jaffe ES, Theile J, Vardiman JW (eds). World Health Organization Classification of Tumours. Pathology and Genetics of Tumours of Haematopoietic and Lymphoid Tissues. IARC Press: Lyon, France, 2008:51–53.

4. Chusid MJ, Dale DC, West BC, Wolff SM. The hypereosinophilic syndrome. Analysis of fourteen cases with review of the literature. Medicine. 1975;54:1–27.

5. Tefferi A, Patnaik MM, Pardanani A. Eosinophilia: secondary, clonal and idiopathic. Br J Haematol. 2006;133:468–492.

6. Ganeva M, Gancheva T, Lazarova R, et al. Carbamazepine-induced drug reaction with eosinophilia and systemic symptoms (DRESS) syndrome: report of four cases and brief review. Int J Dermatol. 2008;47:853–860.

7. Campos LE, Pereira LF. Pulmonary eosinophilia. J Bras Pneumol. 2009;35:561–573.

8. Mendez-Sanchez N, Chavez-Tapia NC, Vazquez-Elizondo G, Uribe M. Eosinophilic gastroenteritis: a review. Dig Dis Sci. 2007;52:2904–2911.

9. Kawasaki A, Mizushima Y, Matsui S, Hoshino K, Yano S, Kitagawa M. A case of T-cell lymphoma accompanying marked eosinophilia, chronic eosinophilic pneumonia and eosinophilic pleural effusion. A case report. Tumori. 1991;77:527–530.

10. Endo M, Usuki K, Kitazume K, Iwabe K, Okuyama Y, Urabe A. Hypereosinophilic syndrome in Hodgkin's disease with increased granulocyte-macrophage colony-stimulating factor. Ann Hematol. 1995;71:313–314.

11. Catovksy D, Bernasconi C, Verdonck PJ, et al. The association of eosinophilia with lymphoblastic leukaemia or lymphoma: a study of seven patients. Br J Haematol. 1980;45:523–534.

12. Pardanani A, Reeder T, Li CY, Tefferi A. Eosinophils are derived from the neoplastic clone in patients with systemic mastocytosis and eosinophilia. Leuk Res. 2003;27:883–885.

13. Le Beau MM, Larson RA, Bitter MA, Vardiman JW, Golomb HM, Rowley JD. Association of inversion 16 with abnormal marrow eosinophils in acute myelomonocytic leukemia. N Engl J Med. 1983;309:630–636.

14. Swirsky DM, Li YS, Matthews JG, Flemans RJ, Rees JKH, Hayhoe FGJ. 8;21 translocation in acute granulocytic leukemia: cytological, cytochemical, and clinical features. Br J Haematol. 1984;56:199–213.

15. Matsushima T, Murakami H, Kim K, et al. Steroidresponsive pulmonary disorders associated with myelodysplastic syndromes with der(1q;7p) chromosomal abnormality. Am J Hematol. 1995;50:110–115.

16. Forrest DL, Horsman DE, Jensen CL, et al. Myelodysplastic syndrome with hypereosinophilia and a nonrandom chromosome abnormality dic(1;7): confirmation of eosinophil clonal involvement by fluorescence in situ hybridization. Cancer Genet Cytogenet. 1998;107:65–68.

17. Roufosse F, Cogan R, Goldman M. The hypereosinophilic syndrome revisited. Annu Rev Med. 2003;54:169–184.

18. Klion AD, Noel P, Akin C, et al. Elevated serum tryptase levels identify a subset of patients with a myeloproliferative variant of idiopathic hypereosinophilic syndrome associated with tissue fibrosis, poor prognosis, and imatinib responsiveness. Blood. 2003;101:4660–4666.

19. Gotlib J, Cools J. Five years since the discovery of the FIPL1-PDGFRA: what we have learned about the fusion and other molecularly defined eosinophilias. Leukemia. 2008; 22:1999–2010.

20. Jovanovic JV, Score J, Waghorn K, Cilloni D, Gottardi E, Metzgeroth G, et al. Low-dose imatinib mesylate leads to rapid induction of major molecular responses

and achievement of complete molecular remission in FIP1L1-PDGFRA-positive chronic eosinophilic leukemia. Blood. 2007;109:4635–4640.

21. Pardanani A, Brockman SR, Paternoster SF, Flynn HC, Ketterling RP, Lasho TL, et al. FIP1L1-PDGFRA fusion: prevalence and clinicopathologic correlates in 89 consecutive patients with moderate to severe eosinophilia. Blood. 2004;104: 3038–3045.

22. Pardanani A, Ketterling RP, Li CY, Patnaik MM, Wolanskyj AP, Elliott MA, et al. FIP1L1-PDGFRA in eosinophilic disorders: prevalence in routine clinical practice, long-term experience with imatinib therapy, and a critical review of the literature. Leuk Res. 2006;30:965–970.

23. Cools J, DeAngelo DJ, Gotlib J, Stover EH, Legare RD, Cortes J, et al. A tyrosine kinase created by fusion of the PDGFRA and FIP1L1 genes as a therapeutic target of imatinib in idiopathic hypereosinophilic syndrome. N Engl J Med. 2003;348:1201–1214.

24. Griffin JH, Leung J, Bruner RJ, Caligiuri MA, Briesewitz R. Discovery of a fusion kinase in EOL-1 cells and idiopathic hypereosinophilic syndrome. Proc Natl Acad Sci U S A. 2003;100:7830–7835.

25. Pardanani A, Ketterling RP, Brockman SR, Flynn HC, Paternoster SF, Shearer BM, et al. CHIC2 deletion, a surrogate for FIP1L1-PDGFRA fusion, occurs in systemic mastocytosis associated with eosinophilia and predicts response to imatinib mesylate therapy. Blood. 2003;102:3093–3096.

26. Trempat P, Villalva C, Laurent G, Armstrong F, Delsol G, Dastugue N, et al. Chronic myeloproliferative disorders with rearrangement of the platelet-derived growth factor alpha receptor: a new clinical target for STI571/Glivec. Oncogene. 2003;22:5702–5706.

27. Baxter EJ, Hochhaus A, Bolufer P, Reiter A, Fernandez JM, Senent L, et al. The t(4;22)(q12;q11) in atypical chronic myeloid leukaemia fuses BCR to PDGFRA. Hum Mol Genet. 2002;11:1391–1397.

28. Score J, Curtis C, Waghorn K, Stalder M, Jotterand M, Grand FH, et al. Identification of a novel imatinib responsive KIF5B-PDGFRA fusion gene following screening for PDGFRA overexpression in patients with hypereosinophilia. Leukemia. 2006;20:827–832.

29. Walz C, Curtis C, Schnittger S, Schultheis B, Metzgeroth G, Schoch C, et al. Transient response to imatinib in a chronic eosinophilic leukemia associated with ins(9;4)(q33;q12q25) and a CDK5RAP2-PDGFRA fusion gene. Genes Chromosomes Cancer. 2006;45:950–956.

30. Curtis CE, Grand FH, Musto P, Clark A, Murphy J, Perla G, et al. Two novel imatinib-responsive PDGFRA fusion genes in chronic eosinophilic leukaemia. Br J Haematol. 2007;138:77–81.

31. Hidalgo-Curtis C, Apperley JF, Start A, Jeng M, Gotlib J, Chase A, et al. Fusion of PDGFRB to two distinct loci at 3p21 and a third at 12q13 in imatinib-respensive myclopdiferative neoplasms. Br J Haematol. 2010; 148: 268–273.

32. Walz C, Metzgeroth G, Haferlach C, Schmitt-Graeff A, Fabarius A, Hagen V, et al. Characterization of three new imatinib-responsive fusion genes in chronic myeloproliferative disorders generated by disruption of the platelet-derived growth factor receptor beta gene. Haematologica. 2007;92:163–169.

33. Rosati R, La Starza R, Luciano L, Gorello P, Matteucci C, Pierini V, et al. TPM3/PDGFRB fusion transcript and its reciprocal in chronic eosinophilic leukemia. Leukemia. 2006;20:1623–1624.

34. Wilkinson K, Velloso ER, Lopes LF, Lee C, Aster JC, Shipp MA, et al. Cloning of the t(1;5)(q23;q33) in a myeloproliferative disorder associated with eosinophilia: involvement of PDGFRB and response to imatinib. Blood. 2003;102:4187–4190.

35. Ross TS, Bernard OA, Berger R, et al. Fusion of Huntington interacting protein 1 to platelet-derived growth factor beta receptor (PDGFbetaR) in chronic myelomonocytic leukemia with t(5;7)(q33;q11.2). Blood. 1998;91:4419–4426.

36. Schwaller J, Anastasiadou E, Cain D, et al. H4/D10S170, a gene frequently rearranged in papillary thyroid carcinoma, is fused to the platelet-derived growth factor receptor beta gene in atypical chronic myeloid leukemia with t(5;10) (q33;q22). Blood. 2001;97:3910–3918.

37. Kulkarni S, Heath C, Parker S, et al. Fusion of H4/D10S170 to the platelet-derived growth factor receptor beta in BCR-ABL negative myeloproliferative disorders with a t(5;10)(q33;q21). Cancer Res. 2000;60:3592–3598.

38. Vizmanos JL, Novo FJ, Roman JP, et al. NIN, a gene encoding a CEP110-like centrosomal protein, is fused to PDGFRB in a patient with a t(5;14)(q33;q24) and an imatinib-responsive myeloproliferative disorder. Cancer Res. 2004;64:2673–2676.

39. Levine RL, Wadleigh M, Sternberg DW, et al. KIAA1509 is a novel PDGFRB fusion partner in imatinib-responsive myeloproliferative disease associated with a t(5;14)(q33;q32). Leukemia. 2005;19:27–30

40. Abe A, Emi N, Tanimoto M, et al. Fusion of the platelet-derived growth factor beta receptor to a novel gene CEV14 in acute myelogenous leukemia after clonal evolution. Blood. 1997;90:4271–4277.

41. Grand FH, Burgstaller S, Kuhr T, et al. P53-binding protein 1 is fused to the platelet-derived growth factor receptor beta in a patient with a t(5;15)(q33;q22) and an imatinib-responsive eosinophilic myeloproliferative disorder. Cancer Res. 2004;64:7216–7219.

42. La Starza R, Rosati R, Roti G, Gorello P, Bardi A, Crescenzi B. A new NDE1/PDGFRB fusion transcript underlying chronic myelomonocytic leukaemia in Noonan syndrome. Leukemia. 2007;21:830–833.

43. Magnusson MK, Meade KE, Brown KE, et al. Rabaptin-5 is a novel fusion partner to platelet-derived growth factor receptor beta in chronic myelomonocytic leukemia. Blood. 2001;98:2518–2525.

44. Morerio C, Acquila M, Rosanda C, et al. HCMOGT-1 is a novel fusion partner to PDGFRB in juvenile myelomonocytic leukemia with t(5;17)(q33;p11.2). Cancer Res. 2004;64:2649–2651.

45. Golub TR, Barker GF, Lovett M, Gilliland DG. Fusion of PDGF receptor beta to a novel ets-like gene, tel, in chronic myelomonocytic leukemia with t(5;12) chromosomal translocation. Cell. 1994;77:307–316.

46. Xiao S, Nalabolu SR, Aster JC, Ma J, Abruzzo L, Jaffe ES, et al. FGFR1 is fused with a novel zinc-finger gene, ZNF198, in the t(8;13) leukaemia/lymphoma syndrome. Nat Genet. 1998;18:84–87.

47. Reiter A, Sohal J, Kulkarni S, Chase A, Macdonald DH, Aguiar RC, et al. Consistent fusion of ZNF198 to the fibroblast growth factor receptor-1 in the t(8;13)(p11;q12) myeloproliferative syndrome. Blood. 1998;92:1735–1742.

48. Popovici C, Adelaide J, Ollendorff V, et al. Fibroblast growth factor receptor 1 is fused to FIM in stem-cell myeloproliferative disorder with t(8;13). Proc Natl Acad Sci U S A. 1998;95:5712–5717.

49. Smedley D, Hamoudi R, Clark J, et al. The t(8;13)(p11;q11-12) rearrangement associated with an atypical myeloproliferative disorder fuses the fibroblast growth factor receptor 1 gene to a novel gene RAMP. Hum Mol Genet. 1998;7:637–642.

50. Guasch G, Mack GJ, Popovici C, et al. FGFR1 is fused to the centrosome-associated protein CEP110 in the 8p12 stem cell myeloproliferative disorder with t(8;9) (p12;q33). Blood. 2000;95:1788–1796

51. Popovici C, Zhang B, Gregoire MJ, et al. The t(6;8)(q27;p11) translocation in a stem cell myeloproliferative disorder fuses a novel gene, FOP, to fibroblast growth factor receptor 1. Blood. 1999;93:1381–1389.

52. Demiroglu A, Steer EJ, Heath C, et al. The t(8;22) in chronic myeloid leukemia fuses BCR to FGFR1: transforming activity and specific inhibition of FGFR1 fusion proteins. Blood. 2001;98:3778–3783.

53. Belloni E, Trubia M, Gasparini P, et al. 8p11 myeloproliferative syndrome with a novel t(7;8) translocation leading to fusion of the FGFR1 and TIF1 genes. Genes Chromosomes Cancer. 2005;42:320–325.

54. Walz, C., Chase A., Weisser, A., et al. The t(8;17)(p11;q25) in the 8p11 myeloproliferative syndrome fuses MYO18A to FGFR1. Leukemia. 2005; 19:1005–1009.

55. Guasch G, Popovici C, Mugneret F, et al. Endogenous retroviral sequence is fused to FGFR1 kinase in the 8p12 stem-cell myeloproliferative disorder with t(8;19) (p12;q13.3). Blood. 2003;101:286–288.

56. Grand EK, Grand FH, Chase AJ, et al. Identification of a novel gene, FGFR1OP2, fused to FGFR1 in 8p11 myeloproliferative syndrome. Genes Chromomosomes Cancer. 2004;40:78–83.

57. Vandenberghe P, Wlodarska I, Michaux L, Zachee P, Boogaerts M, Vanstraelen D, et al. Clinical and molecular features of FIP1L1-PDFGRA (+) chronic eosinophilic leukemias. Leukemia. 2004;18:734–742.

58. Maric I, Robyn J, Metcalfe DD, Fay MP, Carter M, Wilson T, et al. KIT D816V-associated systemic mastocytosis with eosinophilia and FIP1L1/PDGFRA-associated chronic eosinophilic leukemia are distinct entities. J Allergy Clin Immunol. 2007;120:680–687.

59. Metzgeroth G, Walz C, Score J, Siebert R, Schnittger S, Haferlach C, et al. Recurrent finding of the FIP1L1-PDGFRA fusion gene in eosinophilia-associated acute myeloid leukemia and lymphoblastic T-cell lymphoma. Leukemia. 2007;21:1183–1188.

60. Roufosse F, Cogan E, Goldman M. Recent advances in pathogenesis and management of hypereosinophilic syndromes. Allergy. 2004;59:673–689.

61. Cogan E, Schandene L, Crusiaux A, Cochaux P, Velu T, Goldman M. Brief report: clonal proliferation of type 2 helper T cells in a man with the hypereosinophilic syndrome. N Engl J Med. 1994;330:535–538.

62. Simon HU, Yousefi S, Dommann-Scherrer CC, et al. Expansion of cytokine-producing CD4-CD8- T cells associated with abnormal Fas expression and hypereosinophilia. J Exp Med. 1996;183:1071–1082.

63. Brugnoni D, Airo P, Rossi G, et al. CD4+ T-cell population able to secrete large amounts of interleukin-5. Blood. 1996;87:1416–1422.

64. Roufosse F, Schandene L, Sibille C, et al. T-cell receptor-independent activation of clonal Th2 cells associated with chronic hypereosinophilia. Blood. 1999;94:994–1002.

65. Bank I, Amariglio N, Reshef, A, et al. The hypereosinophilic syndrome associated with CD4+CD3- helper type 2 (Th2) lymphocytes. Leuk Lymphoma. 2001;42:123–133.

66. Simon HU, Plotz SG, Dummer R, Blaser K. Abnormal clones of T cells producing interleukin-5 in idiopathic hypereosinophilia. N Eng J Med. 1999;341:1112–1120.

67. Brugnoni D, Airo P, Tosoni C, et al. CD3-CD4+ cells with a Th2-like pattern of cytokine production in the peripheral blood of a patient with cutaneous T cell lymphoma. Leukemia. 1997;11:1983–1985.

68. Roufosse F, Schandene L, Sibille C, et al. Clonal Th2 lymphocytes in patients with the idiopathic hypereosinophilic syndrome. Br J Haematol. 2000;109:540–548.

69. Kitano K, Ichikawa N, Shimodaira S, et al. Eosinophilia associated with clonal T-cell proliferation. Leuk Lymphoma. 1997;27:335–342.

70. Roufosse F. Hypereosinophilic syndrome variants: diagnostic and therapeutic considerations. Haematologica. 2009;94:1188–1193.

71. Helbig G, Wieczorkiewicz A,1, Dziaczkowska-Suszek J, et al. T-cell abnormalities are present at high frequencies at high frequencies in patients with hypereosinophilic syndrome. Haematologica. 2009;94:1236–1241.

72. Schaller JL, Burkland GA. Case report: rapid and complete control of idiopathic hypereosinophilia with imatinib mesylate. MedGenMed. 2001;3:9.

73. Gleich GJ, Leiferman KM, Pardanani A, Tefferi A, Butterfield JH. Treatment of hypereosinophilic syndrome with imatinib mesilate. Lancet. 2002;359:1577–1578.

74. Ault P, Cortes J, Koller C, Kaled ES, Kantarjian H. Response of idiopathic hypereosinophilic syndrome to treatment with imatinib mesylate. Leuk Res. 2002;26:881–884.

75. Nolasco I, Carvalho S, Parreira A. Rapid and complete response to imatinib mesylate (STI-571) in a patient with idiopathic hypereosinophilia. Blood. 2002;100:346b [abstract].

76. Gotlib J, Malone JM, DeAngelo DJ, Stone RM, Gilliland DG, Clark J, et al. Imatinib mesylate (GLEEVEC™) induced rapid and complete hematologic remissions in patients with idiopathic hypereosinophilic syndrome (HES) without evidence of BCR-ABL or activating mutations in c-KIT and platelet derived growth factor receptor-beta. Blood. 2002. 100:798a [Abstract 3152].

77. Klion AD, Robyn J, Akin C, Noel P, Brown M, Law M, et al. Molecular remission and reversal of myelofibrosis in response to imatinib mesylate treatment in patients with the myeloproliferative variant of hypereosinophilic syndrome. Blood. 2004;103:473–478.

78. Baccarani M, Cilloni D, Rondoni M, Ottaviani E, Messa F, Merante S, et al. The efficacy of imatinib mesylate in patients with FIP1L1-PDGFRalpha-positive hypereosinophilic syndrome. Results of a multicenter prospective study. Haematologica. 2007;92:1173–1179.

79. Jovanovic JV, Score J, Waghorn K, Cilloni D, Gottardi E, Metzgeroth G, et al. Low-dose imatinib mesylate leads to rapid induction of major molecular responses and achievement of complete molecular remission in FIP1L1-PDGFRA-positive chronic eosinophilic leukemia. Blood. 2007;109:4635–4640.

80. Klion AD, Robyn J, Maric I, Fu W, Schmid L, Lemery S, et al. Relapse following discontinuation of imatinib mesylate therapy for FIP1L1/PDGFRA-positive chronic eosinophilic leukemia: implications for optimal dosing. Blood. 2007;110:3552–3556.

81. Pardanani A, Ketterling RP, Li CY, Patnaik MM, Wolanskyj AP, Elliott MA, et al. FIP1L1-PDGFRA in eosinophilic disorders: prevalence in routine clinical practice, long-term experience with imatinib therapy, and a critical review of the literature. Leuk Res. 2006;30:965–970.

82. Helbig G, Stella-Hołowiecka B, Majewski M, Całbecka M, Gajkowska J, Klimkiewicz R, et al. A single weekly dose of imatinib is sufficient to induce and maintain remission of chronic eosinophilic leukaemia in FIP1L1-PDGFRA-expressing patients. Br J Haematol. 2008;141:200–204.

83. Cross DM, Cross NC, Burgstaller S, et al. Durable responses to imatinib in patients with PDGFRB fusion gene-positive and BCR-ABL-negative chronic myeloproliferative disorders. Blood. 2007;109:61–64.

84. Chen J, DeAngelo DJ, Kutok JL, et al. PKC412 inhibits the zinc finger 198-fibroblast growth factor receptor 1 fusion tyrosine kinase and is active in treatment of stem cell myeloproliferative disorder. Proc Natl Acad Sci U S A. 2004;101:14479–14484.

85. Pardanani A, Reeder T, Porrata L, et al. Imatinib therapy for hypereosinophilic syndrome and other eosinophilic disorders. Blood. 2003;101:3391–3397.

86. Pitini V, Arrigo C, Azzarello D, et al. Serum concentration of cardiac troponin T in patients with hypereosinophilic syndrome treated with imatinib is predictive of adverse outcomes. Blood. 2003;102:3456–3457.

87. Von Bubnoff N, Sandherr M, Schlimok G, et al. Myeloid blast crisis evolving during imatinib treatment of an FIP1L1-PDGFRalpha-positive chronic myeloproliferative disease with prominent eosinophilia. Leukemia. 2004;19:286–287.

88. Ohnishi H, Kandabashi K, Maeda Y, Kawamura M, Watanabe T. Chronic eosinophilic leukaemia with FIP1L1-PDGFRA fusion and T674I mutation that evolved from Langerhans cell histiocytosis with eosinophilia after chemotherapy. Br J Haematol. 2006;134:547–549.

89. Lierman E Michaux L, Beullens E, et al. FIP1L1-PDGFRalpha D842V, a novel panresistant mutant, emerging after treatment of FIP1L1-PDGFRalpha T674I eosinophilic leukemia with single agent sorafenib. Leukemia. 2009;23:845–851.

90. Simon D, Salemi S, Yousefi S, Simon HU. Primary resistance to imatinib in Fip1-like 1-platelet-derived growth factor receptor alpha-positive eosinophilic leukemia. J Allergy Clin Immunol. 2008;121:1054–1056.

91. Bradeen HA, Eide CA, O'Hare T, Johnson KJ, Willis SG, Lee FY, et al. Comparison of imatinib mesylate, dasatinib (BMS-354825), and nilotinib (AMN107) in an N-ethyl-N-nitrosourea (ENU)-based mutagenesis screen: high efficacy of drug combinations. Blood. 2006;108:2332–2338.

92. Cools J, Stover EH, Boulton CL, Gotlib J, Legare RD, Amaral SM, et al. PKC412 overcomes resistance to imatinib in a murine model of FIP1L1-PDGFRalpha-induced myeloproliferative disease. Cancer Cell. 2003;3:459–469.

93. Lierman E, Folens C, Stover EH, Mentens N, Van MH, Scheers W, et al. Sorafenib is a potent inhibitor of FIP1L1-PDGFRalpha and the imatinib-resistant FIP1L1-PDGFRalpha T674I mutant. Blood. 2006;108:1374–1376.

94. Stover EH, Chen J, Lee BH, Cools J, McDowell E, Adelsperger J, et al. The small molecule tyrosine kinase inhibitor AMN107 inhibits TEL-PDGFRbeta and FIP1L1-PDGFRalpha in vitro and in vivo. Blood. 2005;106:3206–3213.

95. von Bubnoff N, Gorantla SP, Thone S, Peschel C, Duyster J. The FIP1L1-PDGFRA T674I mutation can be inhibited by the tyrosine kinase inhibitor AMN107 (nilotinib). Blood. 2006;107:4970–4971.

96. Ackerman SJ, Butterfield JH. Eosinophilia, eosinophil-associated diseases, chronic eosinophilic leukemia, and the hypereosinophilic syndromes. In: Hematology, 4th Ed. Hoffman R, Benz Jr. E, Shattil SJ, Furie B, Cohen HJ, Silberstein LE, McGlave P (eds). Churchill Livingstone: Philadelphia, 2005:763–786.

97. Brito-Babapulle F. The eosinophilias, including the idiopathic hypereosinophilic syndrome. Br J Haematol. 2003;121:203–223.

98. Weller PF, Bubley GJ. The idiopathic hypereosinophilic syndrome. Blood. 1994;83:2759–2779.

99. Gotlib J, Cools J, Malone JM, et al. The FIP1L1-PDGFRα fusion tyrosine kinase in hypereosinophilic syndrome and chronic eosinophilic leukemia: implications for diagnosis, classification, and management. Blood. 2004;103:2879–2891.

100. Fauci AS, Harley JB, Roberts WC, Ferrans VJ, Gralnick HR, Bjornson BH. NIH conference. The idiopathic hypereosinophilic syndrome. Clinical, pathophysiologic, and therapeutic considerations. Ann Intern Med. 1982;97:78–92.

101. Parrillo JE, Fauci AS, Wolff SM. Therapy of the hypereosinophilic syndrome. Ann Intern Med. 1978;89:167–172.

102. Prin L, Lefebvre P, Gruart V, et al. Heterogeneity of human eosinophil glucocorticoid receptor expression in hypereosinophilic patients: absence of detectable receptor correlates with resistance to corticotherapy. Clin Exp Immunol. 1989;78:383–389.

103. Chusid MJ, Dale DC. Eosinophilic leukemia. Remission with vincristine and hydroxyurea. Am J Med. 1975;59:297–300.

104 Cofrancesco E, Cortellaro M, Pogliani E, Boschetti C, Salavatore M, Polli EE. Response to vincristine treatment in a case of idiopathic hypereosinophilic syndrome with multiple clinical manifestations. Acta Haematol. 1984;72:21–25.

105. Sakamoto K, Erdreich-Epstein A, deClerck Y, Coates T. Prolonged clinical response to vincristine treatment in two patients with hypereosinophilic syndrome. Am J Pediatr Hematol Oncol. 1992;14:348–351.

106. Lee JH, Lee JW, Jang CS, et al. Successful cyclophosphamide therapy in recurrent eosinophilic colitis associated with hypereosinophilic syndrome. Yonsei Med J. 2002;43:267–270.

107. Smit AJ, van Essen LH, de Vries EG. Successful long-term control of idiopathic hypereosinophilic syndrome with etoposide. Cancer. 1991;67:2826–2827.

108. Bourrat E, Lebbe C, Calvo F. Etoposide for treating the hypereosinophilic syndrome. Ann Intern Med. 1994;121:899–900.

109. Zabel P, Schlaak M. Cyclosporin for hypereosinophilic syndrome. Ann Hematol. 1991;62:230–231.

110. Nadarajah S, Krafchik B, Roifman C, Horgan-Bell C. Treatment of hypereosinophilic syndrome in a child using cyclosporine: implication for a primary T-cell abnormality. Pediatrics. 1997;99:630–633.

111. Ueno NT, Zhao S, Robertson LE, Consoli U, Andreeff M. 2-chlorodeoxyadenosine therapy for idiopathic hypereosinophilic syndrome. Leukemia. 1997;11:1386–1390.

112. Quiquandon I, Claisse JF, Capiod JC, Delobel J, Prin L. Alpha-interferon and hypereosinophilic syndrome with trisomy 8: karyotypic remission. Blood. 1995;85:2284–2285.

113. Luciano L, Catalano L, Sarrantonio C, Guerriero A, Califano C, Rotoli B. αIFN-induced hematologic and cytogenetic remission in chronic eosinophilic leukemia with t(1;5). Haematologica. 1999;84:651–653.

114. Yamada O, Kitahara K, Imamura K, Ozasa H, Okada M, Mizoguchi H. Clinical and cytogenetic remission induced by interferon-α in a patient with chronic eosinophilic leukemia associated with a unique t(3;9;5) translocation. Am J Hematol. 1998;58:137–141.

115. Malbrain ML, Van den Bergh H, Zachee P. Further evidence for the clonal nature of the idiopathic hypereosinophilic syndrome: complete haematological and cytogenetic remission induced by interferon-alpha in a case with a unique chromosomal abnormality. Br J Haematol. 1996;92:176–183.

116. Butterfield JH, Gleich GJ. Response of six patients with idiopathic hypereosinophilic syndrome to interferon alpha. J Allergy Clin Immunol. 1994;94:1318–1326.

117. Ceretelli S, Capochiani E, Petrini M. Interferon-alpha in the idiopathic hypereosinophilic syndrome: consideration of five cases. Ann Hematol. 1998;77:161–164.

118. Yoon TY, Ahn GB, Chang SH. Complete remission of hypereosinophilic syndrome after interferon-alpha therapy: report of a case and literature review. J Dermatol. 2000;27:110–115.

119. Broxmeyer HE, Lu L, Platzer E, Feit C, Juliano L, Rubin BY. Comparative analysis of the influences of human gamma, alpha and beta interferons on human multipotential (CFU-GEMM), erythroid (BFU-E), and granulocyte-macrophage (CFU-GM) progenitor cells. J Immunol. 1983;131:1300–1305.

120. Schandene L, Del Prete GF, Cogan E, et al. Recombinant interferon-alpha selectively inhibits the production of interleukin-5 by human CD4+ T cells. J Clin Invest. 1996;97:309–315.

121. Aldebert D, Lamkhioued B, Desaint C, et al. Eosinophils express a functional receptor for interferon alpha: inhibitory role of interferon alpha on the release of mediators. Blood. 1996;87:2354–2360.

122. Hart TK, Cook RM, Zia-Amirhosseini P, et al. Preclinical efficacy and safety of mepolizumab (SB—240563), a humanized monoclonal antibody to IL-5, in cynomolgus monkeys. J Allergy Clin Immunol. 2001;108:250–257.

123. Plotz SG, Simon HU, Darsow U, et al. Use of an anti-interleukin-5 antibody in the hypereosinophilic syndrome with eosinophilic dermatitis. N Engl J Med. 2003;349:2334–2339.

124. Garrett JK, Jameson SC, Thomson B, et al. Anti-interleukin-5 (mepolizumab) therapy for hypereosinophilic syndrome. J Allergy Clin Immunol. 2004;113:115–119.

125. Klion AD, Law MA, Noel P, Kim YJ, Haverty TP, Nutman TB. Safety and efficacy of the monoclonal anti-interleukin-5 antibody SCH55700 in the treatment of patients with hypereosinophilic syndrome. Blood. 2004;103:2939–2941.

126. Rothenberg ME, Klion AD, Roufosse FE, et al. Treatment of patients with the hypereosinophilic syndrome with mepolizumab. New Engl J Med. 2008;358:1215–1228.

127. Mehr S, Rego S, Kakakios A, Kilham H, Kemp A. Treatment of a case of pediatric hypereosinophilic syndrome with anti-interleukin-5. J Pediatr. 2009;155:289–291.

128. Pitini V, Teti D, Arrigo C, Righi M, et al. Alemtuzumab therapy for refractory idiopathic hypereosinophilic syndrome with abnormal T-cells: a case report. Br J Haematol. 2004;127:477.

129. Sefcick, A, Sowter D, DasGupta E, Russell NH, Byrne JL. Alemtuzumab therapy for refractory idiopathic hypereosinophilic syndrome. Br J Haematol. 2004;124:558–559.

130. Verstovsek S, Tefferi A, Kantarjian H, et al. Alemtuzumab therapy for hypereosinophilic syndrome and chronic eosinophilic leukemia. Clin Cancer Res. 2009;15:368–373.

131. Vazquez L, Caballero D, Canizo CD, et al. Allogeneic peripheral blood cell transplantation for hypereosinophilic syndrome with myelofibrosis. Bone Marrow Transplant. 2000;25:217–218.

132. Chockalingam A, Jalil A, Shadduck RK, Lister J. Allogeneic peripheral blood stem cell transplantation for hypereosinophilic syndrome with severe cardiac dysfunction. Bone Marrow Transplant. 1999;23:1093–1094.

133. Basara N, Markova J, Schmetzer B, et al. Chronic eosinophilic leukemia: successful treatment with an unrelated bone marrow transplantation. Leuk Lymphoma. 1998;32:189–193.

134. Sigmund DA, Flessa HC. Hypereosinophilic syndrome: successful allogeneic bone marrow transplantation. Bone Marrow Transplant. 1995;15:647–648.

135. Esteva-Lorenzo FJ, Meehan KR, Spitzer TR, Mazumder A. Allogeneic bone marrow transplantation in a patient with hypereosinophilic syndrome. Am J Hematol. 1996;51:164–165.

136. Sadoun A, Lacotte L, Delwail V, et al. Allogeneic bone marrow transplantation for hypereosinophilic syndrome with advanced myelofibrosis. Bone Marrow Transplant. 1997;19:741–743.

137. Juvonen E, Volin L, Kopenen A, Ruutu T. Allogeneic blood stem cell transplantation following non-myeloablative conditioning for hypereosinophilic syndrome. Bone Marrow Transplant. 2002;29:457–458.

138. Ueno NT, Anagnostopoulos A, Rondon G, et al. Successful non-myeloablative allogeneic transplantation for treatment of idiopathic hypereosinophilic syndrome. Br J Haematol. 2002;119:131–134.

139. Halaburda K, Prejzner W, Szatkowski D, Limon J, Hellmann A. Allogeneic bone marrow transplantation for hypereosinophilic syndrome: long-term follow-up with eradication of FIP1L1-PDGFRA fusion transcript. Bone Marrow Transplant. 2006;319–320.

140. Radford DJ, Garlick RB, Pohlner PG. Multiple valvar replacement for hypereosinophilic syndrome. Cardiol Young. 2002;12:67–70.

141. Harley JB, McIntosh XL, Kirklin JJ, et al. Atrioventricular valve replacement in the idiopathic hypereosinophilic syndrome. Am J Med. 1982;73:77–81.

142. Hendren WG, Jones EL, Smith MD. Aortic and mitral valve replacement in idiopathic hypereosinophilic syndrome. Ann Thorac Surg. 1988; 46:570–571.

143. Cameron J, Radford DJ, Howell J, O'Brien MF. Hypereosinophilic heart disease. Med J Aust. 1985;143:408–410.

144. Weyman AE, Rankin R, King H. Loeffler's endocarditis presenting as mitral and trucuspid stenosis. Am J Cardiol. 1977;40:438–444.

145. Chandra M, Pettigrew RI, Eley JW, Oshinski JN, Guyton RA. Cine-MRI-aided endomyocardectomy in idiopathic hypereosinophilic syndrome. Ann Thorac Surg. 1996;62:1856–1858.

146. Spry CJ, Davies J, Tai PC, Olsen EG, Oakley CM, Goodwin JF. Clinical features of fifteen patients with the hypereosinophilic syndrome. Q J Med. 1983;52:1–22.

147. Moore PM, Harley JB, Fauci AS. Neurologic dysfunction in the idiopathic hypereosinophilic syndrome. Ann Intern Med. 1985;102:109–114.

148. Johnson AM, Woodcock BE. Acute aortic thrombosis despite anticoagulant therapy in idiopathic hypereosinophilic syndrome. J R Soc Med. 1998;91:492–493.

Chapter 11

Pathogenesis, Diagnosis, Classification, and Management of Systemic Mastocytosis

Animesh Pardanani and Ayalew Tefferi

Keywords: Mast cell • Myeloproliferative neoplasm • KIT mutations

Introduction

Mast cell disease (MCD) or mastocytosis is a heterogenous disorder characterized by the abnormal growth and accumulation of morphologically and immunophenotypically abnormal mast cells in one or more organs. The clinical presentation of mastocytosis is diverse, and many patients do not fit the classical description – namely, a variably long history of urticaria pigmentosa (UP), followed by the insidious onset of flushing, cramping abdominal pain, diarrhea, and bone pain [1–3]. Other disease manifestations include osteopenia, hepatosplenomegaly, and abnormalities of blood and bone marrow (BM). Unlike pediatric cases, most adults with UP-like skin lesions have systemic disease (i.e., systemic mastocytosis [SM]) at presentation, a condition generally confirmed by means of a BM biopsy [4]. Diagnosis requires BM examination including immunohistochemical stains for mast cell tryptase or CD117 (KIT receptor). More sensitive techniques to detect clonal mast cells include immunophenotyping for CD25 or mutation screening for the *KIT* D816V mutation.

Pathogenesis

KIT Mutations

The interaction between the cytokine stem cell factor (SCF) (also known as c-Kit-ligand, mast cell growth factor, or steel factor) and its cognate receptor, c-Kit (KIT) plays a key role in regulating mast cell proliferation, maturation, adhesion, chemotaxis, and survival [5]. KIT is expressed on hematopoietic progenitors and is downregulated upon their differentiation into mature cells of all lineages, except mast cells, which retain high levels of cell surface KIT expression [6]. Consequently, gain-of-function mutations in *KIT*, particularly the D816V mutation, have been found to occur frequently in

SM patients [7]. While activating *KIT* mutations are clearly associated with human mastocytosis, they do not occur universally, and the question as to whether individual mutations are necessary and sufficient to cause mast cell transformation remains currently unsettled. The murine homologs of human *KIT*D816V (kinase domain) and *KIT*V560G (juxtamembrane domain) mutations, namely *KIT*D814Y and *KIT*V559G, have been shown to induce ligand-independent growth of interleukin-3-dependent cell lines, including the mast cell line IC2, pro-B-type Ba/F3 cells, and myeloid FDC-P1 cells in vitro; the transformed cells exhibit a more mature phenotype consistent with mast cell differentiation and have the ability to form mastocytomas in syngeneic DBA/2 mice or nude athymic mice [8–10]. These experiments do not, however, provide direct confirmation of the full neoplastic transformation potential of activating KIT mutations since the cytokine-dependent cell lines are immortalized and have acquired, *a priori*, the capacity to self-renew by unknown events. In other studies, however, introduction of *KIT*D814Y or *KIT*V559G mutations into murine hematopoietic progenitor cells induced the growth of both mast cell and non-mast cell lineage colonies in a factor-independent fashion [11]. Transplantation of the *KIT*D814Y-infected, and to a lesser extent *KIT*V559G-infected, BM cells into mast cell-deficient irradiated *W/W^v* mice resulted in the development of leukemia of an immature B-lymphoid phenotype [11]. Furthermore, transgenic mice expressing *KIT*D814Y developed either leukemia of lymphoid phenotype or lymphoma. While these data confirm the oncogenic potential of *KIT*D814Y, and to a lesser extent *KIT*V559G, they also indicate that their transforming effects may not be confined to mast cell lineage cells; it is possible that full transformation of nonlymphoid cells and development of non-lymphoid malignancies, including mast cell neoplasia, require the presence of cooperating mutations in other genes, in addition to constitutively activated KIT receptor. In another study, human *KIT*D816V was introduced into early hematopoietic progenitors from murine fetal liver; induction of megakaryocytic differentiation was observed in the absence of cytokines, while increased mast cell differentiation was seen in the presence of SCF (an effect also seen with wild-type KIT) [12]. The *KIT*D816V-infected cells, however, were not transformed, as assessed by their inability to proliferate extensively in liquid culture, to form colonies in semi-solid medium, or give rise to cell lines on prolonged culture, thus suggesting that *KIT*D816V is not a sufficient transforming stimulus in primary hematopoietic cells but instead leads to survival and maturation of cells whose phenotype is influenced by the presence of SCF. Similarly, expression of *KIT*D816V in Ba/F3 cells induced cluster formation in suspension culture as well as expression of mast cell-differentiation antigens, but was unable to induce factor-independent cell proliferation [13]. Thus, it is possible that *KIT*D816V may promote cell differentiation and maturation rather than serve as a potent proliferative signal for human mast cells. This hypothesis is supported by observations in a transgenic mouse model, wherein *KIT*D816V was expressed under the control of the chymase promoter, specifically in mast cells [14]. A proportion of transgenic mice developed an abnormal accumulation of mast cells at 12–18 months of age, ranging from localized and indolent mast cell hyperplasia to an invasive mast cell tumor. Furthermore, BM-derived mast cells from transgenic animals became growth factor independent and were capable of long-term survival. Overall, these data suggest that *KIT*D816V was necessary but not sufficient for the full neoplastic transformation of mast cells; the latter requires acquisition of additional somatic mutations, and the nature, timing, and clonal dominance of these additional events play an important role in dictating the clinical phenotype of the disease. Thus, it is possible that *KIT*D816V as a single "hit" may explain the pathology and clinical course of indolent mastocytosis but not of the more aggressive disease variants.

Furitsu et al. first demonstrated constitutive phosphorylation of KIT receptor expressed on HMC 1 cells, an immature MC line derived from a patient with mast cell leukemia, and described the presence of 2 mutations in the *KIT* gene (V560G and D816V) in this cell line [15]. Soon after this report, Nagata et al. published the first report of the *KIT*D816V mutation in human SM [16]. Since then, other KIT mutations, either replacement of D816 with a non-valine residue (e.g., D816Y [17], D816F [17], D816H [18], and D820G [19]) or mutations in other domains (extracellular [20], transmembrane [21, 22] or juxtamembrane [23, 24]) have also been identified in MCD. The latter mutations include F522C, A533D, K509I, del419, and V559A, many of which are representative of rare alleles detected in germline DNA in several cohorts of familial mastocytosis (reviewed by Akin) [25]. Interestingly, several kindreds with combined familial gastrointestinal stromal tumors (GIST) and mastocytosis, both of which are associated with gain-of-function *KIT* mutations, have also now been described [20].

TET2 Mutations

TET2 (TET oncogene family member 2) is a putative tumor suppressor gene located at chromosome 4q24. *TET2* mutations were first described in patients with *JAK2*V617F-positive myeloproliferative neoplasms (MPNs) [26]. Subsequently, the same mutations were found in *JAK2*V617F-negative MPN [27]. *TET2* mutations have since been described in other myeloid malignancies including SM, myelodysplastic syndromes (MDS), and acute myeloid leukemia (AML) [28–30]. Mutational frequency in SM was approximately 29%, and the presence of *TET2* mutations in SM was associated with monocytosis. In this preliminary study, *TET2* mutations cosegregated with *KIT*D816V and did not appear to affect survival in SM.

FIP1L1-PDGFRA Mutation

Results from an ~800-kb interstitial deletion of chromosome 4q12, thereby generating a constitutively active PDGFRA tyrosine kinase [31]. Patients harboring this mutation have a stem cell-derived clonal myeloproliferation that is characterized by eosinophilia, elevated serum tryptase level, and BM infiltration by morphologically and immunophenotypically abnormal mast cells, which often do not form the pathognomonic clusters seen in *KIT*-mutated SM [32–37]. It should be emphasized that the 2008 World Health Organization (WHO) document distinguishes this particular entity from *KIT*-mutated SM, given its association with a unique molecular lesion that is sensitive to inhibition by imatinib mesylate therapy, and it is, consequently, now classified under the "Myeloid and lymphoid neoplasms with eosinophilia and abnormalities of *PDGFRA, PDGFRB, or FGFR1*" category [38].

Diagnosis and Classification

Current diagnosis and classification of SM and its distinction from other myeloid malignancies associated with BM mastocytosis remain challenging for both clinicians and hematopathologists. The diagnosis of SM is based on identification of neoplastic MC by morphological, immunophenotypic, and/or genetic (molecular) criteria in various organs (Fig. 11.1). The current approach to diagnosis in SM starts with a BM examination since this site is almost universally involved in adult MCD, and histological diagnostic criteria for non-BM, extra-cutaneous organ involvement in SM have not been firmly established or widely accepted as of yet. BM examination also allows detection of a second hematologic neoplasm, if present [39]. In general, MC may not be readily recognized by standard dyes such as Giemsa, particularly when MC exhibit significant hypo granulation or abnormal nuclear morphology. Among the immunohistochemical markers, tryptase is the most sensitive, given that virtually all MC, irrespective of their stage of maturation, activation status, or tissue of localization, express this marker and, consequently, allows for detection of even small and/or immature MC infiltrates [40–42]. It must be emphasized, however, that tryptase, nor KIT/CD117 immunostaining, is able to distinguish between normal and neoplastic MC [43]. Neoplastic MC generally express CD25 and/or CD2, and the abnormal expression of at least one of these two antigens counts as a minor criterion toward the diagnosis of SM as per the WHO system [44]. Expression of CD2 on MC, as assessed by either flow cytometry or immunostaining, has been noted to be variable in SM, and consequently, CD25 expression may be more reliable marker for neoplastic MC [45, 46]. The aforementioned immunostaining and immunophenotyping studies enhance the morphological and immunophenotypic distinction between normal (round and CD25-negative) and abnormal (spindle-shaped and CD25-positive) mast cells, respectively [41, 46]. In addition, in the presence of blood eosinophilia, screening for *FIP1L1-PDGFRA*, using either FISH or RT-PCR, is warranted [35]. In contrast, conventional cytogenetics analysis

Diagnostic algorithm for systemic mastocytosis (SM)

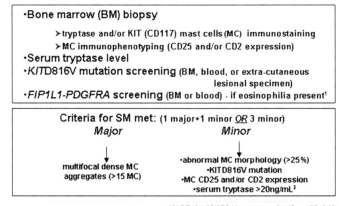

Fig. 11.1 Diagnostic algorithm for systemic mastocytosis as per the World Health Organization proposal

generally permits identification of cases of BM mastocytosis associated with a *PDGFRB* rearrangement (i.e., chromosomal translocations involving 5q31–32) [47]. Mutation screening for *KIT*D816V and measurement of serum tryptase or urinary histamine metabolites are complementary tools for the diagnosis of MCD [7, 48–50]. A recent study found a significant positive correlation between serum tryptase level and BM MC burden in indolent SM (ISM) patients [51]; similarly, aggressive SM (ASM) patients exhibited a higher median serum tryptase level as compared to ISM patients [1]. Of note, there is a high correlation between *KIT* mutation detection and the proportion of lesional cells in the sample, as well as the sensitivity of the screening method employed (reviewed by Akin) [25]. Sensitivity of detection may be enhanced by enriching lesional MC by laser capture microdissection, or magnetic bead- or FACS-based cell sorting, respectively [52, 53], or through the use of highly sensitive PCR techniques [54].

The 2008 WHO classification system for myeloid malignancies considers MCD a MPN and SM as a subcategory of MCD with BM involvement [38, 55, 56]. After establishing the presence of abnormal BM mast cells, it is important to strictly follow the revised WHO criteria for accurately diagnosing and classifying SM (Fig. 11.1 and Table 11.1). Use of the term SM is appropriate, provided BM mastocytosis is the prominent feature in terms of both BM histology and clinical presentation. At the same time, the WHO document distinguishes the usually *KIT*-mutated SM from myeloid neoplasms associated with BM mastocytosis and *PDGFR* mutations (e.g., *FIP1L1-PDGFRA, PRKG2-PDGFRB*) [32–37]. The latter are often associated with eosinophilia or basophilia and are sensitive to treatment with imatinib mesylate. WHO-defined SM is sometimes associated with a clonally related second myeloid neoplasm, which is not surprising, considering its origin as a stem cell disease with multilineage clonal involvement [39, 57, 58]. Conversely, an otherwise well-defined myeloid malignancy, such as MDS or a non-MCD MPN, might harbor neoplastic mast cells [59].

The WHO classification system for hematologic malignancies recognizes several categories of mastocytosis including [38]:

(a) Cutaneous mastocytosis (limited to the skin and variants include UP, cutaneous mastocytoma, diffuse cutaneous mastocytosis, and telangiectasia macularis eruptiva perstans)
(b) Extra-cutaneous mastocytoma (unifocal non-destructive mast cell tumor with low-grade cellular atypia)
(c) Mast cell sarcoma (destructive unifocal mast cell tumor with poorly differentiated mast cells)
(d) Systemic mastocytosis (SM), which always involves the BM and is the predominant form of mastocytosis in adults

The WHO system subclassifies SM into four subcategories:

1. *Indolent systemic mastocytosis (ISM)*: comprises the largest SM subgroup [1, 51]. Compared to other SM subgroups, ISM patients are significantly younger and two-thirds or more have UP-like skin lesions, mast cell mediator release symptoms (MCMRS), and/or gastrointestinal symptoms. The life expectancy of ISM patients is not significantly different than that of the age- and sex-matched U.S. control population (Fig. 11.2). The WHO system recognizes two provisional ISM subvariants: smoldering SM (SSM) and

Table 11.1 Current WHO classification of systemic mastocytosis (SM) [38].

Indolent systemic mastocytosis (ISM)

Meets criteria for SM. No "C" findings (see below). No evidence of AHNMD.

Bone marrow mastocytosis (BMM)

As above (ISM) with BM involvement, but no skin lesions

Smoldering systemic mastocytosis (SSM)

As above (ISM), but with two or more "B" findings but no "C" findings

Systemic mastocytosis with associated clonal hematological non-mast cell lineage disease (AHNMD)

Meets criteria for SM *and* criteria for AHNMD as a distinct entity in the WHO classification

Aggressive systemic mastocytosis (ASM)

Meets criteria for SM. One or more "C" findings. No evidence of mast cell leukemia.

Lymphadenopathic mastocytosis with eosinophilia

Mast cell leukemia

Meets criteria for SM. BM biopsy shows a diffuse infiltration, usually compact, by atypical, immature MC. BM smears show ≥20% MC. In typical MCL, MC account for ≥10% of peripheral blood white cells. Rare variant: aleukemic MCL.

Mast cell sarcoma

Unifocal MC tumor. No evidence of SM. Destructive growth pattern. High-grade cytology.

Extra-cutaneous mastocytoma

Unifocal MC tumor. No evidence of SM. No skin lesions. Non-destructive growth pattern. Low-grade cytology.

"B" findings

- BM biopsy showing >30% infiltration by MC (focal, dense aggregates) and/or serum total tryptase level >200 ng/mL
- Signs of dysplasia or myeloproliferation, in non-MC lineage(s), but insufficient criteria for definitive diagnosis of a hematopoietic neoplasm (AHNMD), with normal or slightly abnormal blood counts.
- Hepatomegaly without impairment of liver function, palpable splenomegaly without hypersplenism, and/or lymphadenopathy on palpation or imaging.

"C" findings

- BM dysfunction manifested by one or more cytopenia (ANC < 1.0×10^9/L, Hb < 10 g/dL, or platelets <100×10^9/L), but no obvious non-MC hematopoietic malignancy.
- Palpable hepatomegaly with impairment of liver function, ascites, and/or portal hypertension.
- Skeletal involvement with large osteolytic lesions and/or pathological fractures.
- Palpable splenomegaly with hypersplenism.
- Malabsorption with weight loss due to GI MC infiltrates.

BM bone marrow, *WHO* World Health Organization, *MC* mast cells, *ANC* absolute neutrophil count, *Hb* hemoglobin, *ng* nanograms, *mL* milliliter, *L* liter, *dL* deciliter, *GI* gastrointestinal

isolated BM mastocytosis (BMM) [38]. SSM is characterized by a higher burden of MC defined by the presence of >=2 "B-findings" (Table 11.1). In the Mayo Clinic series of 159 ISM patients, 22 (14%) had SSM, 36 (23%) BMM, and the remaining 101 (63%) did not fit in with either category (ISM-other). *KIT*D816V and *JAK2*V617F were detected in 78% and 0% of ISM patients, respectively, and *KIT*D816V prevalence was not significantly different amongst the ISM subgroups. SSM patients were significantly older than other ISM subgroups and exhibited a significantly inferior survival (median 120 months) as compared to those with ISM-other (median 301 months) or BMM (not reached). In a multivariable analysis, advanced age was the primary determinant of inferior survival and accounted for the marked difference in survival between SSM and the other two groups. The overall risk of transformation to acute leukemia or ASM was low (<1% and 3%, respectively) but was significantly higher in SSM (18%).

2. *Systemic mastocytosis with associated clonal hematological non-mast cell lineage disease (SM-AHNMD)*: While the pathophysiologic relationship between the "SM" and "AHNMD" components of SM-AHNMD remains to be precisely delineated, lineage distribution studies of the *KIT*D816V mutation suggest clonal origination from a common stem cell [7, 53, 60]; in some cases, however, the two develop concomitantly [61]. SM-AHNMD is the second most common subtype of SM-affected patients [39, 57, 58]. In the recent Mayo Clinic study of 138 SM-AHNMD patients, 123 (89%) had an associated myeloid neoplasm: 55 (45%) had SM-MPN, 36 (29%) SM-CMML, and 28 (23%) SM-MDS [57]. There was a high prevalence (34%) of associated eosinophilia ($>= 1.5 \times 10^9$/L), especially in those with SM-MPN; however, clinical outcome was similar between SM-MPN patients with or without eosinophilia. Abnormal karyotype was present in 18%, 25%, and 41% of patients with SM-MPN, SM-CMML, and SM-MDS, respectively. *JAK2*V617F prevalence was 12% and was virtually exclusively seen in SM-MPN (33%). In the aforementioned study, overall median survival of SM-AHNMD patients was 2 years (Fig. 11.2). SM-MPN patients had a significantly longer median survival (31 months) as compared to patients with SM-CMML (15 months), SM-MDS (13 months), or SM-AL (11 months) patients. Leukemic transformation (13% overall) was seen more frequently in SM-MDS (29%), as compared to SM-MPN (11%) or SM-CMML (6%).

3. *Aggressive systemic mastocytosis (ASM):* In the aforementioned Mayo Clinic cohort, 41 (12%) patients had ASM [1]. Patients with ASM frequently display constitutional symptoms, hepatosplenomegaly, lymphadenopathy, anemia, and thrombocytopenia. An abnormal karyotype and *KIT*D816V were noted in 20% and 82% of ASM patients, respectively. None of the patients with ASM harbored *JAK2*V617F. Overall median survival in ASM was 41 months (Fig. 11.2) and leukemic transformation occurred in 2 patients (5%).

4. *Mast cell leukemia (MCL):* is relatively rare [1]; patients generally exhibit extensive BM infiltration with neoplastic MC, and the prognosis is dismal with median survival of only 2 months (Fig. 11.2).

The marked clinical heterogeneity of SM makes it a challenge to classify this disease. Recently, several limitations of the current classification have been recognized [62], including the following:

(a) Unlike the case with blast phase chronic myelogenous leukemia (CML) or leukemic conversion of *BCR-ABL1*-negative MPN, most MCL cases develop de novo rather than represent transformation of pre-existing SM. Such was the case in the majority of MCL cases identified in a recent review of 342 MCD patients [1]. The mere presence of *KIT*D816V in some MCL cases (the sole MCL case tested in the aforementioned study

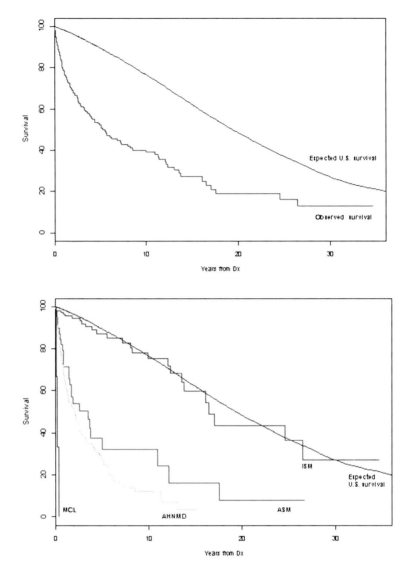

Fig. 11.2 Overall survival of systemic mastocytosis patients. (**a**) The observed Kaplan–Meier survival for systemic mastocytosis patients compared with the expected age- and sex-matched US population's survival. (**b**) The observed Kaplan–Meier survival for systemic mastocytosis patients classified by disease type ISM, ASM, AHNMD, and MCL compared with the expected age- and sex-matched US population's survival for the entire cohort. AHNMD, associated clonal hematological non-mast cell lineage disease. *ASM* aggressive systemic mastocytosis, *ISM* indolent systemic mastocytosis

was negative for the mutation) does not justify the status quo since the pathogenetic contribution of *KIT*D816V in SM and its utility as a therapeutic target is uncertain and definitely not as well defined as it is for *BCR-ABL1* or *FIP1L1-PDGFRA*. From a practical standpoint, the clinical features and treatment of MCL are more akin to acute leukemia than SM.

(b) The clinical relevance of the SM-AHNMD subcategory has not been convincingly made, since the SM component is often not the dominant process from the standpoint of clinical features, diagnosis, BM histology, or treatment. Again, for the reasons outlined above, the presence of *KIT*D816V should not be used as an excuse to lump together a clinico-pathologically heterogenous group of diseases that are prognostically diverse. The observations from a recent review of 123 cases with SM associated with other myeloid malignancies underscore this point [57].

(c) The current proposal fails to address the prognostic relevance of the provisional ISM subvariants, smoldering SM (SSM) and BM mastocytosis (BMM).

Based on the aforementioned points, a recent proposal has advocated revision of the current SM classification (Table 11.2) [62] as follows:

(a) MCL should be eliminated as a subcategory of SM and instead be included under the WHO category of "Acute myeloid leukemia (AML) and related myeloid neoplasms". The frequent occurrence of *KIT*D816V may be emphasized by naming the entity "MCL with *KIT*D816V" similar to other entities in the "AML with recurrent genetic abnormalities" subcategory. Similarly, "myelomastocytic leukemia" and "AML with BM mastocytosis" (i.e., SM-AML) can be included in the same "AML and related myeloid neoplasms" category.

(b) SM-AHNMD should be eliminated as a subcategory of SM; instead, "SM-chronic myelomonocytic leukemia" (SM-CMML) and "SM-myelodysplastic syndrome" (SM-MDS) should be placed under the WHO category of "Myelodysplastic/Myeloproliferative neoplasms" (MDS/MPN), given their similar prognosis and morphologic characteristics. In contrast, there is a firm basis for adopting a "SM-MPN" subcategory; it has been recognized since at least the early 1980s that a proportion of SM patients have BM features that are consistent with a coexisting MPN that is otherwise unclassifiable [63]. The rare cases of SM with associated

Table 11.2 Proposed revised classification of systemic mastocytosis (SM).

Indolent systemic mastocytosis (ISM)
Meets criteria for SM
No "C" findings
No evidence of SM-MDS, SM-CMML, SM-AL, or AML with BM mastocytosis
Minimal or no MPN features

Smoldering systemic mastocytosis (SSM)
As above for "ISM"
Two or more "B" findings

Aggressive systemic mastocytosis (ASM)
Meets criteria for SM
No evidence of SM-MDS, SM-CMML, SM-AL, or AML with BM mastocytosis
One or more "C" findings
MPN features allowed

Systemic mastocytosis associated with myeloproliferative neoplasm, unclassifiable (SM-MPN)
No "C" findings

SM systemic mastocytosis, *MPN* myeloproliferative neoplasm, *MDS* myelodysplastic syndrome, *CMML* chronic myelomonocytic leukemia, *AL* acute leukemia, *AML* acute myeloid leukemia, *BM* bone marrow

lymphoid or plasma cell neoplasm can be classified in the relevant category as, for example, "multiple myeloma with BM mastocytosis".

(c) Given its significantly worse prognosis and different age distribution, as demonstrated in a recent study of 159 cases with ISM [51], SSM should be separated from ISM as a distinct entity. In contrast, the clinical relevance of retaining the provisional entity "BMM" as an ISM subvariant is limited and can be removed.

The motivation for this proposal for revision is to move toward a more clinician-friendly and prognostically relevant classification system that is practical and clinically useful.

Treatment

Life expectancy in ISM is not significantly different than that of the control population (Fig. 11.2) [1], but quality of life might be affected by symptomatic/cosmetically unacceptable skin disease or mast cell mediator release symptoms (MCMRS) such as frequent syncopal episodes and gastrointestinal disturbances. ASM is characterized by organ impairment as a result of mast cell infiltration (e.g., cytopenias, hepatosplenomegaly with liver function test abnormalities, bone fractures from severe osteopenia or lytic bone lesions, cachexia from malabsorption) [1]. Clinical manifestations in SM-AHNMD are often influenced by the non-mast cell lineage component of the disease and include cytosis or cytopenia and hepatosplenomegaly. Presence of MCMRS or organ dysfunction due to direct MC infiltration is the main indication for treatment. Current therapy in SM includes observation alone, local therapy for cutaneous disease, use of anti-MCMRS drugs (e.g., anti-histamines), and cytoreductive therapy (Fig. 11.3) [64]. Management of MCMRS includes avoidance of MCMRS triggering factors and use of histamine antagonists and cromolyn sodium. Phototherapy is sometimes useful for skin disease, including UP. Refractory cases of both MCMRS and skin disease might sometimes require treatment with cytoreductive agents that are often used in the setting of ASM and SM-AHNMD. Cytoreductive agents used in SM include interferon-alpha (IFNα) [65–68], 2-chlorodeoxyadenosine (2-CdA) [69–71], and imatinib mesylate (IM) [72–74], while hydroxyurea (HU) is often utilized in the setting of SM-AHNMD.

With regard to cytoreductive therapy, data were recently reported from a retrospective analysis of 80 SM patients at Mayo Clinic who received a cytoreductive drug and were evaluable for response [75]. Forty-seven patients received IFN-α with or without prednisone; the median weekly dose was 15 MU per week (range 3.5–30 MU per week) and the initial dose of prednisone ranged from 20 to 60 mg per day with a slow tapering over weeks or months in some patients. In 40 evaluable patients, the overall response rate (ORR) was 53% (ISM and ASM 60%; SM-AHNMD 45%). Overall median duration of response was 12 months (range 1–67 months). Responses were not significantly different when comparing patients who did and did not receive prednisone. Absence of systemic mediator-related symptoms was significantly associated with inferior response to IFN-α; 41% vs. 77%, respectively. Major toxicities included fatigue, depression and thrombocytopenia.

HU use was largely restricted to SM-AHNMD patients ($n = 28$) at a dose ranging from 500 mg every other day to 2,000 mg per day. Twenty-six patients were

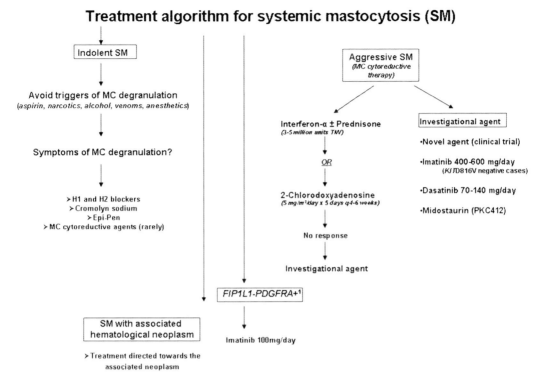

Fig. 11.3 Treatment algorithm for systemic mastocytosis

evaluable for response with ORR of 19%, reflected by control of thrombocytosis, leukocytosis, and/or hepatosplenomegaly. Median duration of response was 31.5 months (range 5–50 months); the major toxicity was myelosuppression.

IM was administered to 27 SM patients (*FIP1L1-PDGFRA* patients were excluded for this analysis); the median starting dose was 400 mg per day (range 100–400 mg per day), and the maintenance dose in responding patients ranged from 200 to 400 mg per day. In 22 evaluable patients, the ORR was 18% (ORR in ISM, ASM, and SM-AHNMD was 14%, 50%, and 9%, respectively), and median duration of response was 19.6 months (range 9–69 months). The majority (86%) of IM-treated patients were *KIT*D816V positive – ORR in mutation-positive and -negative patients was 17% and 33%, respectively. None of the six patients with SM associated with eosinophilia responded to IM treatment; all were *KIT*D816V positive. Major toxicities included diarrhea and peripheral edema; two patients developed interstitial pneumonitis.

2-CdA was administered to 26 patients (8 as first line); the dose was 5 mg/m^2 per day or 0.13–0.17 mg/kg per day for 5 days as a 2-h intravenous (IV) infusion, and median number of treatment cycles was 3 (range 1–9). Treatment response was evaluable in 22 patients and the ORR was 55% (ORR in ISM, ASM, and SM-AHNMD was 56%, 50%, and 55%, respectively). Median duration of response was 11 months (range 3–74 months). Presence of circulating immature myeloid cells was significantly associated with inferior response to 2-CdA (0 vs. 75%). Major toxicities were myelosuppression and infection. In the overall cohort (n = 80), treatment response was not significantly different based on *KIT*D816V or *TET2* mutational status.

Although several drugs have shown in vitro anti-KIT activity [76–80], the immediately most relevant in terms of clinical development include the tyrosine kinase inhibitors IM, nilotinib, dasatinib, masitinib, and PKC412. Overall, IM has limited activity in unselected SM patients; this is consistent with in vitro experiments, which show that IM inhibits wild-type KIT and KIT mutants with transmembrane (F522C) and juxtamembrane (V559G and V560G) but not kinase (D816V or D814V) domain mutations [22, 81, 82]. Similarly, not all juxtamembrane mutations are sensitive to IM (e.g., V559I) [83]. Our data suggest that IM is of limited benefit in SM therapy and is discordant with the results of another study that suggested an ORR of 36% in *KIT*D816V-positive SM patients [73]. In yet another study of 20 SM patients treated with IM, only one *KIT*D816V-negative patient responded while 6 other patients reported symptomatic improvement [74]. Nilotinib is more potent than IM in its in vitro anti-*BCR-ABL* activity but appears to be similarly ineffective against *KIT*D816V [84]. Another study, however, suggested a more potent activity of nilotinib against *KIT*D816V [85].

Dasatinib has shown potent anti-KIT activity in mast cells and leukemia cell lines with different *KIT* mutants including D816V [86, 87]. Furthermore, dasatinib might synergize with both PKC412 and chemotherapy in this regard [88–90]. In the largest study of dasatinib therapy in SM [91], the drug was given at a starting dose of 70 mg PO bid to 33 SM patients:18 indolent, 9 aggressive, and 6 with associated non-mast cell myeloid neoplasm. Two (6%) patients, both of whom were D816V negative, achieved complete remission. Nine (27%) patients experienced symptomatic improvement. However, grade 3 toxicities were observed in 19 (58%) patients. In another report [92], 4 SM patients (all *KIT*D816V positive; 2 with ASM, 1 SM-AHNMD, and 1 ISM) were treated with dasatinib at a dose ranging from 50 to 100 mg twice daily. Two patients (1 each with ASM and SM-AHNMD) had a major response, which in the case of the SM-AHNMD patient was accompanied by decrease in the BM MC burden. Both responders experienced an initial exacerbation of MCMRS and rash lasting several days before the benefits of dasatinib therapy became evident.

PKC412 has in vitro activity against cells transformed with kinase domain KIT mutants (D816Y and D816V) [93, 94], and treatment of a patient with MCL who harbored *KIT*D816V resulted in transient clinical benefit [95]. Preliminary data from a clinical trial in SM have been presented [96], wherein oral PKC412 was administered at a daily dose of 100 mg bid to 15 SM patients, 9 of whom had associated non-mast cell myeloid neoplasm. *KIT*D816V mutational frequency was 60%.There was some evidence of clinical activity in 11 (73%) patients including increase in hemoglobin (n = 1) and reduction of ascites (n = 2) or pleural effusion (n = 2). In four patients, the BM mast cell burden was reported to have decreased from 50–60% to 10–15% range. Untoward reactions of PKC412 in the particular study included nausea and vomiting, anemia and thrombocytopenia.

Conflicts of Interest

The authors have no competing financial interests.

References

1. Lim KH, Tefferi A, Lasho TL, et al. Systemic mastocytosis in 342 consecutive adults: survival studies and prognostic factors. Blood. 2009;113:5727–5736.
2. Patnaik MM, Rindos M, Kouides PA, Tefferi A, Pardanani A. Systemic mastocytosis: a concise clinical and laboratory review. Arch Pathol Lab Med. 2007;131:784–791.
3. Travis WD, Li CY, Bergstralh EJ, Yam LT, Swee RG. Systemic mast cell disease. Analysis of 58 cases and literature review. Medicine (Baltimore). 1988;67:345–368.
4. Czarnetzki BM, Koldc G, Schoemann A, Urbanitz S, Urbanitz D. Bone marrow findings in adult patients with urticaria pigmentosa. J Am Acad Dermatol. 1988;18:45–51.
5. Valent P, Spanblochl E, Sperr WR, et al. Induction of differentiation of human mast cells from bone marrow and peripheral blood mononuclear cells by recombinant human stem cell factor/kit-ligand in long-term culture. Blood. 1992;80:2237–2245.
6. Scheijen B, Griffin JD. Tyrosine kinase oncogenes in normal hematopoiesis and hematological disease. Oncogene. 2002;21:3314–3333.
7. Garcia-Montero AC, Jara-Acevedo M, Teodosio C, et al. KIT mutation in mast cells and other bone marrow hematopoietic cell lineages in systemic mast cell disorders: a prospective study of the Spanish Network on Mastocytosis (REMA) in a series of 113 patients. Blood. 2006;108:2366–2372.
8. Hashimoto K, Tsujimura T, Moriyama Y, et al. Transforming and differentiation-inducing potential of constitutively activated c-kit mutant genes in the IC-2 murine interleukin-3-dependent mast cell line. Am J Pathol. 1996;148:189–200.
9. Piao X, Bernstein A. A point mutation in the catalytic domain of c-kit induces growth factor independence, tumorigenicity, and differentiation of mast cells. Blood. 1996;87:3117–3123.
10. Kitayama H, Kanakura Y, Furitsu T, et al. Constitutively activating mutations of c-kit receptor tyrosine kinase confer factor-independent growth and tumorigenicity of factor-dependent hematopoietic cell lines. Blood. 1995;85:790–798.
11. Kitayama H, Tsujimura T, Matsumura I, et al. Neoplastic transformation of normal hematopoietic cells by constitutively activating mutations of c-kit receptor tyrosine kinase. Blood. 1996;88:995–1004.
12. Ferrao PT, Gonda TJ, Ashman LK. Constitutively active mutant D816VKit induces megakayocyte and mast cell differentiation of early haemopoietic cells from murine foetal liver. Leuk Res. 2003;27:547–555.
13. Mayerhofer M, Aichberger KJ, Florian S, et al. c-kit D816V provides a strong signal for myelomastocytic differentiation and cluster formation in murine Ba/F3 Cells. Blood. 2004;104:141a.
14. Zappulla JP, Dubreuil P, Desbois S, et al. Mastocytosis in mice expressing human Kit receptor with the activating Asp816Val mutation. J Exp Med. 2005;202:1635–1641.
15. Furitsu T, Tsujimura T, Tono T, et al. Identification of mutations in the coding sequence of the proto-oncogene c-kit in a human mast cell leukemia cell line causing ligand-independent activation of c-kit product. J Clin Invest. 1993;92:1736–1744.
16. Nagata H, Worobec AS, Oh CK, et al. Identification of a point mutation in the catalytic domain of the protooncogene c-kit in peripheral blood mononuclear cells of patients who have mastocytosis with an associated hematologic disorder. Proc Natl Acad Sci U S A. 1995;92:10560–10564.
17. Longley BJ, Jr, Metcalfe DD, Tharp M, et al. Activating and dominant inactivating c-KIT catalytic domain mutations in distinct clinical forms of human mastocytosis. Proc Natl Acad Sci U S A. 1999;96:1609–1614.
18. Pullarkat VA, Pullarkat ST, Calverley DC, Brynes RK. Mast cell disease associated with acute myeloid leukemia: detection of a new c-kit mutation Asp816His. Am J Hematol. 2000;65:307–309.

19. Pignon JM, Giraudier S, Duquesnoy P, et al. A new c-kit mutation in a case of aggressive mast cell disease. Br J Haematol. 1997;96:374–376.

20. Hartmann K, Wardelmann E, Ma Y, et al. Novel germline mutation of KIT associated with familial gastrointestinal stromal tumors and mastocytosis. Gastroenterology. 2005;129:1042–1046.

21. Tang X, Boxer M, Drummond A, Ogston P, Hodgins M, Burden AD. A germline mutation in KIT in familial diffuse cutaneous mastocytosis. J Med Genet. 2004;41:e88.

22. Akin C, Fumo G, Yavuz AS, Lipsky PE, Neckers L, Metcalfe DD. A novel form of mastocytosis associated with a transmembrane c-kit mutation and response to imatinib. Blood. 2004;103:3222–3225.

23. Beghini A, Tibiletti MG, Roversi G, et al. Germline mutation in the juxtamembrane domain of the kit gene in a family with gastrointestinal stromal tumors and urticaria pigmentosa. Cancer. 2001;92:657–662.

24. Zhang LY, Smith ML, Schultheis B, et al. A novel K509I mutation of KIT identified in familial mastocytosis-in vitro and in vivo responsiveness to imatinib therapy. Leuk Res. 2006;30:373–378.

25. Akin C. Molecular diagnosis of mast cell disorders: a paper from the 2005 William Beaumont Hospital Symposium on Molecular Pathology. J Mol Diagn. 2006;8:412–419.

26. Delhommeau F, Dupont S, Della Valle V, et al. Mutation in TET2 in myeloid cancers. N Engl J Med. 2009;360:2289–2301.

27. Tefferi A, Pardanani A, Lim KH, et al. TET2 mutations and their clinical correlates in polycythemia vera, essential thrombocythemia and myelofibrosis. Leukemia. 2009;23:905–911.

28. Tefferi A, Levine RL, Lim KH, et al. Frequent TET2 mutations in systemic mastocytosis: clinical, KITD816V and FIP1L1-PDGFRA correlates. Leukemia. 2009;23:900–904.

29. Tefferi A, Lim KH, Abdel-Wahab O, et al. Detection of mutant TET2 in myeloid malignancies other than myeloproliferative neoplasms: CMML, MDS, MDS/MPN and AML. Leukemia. 2009;23:1343–1345.

30. Langemeijer SM, Kuiper RP, Berends M, et al. Acquired mutations in TET2 are common in myelodysplastic syndromes. Nat Genet. 2009;41:838–842.

31. Cools J, DeAngelo DJ, Gotlib J, et al. A tyrosine kinase created by fusion of the PDGFRA and FIP1L1 genes as a therapeutic target of imatinib in idiopathic hypereosinophilic syndrome. N Engl J Med. 2003;348:1201–1214.

32. Klion AD, Noel P, Akin C, et al. Elevated serum tryptase levels identify a subset of patients with a myeloproliferative variant of idiopathic hypereosinophilic syndrome associated with tissue fibrosis, poor prognosis, and imatinib responsiveness. Blood. 2003;101:4660–4666.

33. Klion AD, Robyn J, Akin C, et al. Molecular remission and reversal of myelofibrosis in response to imatinib mesylate treatment in patients with the myeloproliferative variant of hypereosinophilic syndrome. Blood. 2004;103:473–478.

34. Pardanani A, Brockman SR, Paternoster SF, et al. FIP1L1-PDGFRA fusion: prevalence and clinicopathologic correlates in 89 consecutive patients with moderate to severe eosinophilia. Blood. 2004;104:3038–3045.

35. Pardanani A, Ketterling RP, Brockman SR, et al. CHIC2 deletion, a surrogate for FIP1L1-PDGFRA fusion, occurs in systemic mastocytosis associated with eosinophilia and predicts response to imatinib mesylate therapy. Blood. 2003;102:3093–3096.

36. Pardanani A, Ketterling RP, Li CY, et al. FIP1L1-PDGFRA in eosinophilic disorders: prevalence in routine clinical practice, long-term experience with imatinib therapy, and a critical review of the literature. Leuk Res. 2006;30:965–970.

37. Robyn J, Lemery S, McCoy JP, et al. Multilineage involvement of the fusion gene in patients with FIP1L1/PDGFRA-positive hypereosinophilic syndrome. Br J Haematol. 2006;132:286–292.

38. Horny HP, Metcalfe DD, Bennett JM, et al. Mastocytosis. In: Swerdlow SH, Campo E, Harris NL, et al., eds. WHO Classification of Tumors of Hematopoietic and Lymphoid Tissues (ed 4th). Lyon: International Agency for Research and Cancer (IARC); 2008:54–63.

39. Horny HP, Sotlar K, Sperr WR, Valent P. Systemic mastocytosis with associated clonal haematological non-mast cell lineage diseases: a histopathological challenge. J Clin Pathol. 2004;57:604–608.

40. Horny HP, Sillaber C, Menke D, et al. Diagnostic value of immunostaining for tryptase in patients with mastocytosis. Am J Surg Pathol. 1998;22:1132–1140.

41. Horny HP, Valent P. Histopathological and immunohistochemical aspects of mastocytosis. Int Arch Allergy Immunol. 2002;127:115–117.

42. Sotlar K, Horny HP, Simonitsch I, et al. CD25 indicates the neoplastic phenotype of mast cells: a novel immunohistochemical marker for the diagnosis of systemic mastocytosis (SM) in routinely processed bone marrow biopsy specimens. Am J Surg Pathol. 2004;28:1319–1325.

43. Jordan JH, Walchshofer S, Jurecka W, et al. Immunohistochemical properties of bone marrow mast cells in systemic mastocytosis: evidence for expression of CD2, CD117/Kit, and bcl-x(L). Hum Pathol. 2001;32:545–552.

44. Valent P, Horny HP, Escribano L, et al. Diagnostic criteria and classification of mastocytosis: a consensus proposal. Leuk Res. 2001;25:603–625.

45. Escribano L, Garcia Montero AC, Nunez R, Orfao A. Flow cytometric analysis of normal and neoplastic mast cells: role in diagnosis and follow-up of mast cell disease. Immunol Allergy Clin North Am. 2006;26:535–547.

46. Pardanani A, Kimlinger T, Reeder T, Li CY, Tefferi A. Bone marrow mast cell immunophenotyping in adults with mast cell disease: a prospective study of 33 patients. Leuk Res. 2004;28:777–783.

47. Walz C, Metzgeroth G, Haferlach C, et al. Characterization of three new imatinib-responsive fusion genes in chronic myeloproliferative disorders generated by disruption of the platelet-derived growth factor receptor beta gene. Haematologica. 2007;92:163–169.

48. Schwartz LB. Clinical utility of tryptase levels in systemic mastocytosis and associated hematologic disorders. Leuk Res. 2001;25:553–562.

49. Schwartz LB, Metcalfe DD, Miller JS, Earl H, Sullivan T. Tryptase levels as an indicator of mast-cell activation in systemic anaphylaxis and mastocytosis. N Engl J Med. 1987;316:1622–1626.

50. Keyzer JJ, de Monchy JG, van Doormaal JJ, van Voorst Vader PC. Improved diagnosis of mastocytosis by measurement of urinary histamine metabolites. N Engl J Med. 1983;309:1603–1605.

51. WHO subvariants of indolent mastocytosis: clinical details and prognostic evaluation in 159 consecutive adults. Blood. 2010 Jan 7;115(1):150–151.

52. Sotlar K, Fridrich C, Mall A, et al. Detection of c-kit point mutation Asp-816 > Val in microdissected pooled single mast cells and leukemic cells in a patient with systemic mastocytosis and concomitant chronic myelomonocytic leukemia. Leuk Res. 2002;26:979–984.

53. Yavuz AS, Lipsky PE, Yavuz S, Metcalfe DD, Akin C. Evidence for the involvement of a hematopoietic progenitor cell in systemic mastocytosis from single-cell analysis of mutations in the c-kit gene. Blood. 2002;100:661–665.

54. Sotlar K, Escribano L, Landt O, et al. One-step detection of c-kit point mutations using peptide nucleic acid-mediated polymerase chain reaction clamping and hybridization probes. Am J Pathol. 2003;162:737–746.

55. Tefferi A, Vardiman JW. Classification and diagnosis of myeloproliferative neoplasms: the 2008 World Health Organization criteria and point-of-care diagnostic algorithms. Leukemia. 2008;22:14–22.

56. Vardiman JW, Thiele J, Arber DA, et al. The 2008 revision of the World Health Organization (WHO) classification of myeloid neoplasms and acute leukemia: rationale and important changes. Blood. 2009;114:937–951.

57. Pardanani A, Lim KH, Lasho TL, et al. Prognostically relevant breakdown of 123 patients with systemic mastocytosis associated with other myeloid malignancies. Blood. 2009;114:3769–3772.

58. Travis WD, Li CY, Yam LT, Bergstralh EJ, Swee RG. Significance of systemic mast cell disease with associated hematologic disorders. Cancer. 1988;62:965–972.

59. Dunphy CH. Evaluation of mast cells in myeloproliferative disorders and myelodysplastic syndromes. Arch Pathol Lab Med. 2005;129:219–222.

60. Akin C, Kirshenbaum AS, Semere T, Worobec AS, Scott LM, Metcalfe DD. Analysis of the surface expression of c-kit and occurrence of the c-kit Asp816Val activating mutation in T cells, B cells, and myelomonocytic cells in patients with mastocytosis. Exp Hematol. 2000;28:140–147.

61. Kim Y, Weiss LM, Chen YY, Pullarkat V. Distinct clonal origins of systemic mastocytosis and associated B-cell lymphoma. Leuk Res. 2007;31:1749–1754.

62. Pardanani A, Tefferi A. Proposal for a revised classification of systemic mastocytosis. Blood. 2010;115:2720–2721.

63. Horny HP, Parwaresch MR, Lennert K. Bone marrow findings in systemic mastocytosis. Hum Pathol. 1985;16:808–814.

64. Tefferi A, Pardanani A. Clinical, genetic, and therapeutic insights into systemic mast cell disease. Curr Opin Hematol. 2004;11:58–64.

65. Casassus P, Caillat-Vigneron N, Martin A, et al. Treatment of adult systemic mastocytosis with interferon-alpha: results of a multicentre phase II trial on 20 patients. Br J Haematol. 2002;119:1090–1097.

66. Kluin-Nelemans HC, Jansen JH, Breukelman H, et al. Response to interferon alfa-2b in a patient with systemic mastocytosis. N Engl J Med. 1992;326:619–623.

67. Butterfield JH. Response of severe systemic mastocytosis to interferon alpha. Br J Dermatol. 1998;138:489–495.

68. Hauswirth AW, Simonitsch-Klupp I, Uffmann M, et al. Response to therapy with interferon alpha-2b and prednisolone in aggressive systemic mastocytosis: report of five cases and review of the literature. Leuk Res. 2004;28:249–257.

69. Kluin-Nelemans HC, Oldhoff JM, Van Doormaal JJ, et al. Cladribine therapy for systemic mastocytosis. Blood. 2003;102:4270–4276.

70. Tefferi A, Li CY, Butterfield JH, Hoagland HC. Treatment of systemic mast-cell disease with cladribine. N Engl J Med. 2001;344:307–309.

71. Pardanani A, Hoffbrand AV, Butterfield JH, Tefferi A. Treatment of systemic mast cell disease with 2-chlorodeoxyadenosine. Leuk Res. 2004;28:127–131.

72. Pardanani A, Elliott M, Reeder T, et al. Imatinib for systemic mast-cell disease. Lancet. 2003;362:535–536.

73. Droogendijk HJ, Kluin-Nelemans HJ, van Doormaal JJ, Oranje AP, van de Loosdrecht AA, van Daele PL. Imatinib mesylate in the treatment of systemic mastocytosis: a phase II trial. Cancer. 2006;107:345–351.

74. Vega-Ruiz A, Cortes JE, Sever M, et al. Phase II study of imatinib mesylate as therapy for patients with systemic mastocytosis. Leuk Res. 2009;33:1481–1484.

75. Lim KH, Pardanani A, Butterfield JH, Li CY, Tefferi A. Cytoreductive therapy in 108 adults with systemic mastocytosis: Outcome analysis and response prediction during treatment with interferon-alpha, hydroxyurea, imatinib mesylate or 2-chlorodeoxyadenosine. Am J Hematol. 2009;84:790–794.

76. Tanaka A, Konno M, Muto S, et al. A novel NF-kappaB inhibitor, IMD-0354, suppresses neoplastic proliferation of human mast cells with constitutively activated c-kit receptors. Blood. 2005;105:2324–2331.

77. Gabillot-Carre M, Lepelletier Y, Humbert M, et al. Rapamycin inhibits growth and survival of D816V-mutated c-kit mast cells. Blood. 2006;108:1065–1072.

78. Pan J, Quintas-Cardama A, Kantarjian HM, et al. EXEL-0862, a novel tyrosine kinase inhibitor, induces apoptosis in vitro and ex vivo in human mast cells expressing the KIT D816V mutation. Blood. 2007;109:315–322.

79. Pan J, Quintas-Cardama A, Manshouri T, Cortes J, Kantarjian H, Verstovsek S. Sensitivity of human cells bearing oncogenic mutant kit isoforms to the novel tyrosine kinase inhibitor INNO-406. Cancer Sci. 2007;98:1223–1225.

80. Dubreuil P, Letard S, Ciufolini M, et al. Masitinib (AB1010), a potent and selective tyrosine kinase inhibitor targeting KIT. PLoS One. 2009;4:e7258.

81. Zermati Y, De Sepulveda P, Feger F, et al. Effect of tyrosine kinase inhibitor STI571 on the kinase activity of wild-type and various mutated c-kit receptors found in mast cell neoplasms. Oncogene. 2003;22:660–664.

82. Akin C, Brockow K, D'Ambrosio C, et al. Effects of tyrosine kinase inhibitor STI571 on human mast cells bearing wild-type or mutated c kit. Exp Hematol. 2003;31:686–692.

83. Nakagomi N, Hirota S. Juxtamembrane-type c-kit gene mutation found in aggressive systemic mastocytosis induces imatinib-resistant constitutive KIT activation. Lab Invest. 2007;87:365–371.

84. Verstovsek S, Akin C, Manshouri T, et al. Effects of AMN107, a novel aminopyrimidine tyrosine kinase inhibitor, on human mast cells bearing wild-type or mutated codon 816 c-kit. Leuk Res. 2006;30:1365–1370.

85. von Bubnoff N, Gorantla SH, Kancha RK, Lordick F, Peschel C, Duyster J. The systemic mastocytosis-specific activating cKit mutation D816V can be inhibited by the tyrosine kinase inhibitor AMN107. Leukemia. 2005;19:1670–1671.

86. Schittenhelm MM, Shiraga S, Schroeder A, et al. Dasatinib (BMS-354825), a dual SRC/ABL kinase inhibitor, inhibits the kinase activity of wild-type, juxtamembrane, and activation loop mutant KIT isoforms associated with human malignancies. Cancer Res. 2006;66:473–481.

87. Shah NP, Lee FY, Luo R, Jiang Y, Donker M, Akin C. Dasatinib (BMS-354825) inhibits KITD816V, an imatinib-resistant activating mutation that triggers neoplastic growth in most patients with systemic mastocytosis. Blood. 2006;108:286–291.

88. Gleixner KV, Mayerhofer M, Sonneck K, et al. Synergistic growth-inhibitory effects of two tyrosine kinase inhibitors, dasatinib and PKC412, on neoplastic mast cells expressing the D816V-mutated oncogenic variant of KIT. Haematologica. 2007;92:1451–1459.

89. Aichberger KJ, Sperr WR, Gleixner KV, Kretschmer A, Valent P. Treatment responses to cladribine and dasatinib in rapidly progressing aggressive mastocytosis. Eur J Clin Invest. 2008;38:869–873.

90. Ustun C, Corless CL, Savage N, et al. Chemotherapy and dasatinib induce long-term hematologic and molecular remission in systemic mastocytosis with acute myeloid leukemia with KIT D816V. Leuk Res. 2009;33:735–741.

91. Verstovsek S, Tefferi A, Cortes J, et al. Phase II study of dasatinib in Philadelphia chromosome-negative acute and chronic myeloid diseases, including systemic mastocytosis. Clin Cancer Res. 2008;14:3906–3915.

92. Purtill D, Cooney J, Sinniah R, et al. Dasatinib therapy for systemic mastocytosis: four cases. Eur J Haematol. 2008;80:456–458.

93. Growney JD, Clark JJ, Adelsperger J, et al. Activation mutations of human c-KIT resistant to imatinib mesylate are sensitive to the tyrosine kinase inhibitor PKC412. Blood. 2005;106:721–724.

94. Gleixner KV, Mayerhofer M, Aichberger KJ, et al. PKC412 inhibits in vitro growth of neoplastic human mast cells expressing the D816V-mutated variant of KIT: comparison with AMN107, imatinib, and cladribine (2CdA) and evaluation of cooperative drug effects. Blood. 2006;107:752–759.

95. Gotlib J, Berube C, Growney JD, et al. Activity of the tyrosine kinase inhibitor PKC412 in a patient with mast cell leukemia with the D816V KIT mutation. Blood. 2005;106:2865–2870.

96. Gotlib J, George TI, Corless C, et al. The KIT tyrosine kinase inhibitor midostaurine (PKC412) exhibits a high response rate in aggressive systemic mastocytosis (ASM): interim results of a Phase II trial. ASH Annual Meeting Abstracts. 2007;110:3536.

Index